ATTENTION-DEFICIT HYPERACTIVITY DISORDER IN ADULTS

ATTENTION-DEFICIT HYPERACTIVITY DISORDER IN ADULTS

■

Paul H. Wender, M.D.

New York   Oxford
OXFORD UNIVERSITY PRESS
1995

Oxford University Press

Oxford   New York
Athens   Auckland   Bangkok   Bombay
Calcutta   Cape Town   Dar es Salaam   Delhi
Florence   Hong Kong   Istanbul   Karachi
Kuala Lampur   Madras   Madrid   Melbourne
Mexico City   Nairobi   Paris   Singapore
Taipei   Tokyo   Toronto

and associated companies in
Berlin   Ibadan

Copyright © 1995 by Paul H. Wender

Published by Oxford University Press, Inc.,
198 Madison Avenue, New York, New York 10016

Library of Congress Cataloging-in-Publication Data
Wender, Paul H., 1934–
Attention-deficit hyperactivity disorder in adults /
Paul H. Wender.
p. cm   Includes bibliographical references.
ISBN 0–19–509227–9
1. Attention-deficit disorder in adults. I. Title.
[DNLM: 1. Attention Deficit Disorder with Hyperactivity—in adulthood.
WL 354 W469a 1995]
RC394.A85W46   1995
616.85'89—dc20
DNLM/DLC
for Library of Congress   94–46139

3 5 7 9 8 6 4 2

Printed in the United States of America
on acid-free paper

For my wife,
Frances L. Burger, M.D.

Acknowledgments

■

Most of the work on ADHD in adults—including the development of diagnostic criteria, the development of the WURS and the TADDS rating scales, and the drug trials—has been performed with my colleagues, particularly Frederick W. Reimherr, M.D., on the TADDS, and David R. Wood, M.D. (who died tragically in 1986 at the age of 43). Other collaborators at different times have included David Bradford, Ph.D., Michael Ebert, M.D., Jean Eden, B.S., David Erickson, Lyn Gardner, Jean Greenwood, Joan Hansen, Leonard W. Jarcho, M.D., Nancy Norwood, David J. Thurman, M.D., Mark Ward, Ph.D., Kuang Wong, M.D., and Richard J. Wyatt, M.D. My editor, Gloria Parloff, was of invaluable assistance in editing and reediting of the manuscript in addition to being a valuable intellectual resource. I have been greatly helped by my indefatigable and exceedingly competent secretary, Jean Eden, who cheerfully typed the many revisions of this manuscript.

To my patients from whom I have learned much—who have been my tutors—and to sufferers from ADHD in the hope that this book will help them and those who treat them to cope with their disease.

Foreword

■

It is a pleasure to write the foreword for this book on Attention-deficit Hyperactivity Disorder (ADHD) in adults. Dr. Wender has been a pioneer in the study of attention deficit disorder for several decades. In particular, he was one of the first clinical research scientists to recognize that this disorder was not simply "outgrown" after puberty. Rather, he suggested that in a substantial number of individuals, the disorder persists into adult life. Moreover, this persistence into adult life may be associated with a significant degree of psychosocial and psychiatric morbidity.

As our diagnostic techniques get better and more epidemiologic studies are done, we have become cognizant of the fact that attention deficit disorder and its various subtypes are one of the most common psychiatric disorders of childhood. The disorder is generally recognizable by toddlerhood, but often is not diagnosed for the first time until grade school. Both retrospective and prospective follow-up studies now suggest that as many as 60 to 70 percent of children with this syndrome have continuing symptomatology in adulthood. About 30 percent no longer seem to demonstrate significant symptomatology, and no differences can be domonstrated with and without treatment in this subgroup later in life. Probably as many as 20 to 30 percent of an initial sample of children with the syndrome will have a significantly negative outcome, with antisocial behavior, substance abuse, and alcoholism as the negative consequences. The middle group who continue to manifest symptoms, but who do not have associated serious psychopathology, such as antisocial behavior and substance abuse, has a "continual display" picture. In these individuals, symptoms of the disorder are present, but in a more developmentally appropriate manner. Many of these will also have comorbid psychiatric disorder. Studies of adults who come for psychiatric evaluation in adulthood and who have the disorder but no previous diagnosis or treatment suggest that the range of comorbid psychopathology in adult life may be quite broad.

Dr. Wender does an excellent job of describing the core signs and symptoms of attention deficit disorder and how they are manifest in adult life. The review of the epidemiology of ADHD and prevalence of ADHD in adults is quite comprehensive and demonstrates how common the problem can be in adults.

While we have well-developed interviews and rating scales that have been shown to be valid and reliable in childhood diagnoses, the diagnosis of ADHD in adults is considerably more difficult. Dr. Wender has been a pioneer in the development of instruments and diagnostic criteria for children and adults with ADHD, many of which are included in the Appendix of this book. For clinicians, this part of the book will be extremely valuable. The discussion of treatment in adults is comprehensive, and again clinicians will benefit greatly from Dr. Wender's discussion. Probably the most unique chapter of the book contains descriptions by the patients themselves of their experiences on stimulant medication. This heretofore has been absent in the literature, and this is true of the literature on children and adolescents as well. In summary, this is a comprehensive, up-to-date, state-of-the-art review of one of our more common psychiatric problems. This book is the starting point for anyone with a serious interest in either clinical treatment of ADHD adults or in research on the topic.

Dennis P. Cantwell, M.D.
Joseph Campbell Professor of Child Psychiatry
UCLA Neuropsychiatric Institute
Department of Psychiatry and Biobehavioral Sciences

Contents

■

1 Introduction   3

2 Signs and Symptoms   13

3 The Prevalence of ADHD in Adults   41

4 Etiology   76

5 Diagnosis of ADHD in Adults   122

6 The Treatment of ADHD in Adults   144

7 The Experiences of Adult ADHD Patients on Stimulants   198

8 Conclusion   228

APPENDIXES
A. Evaluation Measures Frequently Used in Studies   235

B. Parents' Rating Scale   237

C. Utah Criteria for ADHD in Adults   241

D. Wender Utah Rating Scale   245

E. Targeted Attention-deficit Disorder Symptoms
Rating Scale   249

F. ADHD Symptoms and Other Psychiatric Symptoms
in Families of Representative Patients from
the Utah Studies   255

References   259

Name Index   283

Subject Index   287

ATTENTION-DEFICIT HYPERACTIVITY DISORDER IN ADULTS

1

Introduction

■

During the past decade researchers have become convinced that Attention-deficit Hyperactivity Disorder (ADHD), formerly believed to be a psychiatric syndrome of childhood that is outgrown with age, persists into later life and is a *common* psychiatric disorder in adults.

The study of ADHD in adults has led to several conclusions:

- The investigation of ADHD in adults can shed light on the experience of ADHD in children.
- The symptoms of ADHD in adults respond to drug treatment about as frequently and dramatically as they do in children.
- ADHD *may* be "related" to conduct disorders and "learning disorders" in childhood, and ADHD in adults *may* be "related" to the adult psychiatric disorders associated with conduct disorder: antisocial personality disorder, alcohol and substance abuse and, possibly, Briquet's syndrome (somatization disorder), as well as residual "learning difficulties."
- There is reason to believe that ADHD is (usually) genetically transmitted and biologically mediated, and the principles and findings of clinical and molecular genetics can be helpful in understanding, conceptualizing, and defining the syndrome.
- Many of the symptoms of ADHD can be interpreted as the manifestations of decreased monoaminergic—probably dopaminergic—functioning (Wender, 1971, 1972); if this interpretation is correct, ADHD in adulthood should be associated with certain biological correlates.

To provide a context for the presentation of what is known about ADHD in adults, I first discuss ADHD in childhood and issues surrounding it, as well as how thoughts about the syndrome have evolved.

A BRIEF NOSOLOGICAL HISTORY OF ADHD

■

The concepts behind, the criteria for, and the names of the syndrome of Attention-deficit Hyperactivity Disorder have changed frequently. Prior to the third edition of the American Psychiatric Association's *Diagnostic and Statistical Manual of Mental Disorders* (DSM-III, APA, 1980), the syndrome was conceptualized as composed of behavioral, motor, "perceptual," and cognitive impairments. What is now conceptualized as ADHD was variously designated as "minimal brain damage," "minimal brain dysfunction," "minimal cerebral dysfunction," "hyperkinesis," and the "hyperactive child syndrome." The behavioral and cognitive abnormalities associated with the syndrome included, but were not limited to, overactivity, inattentiveness and distractibility, impulsivity, affective lability and moodiness, temper outbursts, "immaturity," poor peer relations, disobedience, defiance, hostility, "acting out" or delinquent behaviors, and "dyslexia" and other "learning problems."

DSM-III separated a cluster of symptoms from this potpourri which it designated as "Attention Deficit Disorder" (ADD), and grouped other behavioral problems under the category of "Conduct Disorder." DSM-III states that the "essential features are signs of developmentally inappropriate inattention and impulsivity." Hyperactivity is frequently present (ADD-H) but not essential for the diagnosis. The identification of ADD as a diagnosis that might or might not be associated with hyperactivity avoided a former oxymoron or linguistic problem—that of the nonhyperactive "hyperactive child." The (frequently) associated features "vary as a function of age and include obstinacy, stubbornness, negativism, bossiness, bullying, increased mood lability, low frustration tolerance, temper outbursts, low self-esteem, and lack of response to discipline." In addition, "Specific Developmental Disorders [SDD, learning disorders] are common." Conduct Disorder was seen as a "complication."

The diagnostic criteria in DSM-III for Attention Deficit Disorder with Hyperactivity are as follows:

The child displays, for his or her mental and chronological age, signs of developmentally inappropriate inattention, impulsivity, and hyperactivity. The signs must be reported by adults in the child's environment, such as parents and teachers. Because the symptoms are typically variable, they may not be observed directly by the clinician. When the reports of teachers and parents conflict, primary consideration should be given to the teacher reports because of greater familiarity with age-appropriate norms. Symptoms typically worsen in situations that require self-application, as in the classroom. Signs of the disorder may be absent when the child is in a new or a one-to-one situation.

The number of symptoms specified is for children between the ages of eight and ten, the peak age range for referral. In younger children, more severe forms of the symptoms and a greater number of symptoms are usually present. The opposite is true of older children.

DSM-III goes on to require at least three of five symptoms of inattention (e.g., "often fails to finish things . . . ," "easily distracted"); three of six symptoms of impulsivity (e.g., "often acts before thinking," "frequently calls out in class"); and at least two of five symptoms of hyperactivity (e.g., "runs about . . . excessively," ". . . fidgets excessively"). DSM-III completes the diagnostic picture by specifying onset before age seven, duration of at least six months, and no presence of schizophrenia, affective disorder, or severe mental retardation.

An important feature of the DSM-III criteria is that the symptoms are grouped under the headings of inattention, impulsivity, and hyperactivity. Many of the diagnostic symptoms are age-related and do not apply to adults—for example, "has difficulty sticking to a play activity," or "frequently calls out in class." DSM-III refers to manifestations of ADD in adults as Attention Deficit Disorder, Residual Type, which includes the following criteria:

A. The individual once met the criteria for Attention Deficit Disorder with Hyperactivity. This information may come from the individual or from others, such as family members.
B. Signs of hyperactivity are no longer present, but other signs of the illness have persisted to the present without periods of remission, as evidenced by signs of both attentional deficits and impulsivity (e.g., difficulty organizing work and completing tasks, difficulty concentrating, being easily distracted, making sudden decisions without thought of the consequences).
C. The symptoms of inattention and impulsivity result in some impairment in social or occupational functioning.
D. Not due to Schizophrenia, Affective Disorder, Severe or Profound

Mental Retardation, or Schizotypal or Borderline Personality Disorders.

Note that the diagnostician may substitute age-appropriate symptoms for the categories of inattention and impulsivity.

DSM-III-R (APA, 1987) introduced several modifications. ADD was rechristened Attention-deficit Hyperactivity Disorder (ADHD) and was classified as one member of a three-member category called Disruptive Behavior Disorders; the two other members were Conduct Disorder and Oppositional Defiant Disorder. Of Disruptive Behavior Disorders, DSM-III-R states: "This subclass of disorders is characterized by behavior that is socially disruptive and is often more distressing to others than to the people with the disorders. . . . Studies have indicated that in both clinic and community samples, the symptoms of these disorders covary to a high degree. In the literature the behaviors that these disorders encompass have been referred to as 'externalizing' symptoms." What had been Attention Deficit Disorder Without Hyperactivity in DSM-III became Undifferentiated Attention Deficit Disorder, which was placed in an "Other" category.

Turning to ADHD, DSM-III-R continues, "The essential features of this disorder are developmentally inappropriate degrees of inattention, impulsiveness, and hyperactivity." However, instead of dividing the symptoms into three groups, DSM-III-R requires the presence of eight of fourteen possible symptoms. These fourteen symptoms are essentially the sixteen symptoms of DSM-III, with slight refinements.

DSM-III and DSM-III-R *defined* ADD-H and ADHD in terms of inattention, impulsivity, and (usually) hyperactivity. The features listed as "associated" were the "left over" signs and symptoms that had previously been lumped under the rubrics of "minimal brain dysfunction" and the "hyperactive child syndrome" but were not included in the revised symptomatic triad.

The associated symptoms include obstinacy, stubbornness, negativism, bossiness, bullying, mood lability, low frustration tolerance, temper outbursts, low self-esteem, and lack of response to discipline. Associated disorders (whose symptoms were *included* in the syndrome of pre-DSM-III days) are Conduct Disorder (CD), Oppositional Defiant Disorder (ODD), and the Specific Developmental Disorders.

DSM-IV (1994) has made the following changes. The main heading under which ADHD falls is now "Attention-Deficit and Disruptive Behavior Disorders." This heading corrects the DSM-III-R scheme, which incorrectly implied that all children with ADHD are disruptive.

In the ADHD section of this major category, a slight stylistic change is being made in the name: Attention-Deficit/Hyperactivity Disorder. DSM-IV now divides the symptoms for ADHD into two groups: *"inattention"* and *"hyperactivity-impulsivity"*; each group contains nine possible symptoms (in the latter group, six symptoms fall under *hyperactivity* and three under *impulsivity*). Using these two groups, *DSM-IV* identifies three subtypes of ADHD:

Attention-Deficit/Hyperactivity Disorder, Combined Type. This subtype should be used if at least six symptoms of inattention and six of hyperactivity-impulsivity have persisted for at least six months. Most children and adolescents have the Combined Type. DSM-IV adds that it is not known whether the same is true of adults with the disorder.

Attention-Deficit/Hyperactivity Disorder, Predominantly Inattentive Type. Used if at least six symptoms of inattention (but fewer than six symptoms of hyperactivity-impulsivity) have persisted for at least six months.

Attention-Deficit/Hyperactivity Disorder, Predominantly Hyperactive-Impulsive Type. Used if at least six symptoms of hyperactivity-impulsivity (but fewer than six symptoms of inattention) have persisted for at least six months.

The important practical consequence of the pre-DSM-III failure to distinguish among Attention-deficit Hyperactivity Disorder, Conduct Disorder, Oppositional Defiant Disorder, and the Specific Developmental Disorders means that the earlier studies, which were based on samples of varying (and unknown) composition, can tell us nothing about the etiology, epidemiology, biological correlates, and natural history or response to treatment of "pure" ADHD, ODD, CD, or SDD. They tell us only something about the mixed syndromes. As Loney and Milich (1982) have observed: "We do not have literature about childhood hyperactivity as such; instead we have literature about childhood externalizing behavior problems (hyperactivity *and* aggression) [or hyperactivity and conduct disorders] that we call a literature about hyperactivity" (p. 143).[1] The important practical point is that these disorders cluster together, and if a child has one he appears more likely to have one or two of the others.

The current construction is illustrated in the Venn diagram (Figure 2.1) in Chapter 2 on signs and symptoms. The diagram is qualitative, not quantitative, and is, I hope, a useful mnemonic. The absence of a name for the conjunction of these three syndromes is based on the notion that they are "co-morbid" rather than varying manifestations of the same disorder—a point that will be discussed later.

ADHD IN ADULTS

∎

Although DSM-III recognized that ADD might persist into adulthood, as Attention Deficit Disorder, Residual Type (ADD,RT), there were few systematically acquired data about the syndrome and DSM-III was understandably vague about its symptoms. There are at least three problems with the description. First is the statement that hyperactivity disappears. Often it does not—it persists but changes its form (more about that later). Second, the use of the word "residual" implies persistence despite partial recovery (analogous to "Schizophrenia, Residual Type"). This is a prejudgment: As I discuss later, in many instances ADHD in adults is a continuation of the same childhood disorder in which many symptoms persist without diminution; the patient copes with the resultant problems in an age-specific way but is still handicapped. For example, the child's temper tantrums and failure to hand in his homework may be paralleled by the ADHD adult's drunken explosion at his family and failure to compile and submit his tax forms on time. Third, many of the descriptors mentioned earlier that are useful in school-age children, such as "has difficulty sticking to a play activity," "has difficulty awaiting turn in games or group situations," or "runs about or climbs on things excessively," are not useful in diagnosing adults—for example, in a 45-year-old professor of comparative literature with ADHD.

DSM-III-R does not specify the criteria for diagnosing ADHD in adults but says that the diagnosis should be given if the patient had ADHD symptoms in childhood or adolescence and if the "condition has persisted." Characteristic adult symptoms are not provided. Using DSM-III criteria, the diagnostician could employ adult instances of inattention, impulsivity, and hyperactivity, such as "takes forever to complete tax forms" or "doesn't pay attention to and keeps interrupting wife."

Since the DSM-III and DSM-III-R criteria (DSM-IV makes no further refinements regarding adults with ADHD) suggest but do not specify symptoms, the diagnostician who suspects ADHD in an adult faces the problem of needing more explicit description. For the researcher who seeks to provide such a description, the most straightforward means would be to examine a group of adults who had been diagnosed with ADHD in childhood. In approaching the research task of identifying ADHD in adults, my colleagues and I did not have that option; we had no such sample available.

I began by studying the parents of ADHD children who described their own childhood as similar to that of their child. Many reported that their problems had continued. They described a recurring list of *symptoms,* and their spouses described a recurring list of maladaptive or unpleasant behaviors or signs. These, together with others I had chosen as characteristic in pre-DSM-III days (Wender, 1971), formed the pool from which we constructed operational adult diagnostic criteria. There remained the problem of whether adults with such symptoms and signs, who could presumably be diagnosed as having ADHD, would have qualified for such a diagnosis in childhood. Our first approach was to query them systematically about their behavior and problems as children. Since their memories were often hazy, we then began to interview *their* parents. Finally, we attempted to quantify their childhood behavior by having their parents rate that behavior on a standardized checklist. The foregoing will be described in detail in Chapter 5 on diagnosis.

THE POLYTHETIC DEFINITION OF ADHD

■

ADHD is *said* to be present if a certain *number* of symptoms is present. In modern terminology, this is a "polythetic" method of categorization. When most of us think about classifying objects, shapes, species, we think, nonreflectively, of *monothetic* definitions: man is a featherless biped, an isosceles triangle is a triangle with two equal sides. However, in medicine we unconsciously employ polythetic definition whenever we employ syndromal definitions, and since the birth of the American Psychiatric Association's DSM-III, psychiatry has used it widely.

A polythetic definition of a disease (or of anything else) might assert that it is present if any two of symptoms A, B, C, D, or E are present. Thus, two patients may have the same disease and have no *outward* symptoms in common. For example, one patient might have the two symptoms A and B while another had C and D or C and E or D and E. A good medical example is rheumatic fever. It is defined to be present if a patient has any two of the five major clinical signs: polyarthritis, carditis, chorea, erythema marginatum, or subcutaneous nodules.[2] The reason this definition is employed is that these symptoms are felt to be the different consequences of infections by various strains of group "A" streptococci. Not only may two individuals have rheumatic fever and completely different signs and symptoms, but also they may have different natural histories: the course of patients with and without carditis differs greatly—the patients with carditis are at increased risk for persistent symptoms.

A more pertinent instance would be DSM-III's ADD-H and ADD without hyperactivity. It is commonly believed, and there are some data to support the belief, that ADD with hyperactivity responds more frequently to stimulant medication than does ADD without hyperactivity. Since DSM-III-R is based on the number rather than the nature of symptoms, it is entirely possible that this observation will be lost. Thus, ADHD may bear some resemblances to rheumatic fever.

A COMMENT ON SYNDROMES, PRECISION, AND RELATED ADHD SYNDROMES

■

I believe that ADHD is a genetically transmitted and biologically mediated group of conditions and that it is virtually certain that the individuals we classify as having ADHD are genetically—and therefore biologically—heterogeneous. I am here hypothesizing that genetically transmitted psychiatric disorders are no different from other genetically transmitted medical disorders. Thus, I believe that ADHD might be like the disorders of hemoglobin synthesis, such as sickle cell disease, hemoglobin C, and the thalassemias, of which there are at least 300 forms, or the more than 200 variants of glucose-6-phosphate dehydrogenase. Another illustrative example of genetic heterogeneity is phenylketonuria, a disorder in which the affected individual cannot hydroxylate phenylalanine to tyrosine. PKU was first demonstrated to have an autosomal recessive pattern of inheritance, which is now regarded as "classical PKU." Currently, more than forty forms of PKU are recognized, based on genetic mutations affecting enzymes involved in the hydroxylation process. In addition, there is a phenocopy of PKU, produced by a fetus's exposure to a previously treated mother who is no longer on a restrictive diet. Similarly, in the case of ADHD, there may be "phenocopies," instances in which the syndrome might be produced by nongenetic effects, such as maternal alcohol or substance abuse, malnutrition, or infection during the pregnancy.

An essential feature of the major psychiatric disorders is that they are *not* defined at the etiological or pathophysiological level. We do not have any method of testing for the presence or absence of ADHD or any of its subgroups. Recognizing that, it is meaningless to define a syndrome on the basis of particular signs and symptoms and then to study the occurrence of others. This has been clearly stated by McKusick: "When one does not have a specifically diagnostic laboratory test or other diagnostic means independent of the clinical phenotype, one cannot list the frequency of occurrence of specific features without falling into circular reasoning" (1969, p. 343).

Aristotle observed, "It is a mark of an educated man to look for precision in things so far as the nature of the subject admits." His observation is not outdated. Accordingly, the findings in the studies of ADHD that will be examined in this book may be highly variable. The prevalence, natural history, response to medication, and biological concomitants may have huge variations—produced by unrecognizable heterogeneity in the population studied. There is no "pure" ADHD and further phenomenological redefining of ADHD cannot be expected to solve the problem. The number of symptoms chosen "to make" the diagnosis is not based on independent characteristics at a different level of discourse (i.e., a pathophysiological foundation). All the studies in this book must be taken with a large grain of salt. Figures (prevalence, outcome, etc.) may be given to two decimal places while we cannot be sure of our figures to one decimal place. We are measuring amoebas with a rubber ruler. This point cannot be made strongly enough and will be repeated throughout this monograph. The diagnostic criteria are provisional (tentative) and will be kept only as long as they are useful.

In sum, Attention-deficit Hyperactivity Disorder is the name of a syndrome, but applying the same name to disorders suffered by a group of individuals does not necessarily mean "they have the same thing." In medicine we realize that syndromes are frequently etiologically heterogeneous. (This is particularly true in the early stages of nosology: Consider "fever," "anemia," and especially "mental retardation.") It would be helpful if, following the example of Bleuler with respect to schizophrenia,[3] we referred to "The Group of ADHDs"; among other consequences, we would expend less effort on trying to select the *exact* signs and symptoms that characterize *the* illness.[4] The syndromal character of this disorder has implications for pathogenesis, such as the phenomena of polygenic determination, genetic heterogeneity, variable penetrance and pleiotropy. These will be discussed in Chapter 4 on etiology.

NOTES

1. A comparable situation in pre-DSM-III psychiatry occurs with respect to the schizophrenias, chronic and acute (or "schizophreniform" disorders). Many instances of the acute schizophrenias are now diagnosed—and *treated*—as major affective disorders with psychosis.

2. American Heart Association: Jones criteria (revised) for guidance in the diagnosis of rheumatic fever. *Circulation* 69:204A, 1984. There are ten possible and distinct symptom patterns: (1) Carditis and Sydenham's Chorea, (2) Carditis and Subcutaneous Nodules, (3) Carditis and Polyarthritis, (4) Carditis and Erythema Marginatum, (5) Sydenham's Chorea and Subcutaneous Nodules, (6) Sydenham's Chorea and Polyarthritis, (7) Sydenham's Chorea and Erythema Marginatum, (8) Subcutaneous Nodules and Polyarthritis, (9) Subcutaneous Nodules and Erythema Marginatum, (10) Polyarthritis and Erythema Marginatum.

3. Bleuler's monograph (1911) is titled *Dementia Praecox or The Group of Schizophrenias;* note the word "group."

4. This point is not novel. The betrayal of thought by language was noted and commented on by the early American semanticist Alexander Bryant Johnson (1836), who observed, "The identity which language implies is responded to by nature very nearly or we could possess no medical science; but the most skillful physician is often defeated by the anomalies of nature. Physicians have long noted the anomalies, and deemed them anomalies of nature. The anomaly is, however, in language which united under one name, as identities, what is only partially identical. Individuality is no anomaly of nature. It is nature's regular production, and boundless richness" (1959, p. 80).

2

Signs and Symptoms

■

In developing an understanding of Attention-deficit Hyperactivity Disorder in adults, it is useful to review briefly the nature of ADHD in children and then to examine the adult versions of ADHD symptoms in children. I will, therefore, present in this chapter a description of the following characteristics of ADHD, as found in both children and adults: attention difficulties, motor abnormalities (hyperactivity and impaired coordination), impulsivity, disorganization, altered response to social reinforcement, altered interpersonal relations, altered emotionality, stress intolerance, response to medication, and associated syndromes.

ATTENTION DIFFICULTIES

■

CHILDHOOD

ADHD children are described as having a "short attention span," as not sticking with things, as being distractible. Parents report that the child never plays at one game for a long period of time and rushes from one activity to another. As a toddler, the child pulls every toy from the shelf, plays with each desultorily, and then seems at a loss for further things to do. Attentional difficulties may be noticed by parents, but in general they become a salient problem when the ADHD child first attends school. There his[1] inattentiveness produces a recurrent litany of teacher complaints: he "can't stick with things for long," is "always wool gathering or daydreaming," "unmotivated," or "lacking in stick-to-it-tiveness," "can't follow instructions."

At home his mother notices that "he doesn't listen for long . . . he doesn't mind . . . he doesn't remember." The parents must hover over the child to get him to do what they want. Told once to eat with his fork and not his hands, he complies, but a few seconds later he is eating with his hands again. He may begin his homework as requested but fail to complete it unless the parents nag him. The child may not necessarily disobey instructions, but in the middle of an assigned job he starts doing something else. His room is half restored to order; the lawn is half mowed. Sometimes the child appears to remember but is reluctant to comply. At other times he appears to be distracted from the task at hand. As a consequence of decreased attentiveness, the child is told repeatedly by teachers that he could do well if he wanted to but that he doesn't want to. This is often capped by comparing him unfavorably with a previously taught, virtuous, hard-working sibling.

It is important to note that like hyperactivity, distractibility is not always present. Often when the child receives individual attention, he can attend well for a while. The teacher may report that he "does well with one-on-one attention." A psychologist may note that the child can attend during testing. A pediatrician may observe that the child was attentive during the brief office examination. They are all correct, but what is important is not how the child can pay attention when an adult is exerting the maximum effort to get him to do so or when he feels ill at ease in a new setting. If the examiner does not realize the potential variability of such behavior, he or she may incorrectly come to the conclusion that the child is perfectly fine and that the parents and teacher are overreacting.

Furthermore, the child *can* often pay attention to material *he* finds interesting. He follows Saturday morning TV cartoons and advertisements; he may read and reread books about dinosaurs, earthquakes, typhoons, tidal waves, volcanoes, war, and other natural and unnatural disasters; and his interests may even appear perseverative. In these instances, his attention is not under what might be called "social control." Unlike the "obedient" child, his attention lags when he is requested to attend to, say, fractions and spelling. (A clear-cut example of the relationship between attention and interest was that of a ten-year-old boy with an IQ of 142 who obtained C's and D's in school while in his spare time he bought used lawn mowers, rebuilt their motors, and sold them for a substantial profit.)

As the ADHD child grows older, he often continues to have less ability to focus his attention where he *has* to, even though the pressures are now internalized—when he himself insists that he do certain necessary and uninteresting things. That attention increases with age and that attention and interest are closely related are not novel observations. William James observes in his *Principles of Psychology*, "My experience is what I *agree* to attend to" and "Interest alone gives accent" (1890, p. 402, my emphasis). He also addresses the normal ("physiological") inattentiveness of childhood, saying

> childhood is characterized by great active energy, and has few organized interests by which to meet new impressions and decide whether they are worthy of notice or not, and the consequence is that extreme mobility of the attention with which we are all familiar in children, and which makes their first lessons such rough affairs. . . . This reflexive and passive character of the attention . . . makes the child seem to belong less to himself than to every object which happens to catch notice, [and] is the first thing which the teacher must overcome. It never is overcome in *some people, whose work, to the end of life, gets done in the interstices of their mind-wandering.* (p. 417, my emphasis)

ADULTHOOD

In adulthood, only a small fraction of ADHD patients mention attentional difficulties spontaneously. Apparently the major reason for this is that our patients are no longer in school or in occupations that routinely require the ability to focus attention steadily for long periods of time. However, the ADHD adult continues to have less ability to focus his attention when that is necessary. Because many ADHD adults have learned that they do poorly in situations requiring constant and careful attention to detail, they have sought jobs—such as non-clerical work—without such requirements in order to reduce the stress upon themselves.

The ADHD adult who is still in technical school or college may have persistent attentional problems that continue to interfere with his performance, and he will be the same "underachiever" at 30 that he was at 7. Such a subject usually reports that he has difficulty keeping his "mind on" reading materials in which he is not interested or in performing necessary tasks that he finds boring. He relates that when confronted by stern necessity, he can stay at a desk for five or ten minutes, but then he must get up and walk around for a few minutes before continuing. (If a patient reads much less than expected for his or her level of education, one suspects the persistence of ADHD or a developmental reading disorder.)

Regardless of the demands of school and job, attentional difficulties manifest themselves elsewhere in the life of the ADHD adult. For example, he may rarely be able to sit through a television program or a movie. Attentional difficulties often also interfere with personal relationships. The ADHD adult may find it as difficult to keep his mind on his wife's conversation as he did on his teacher's lectures. His inattentiveness is often compounded by impulsivity, so that even when he's listening, he interrupts, annoying his spouse and preventing her from completing her thoughts. Such failures to attend to what his spouse is saying may be incompletely diagnosed (i.e., misdiagnosed as simply a *learned* interactive style) as a "communication problem" by a psychotherapist.

ADHD adults report that they are distractible, which reveals another aspect of attention problems. Such ADHD sufferers learn that the best way to minimize distractions is to seek a place with no visual stimuli that is as quiet as possible. One medical student would retire to a small locked room in the library in the early morning hours to obtain what was virtually an anechoic chamber.

Attentional difficulties are also associated with problems of short-term memory. Patients state that even when they force themselves to look systematically at the page (which is, of course, different from concentrating on the page!) they retain little or nothing. One skilled machinist had to write down his boss's instructions because otherwise he would forget them. Unfocused attention is associated with frequent complaints of losing or misplacing keys, wallets, purses, and so forth, being late for appointments, and forgetting plans. As in childhood, the ADHD adult is accused of having a mind that "is frequently somewhere else."

As indicated, appropriate choice of occupation and interpersonal relations can minimize problems due to attention. The 30-year-old ADHD male who is an oil rig roustabout or truck driver and who is accepted as a person of few words will obviously have much less difficulty than the ADHD adult who works daily with detail, who must include reading and writing in his usual routines, and who lives among people who want or need to be listened to carefully.

MOTOR ABNORMALITIES: HYPERACTIVITY AND IMPAIRED COORDINATION

■

CHILDHOOD

ADHD children may have both gross and fine motor hyperactivity, kicking their feet, drumming with their fingers, twisting in their seats *and* rushing hither and yon, "driven like a motor." To paraphrase George Orwell,[2] all little boys are hyperactive, but some little boys are more hyperactive than others. Excessive motor activity is not evident on the playground when all the children may be going full speed, but it becomes clear in the classroom, where the children are expected to take their feet off their accelerators or apply the brakes.

There is a predictable developmental sequence for "hyperactivity," which may begin in fetal life. Astute mothers of several children (some of these mothers are hyperactive themselves) sometimes report that the ADHD child began kicking more vigorously in utero than his nonhyperactive sibs. The ADHD child is often described as active and restless in infancy and toddlerhood, "into everything," inadvertently breaking his toys and household objects, and requiring supervision at all times for his own protection as well as the preservation of the household. When he grows older, he is constantly fidgeting, unable to sit still at the dinner table or even in front of the television set. Another manifestation of hyperactivity may be persistent overtalkativeness, sometimes described as "motor mouth."

It is important to emphasize that excessive motor activity is not a necessary diagnostic component of the ADHD syndrome. The attentional deficit and allied problems may occur in children who are normally active or even relatively inactive.

Impaired coordination is present in many but not all ADHD children. The difficulties may be in balance, hand-eye coordination, or fine motor performance. Such children can be slow at learning to button buttons, zip zippers, and tie shoelaces. In kindergarten they have difficulty cutting along or coloring between lines. In elementary school, the child's printing is sometimes legible, but his script is hard to read (handwriting may improve substantially in response to stimulant medication). On the playing field, poor hand-eye coordination affects the children's skill at sports—for example, in baseball these boys are often strike-out artists when *at bat*. Such deficits are quickly identified by their peers, who will pick them last when choosing teams and have them batting ninth and playing right field.

Because ADHD children show these motor problems, repeated attempts have been made to quantify the motor and other neurological signs by neurological examinations. These studies have been primarily concerned with "soft signs" since no one has claimed an appreciably increased frequency of "hard" classical neurological deficits in most ADHD children. The term "soft" has been used variably to characterize three distinct groups of abnormalities: (1) Functions that are age and developmentally dependent; that is, tasks that normal younger children cannot perform and that normal older children *can* perform. An average four-year-old might be expected to stand on one foot for N seconds, while a normal ten-year-old might be expected to do so for $2N$ seconds; if a ten-year-old could stand for only N seconds, he might be said to have a "soft" sign. (2) Abnormalities in neurological function whose neurological basis is unknown. Where is the lesion in a twelve-year-old boy who can sink only one basket out of ten, has a batting average of 0.073, or is "just clumsy" ("all thumbs" or has "two left feet")? (3) Slight abnormalities in "hard" neurological signs, difficult to detect and difficult to measure in replication studies, resulting in poor test-retest reliability. Note the difference between this category and the previous category. Rutter et al. (1970) conducted a study in which they administered a standardized neurological examination to a large sample of normal and neurologically impaired 9- and 10-year-olds. The authors found that "language, speech, motor coordination and constructional abilities can all be assessed with good reliability; in most cases these assessments proved more reliable than assessments of slight abnormalities in reflex and tone" (p. 60).

A major limitation of these and other neurodevelopmental examinations is that motor proficiency increases with age, and a useful examination must be standardized for different ages. Gardner (1979) examined a large sample of "minimally brain dysfunctioned" (MBD) and normal children between the ages of 5 and 15 and thus dealt with the issue of performance changes with age. He found considerable differences between MBD and comparison children on a variety of psychomotor, perceptual, and cognitive tasks, *but* these differences were most marked in the younger children and diminished substantially with age. Thus, as the children became older the mean scores of the MBD children and controls still differed, but there was an increasing degree of overlap between the two groups. One would consequently predict that these and similar tasks, while perhaps diagnostically useful in younger children, would be less diagnostically useful in the differential diagnosis of adult ADHD. It is also important to remember that like motoric "hyperactivity," impaired coordination is frequently not present in ADHD children and is not diagnostically necessary.

ADULTHOOD

"ADHD children grown up"—our patients—continue to manifest signs as adults that indicate they remain hyperactive. In making this statement, I am amplifying DSM-III and DSM-III-R. DSM-III states that in cases of ADD, Residual Type "signs of hyperactivity are no longer present, but other signs of the illness have persisted to the present without periods of remission." DSM-III-R adds that "In older children and adolescents, the most prominent features tend to be excessive fidgeting and restlessness rather than gross motor overactivity." ADHD adults may no longer run about or climb on things excessively, but they continue to be uncomfortable sitting still, dislike being "inactive," and find it difficult to "relax." Some feel comfortable only when they manage to maintain a constant high level of physical activity. They prefer to stand rather than sit and will move—or even run—continually from task to task (see Disorganization in this chapter). Unlike Ferdinand the Bull, they do not want to sit quietly under a cork tree and smell the flowers. They cannot sit and contemplate life.

When such perpetual motion or constant restlessness is present, it is not accompanied by dysphoria. However, forced immobility may cause anxiety. One young lawyer remembered that as a late adolescent he had to run to deplete excess energy so that he could do his homework. He would take several turns around the block in Manhattan, but when night fell he was restricted to his apartment house. At such times he would study for ten or fifteen minutes, build up a full head of steam, rush down 18 flights of stairs and sprint up again to lower his energy level enough to study. As an adult he felt a compulsive need to be active, and if he had been taking neuroleptics, he might have been diagnosed as having akathasia. Another patient described how he "nearly went crazy" when a heavily casted compound fracture of the leg kept him in bed for one month. Many ADHD subjects are unable to persist in sedentary activities, such as watching movies or television, or reading a book. "He can't sit still—he gets up from the table the second dinner is finished . . . he's a jack-in-the-box." In one example, following the forced immobility of a dinner party, the hostess not only took care of the protracted cleaning up but strong-armed all the family members to move the furniture in anticipation of the decorators' arrival three days hence. Once she had begun to clean, she couldn't stop moving and commandeered her non-ADHD family to participate.

Fidgeting and foot movements (known in our research setting as "Wender's sign") are very common signs of hyperactivity in adult ADHD patients—so much so that such patients can usually be diagnosed in the waiting room by a knowledgeable receptionist. The two most common foot motions are the crossed-knee foot jiggle and the unilateral or bilateral toe tap (with heels on or off the floor). My impression is that both occur at a faster frequency than similar movements in non-ADHD adults. I seriously entertain the possibility that this foot movement may be a biological marker for ADHD—or a genetic marker of alcoholism.[3] Interestingly, F. Scott Fitzgerald included similar movements in his description of Jay Gatsby: "He was never quite still; there was always a tapping foot somewhere or the impatient opening and closing of a hand" (Fitzgerald, 1925, p. 64).

Motor function has not been studied in ADHD adults, and tests that have been employed with children have not been standardized with adults and probably would not be useful. Because the motor tests that discriminate between younger ADHD children and controls become increasingly less discriminating in older children, the best one can do is to query the patient about his performance in a number of areas—such as precision work with tools. Frequently, he is still maladroit and inept at various sports, and his handwriting may remain childish (it may be useful to have the patient write cursively to rapid dictation).

IMPULSIVITY

■

CHILDHOOD

Impulsivity is one of the striking characteristics of ADHD children and is manifest in the classroom, in the playground, and in the home. In formal terminology, ADHD children are often said to have a decrease in the ability to "delay gratification" or to have "a low frustration tolerance." They are described as impatient and as rapidly becoming upset when people or things fail to behave as expected. In the classroom, they blurt things out, interrupt others, and commit other disruptive peccadilloes. Outside the classroom, ADHD children are often reckless and manifest no concern for bodily safety. They are likely to jump off the roof with an umbrella parachute, pursue a ball into the street without thinking, or dive into a dry swimming pool before looking. Because they act without thinking, they suffer more than their share of accidents. The frequent reports of injuries (including head injuries) in the histories of these children are often a manifestation of ADHD and not a primary cause of it. One study (Stewart, 1970) found that one out of three or four boys (average age 2 to 7) brought to a hospital for accidental poisoning was diagnosed as "hyperactive."

The relationship between the impulsivity of ADHD and the social transgressions seen in older children and adolescents is unclear. In the older literature the list of related transgressions includes lying, shoplifting, stealing, destructiveness, joyriding, fire setting, early drug and alcohol use, and fighting. However, more recent analyses question whether such transgressions are associated with ADHD or with mixtures of ADHD and conduct disorder (ADHD/CD). Moreover, the earlier studies did not discriminate between ADHD children who impulsively initiate or "go along" with antisocial behavior and CD children whose antisocial activities are a more characteristic part of their behavior.

ADULTHOOD

Adulthood unfortunately provides a much broader scope for impulsive behavior and a much greater opportunity for inflicting serious self-damage. ADHD adults continue to act on the spur of the moment—and to think afterward. As in mania, important decisions are often made without reflection and on the basis of insufficient information. Impulsivity occurs in work, in interpersonal activities, and in problem solving. The ADHD adult quits jobs without thinking of the possible disadvantages of doing so. Subjects frequently give a history of multiple personal relationships and marriages, contracted and ended without reflection. One unsubtle instance of impulsivity occurred in our pemoline study. A patient asked me to compliment him because "I'm getting married." When I said, "I didn't even know there was anybody on the scene," he replied, "There wasn't—we've only known each other for three days." I did compliment him, and then realized he had probably recruited another subject—his wife to be.

DISORGANIZATION

∎

CHILDHOOD

ADHD children are often massively disorganized. Elementary school forms a sensitive detection device for this, and if the evaluator of the putative ADHD patient can obtain any of the patient's early school papers, the diagnosis may make itself. Assignments are not written down or are copied inaccurately. Frequently, they are not finished on time or not done at all. Writing is often placed unsystematically, and a complete composition may be placed in one-quarter of the page. Columnar arrangement of arithmetic calculations is often chaotic. Disorganization is also noticeable in desks, lockers, and at home. Preadolescent boys are not renowned for neatness, but preadolescent ADHD children are often easily distinguished from their "ordinarily sloppy" peers by the degree of their messiness.

ADULTHOOD

The ADHD child's untidiness and failure to plan ahead are given much greater scope in adulthood. Messy school desks become messy desks at work, and overdue, inadequate homework becomes delayed and confused reports and memoranda. One car salesman was not able to see why his wife was apoplectic about his failure to organize and why his boss was about to fire him because his sales records were incomplete for six months. The ADHD child's cluttered bedroom becomes the adult's unkempt home. One despairing husband of an ADHD woman described their refrigerator as having been taken over by a rich collection of bacterial and fungal life that had established itself on six-month-old food, threatened to escape, and might soon be contained only with a flame thrower. His wife, the co-parent of three "hyperactive" children, was a witty, literate, absentminded professor, who had never mastered the art of aligning or sequentially buttoning her invariably stained white blouses.

Disorganization around a household is easy to observe. The housewife with ADHD tells us (or her husband does) that she may start to vacuum, think it would be a good time to bake a cake and mix the ingredients, and then before putting the cake in the oven, decide to do her laundry. Her male counterpart not infrequently has several projects underway simultaneously (e.g., building a deck, paneling the basement, painting a room). Patients' spouses complain of months taken to complete home improvements that could ordinarily be completed by even an inept home improver in two weeks.

ALTERED RESPONSE TO SOCIAL REINFORCEMENT

■

CHILDHOOD

Repeated failure to comply with requests occurs in children with ADHD, Conduct Disorder (CD), and Oppositional Defiant Disorder (ODD), but the quality and style of noncompliance differ among the three groups. "Pure" hyperactive children often fail to do what they are asked, but usually through forgetfulness or distraction. When reminded, they may be both apologetic and, when young, tearful. The ODD child is also noncompliant, but when he refuses to do what is asked he seems to be deliberately provocative, enjoying the discomfort his noncompliance causes others—behavior that could be the childhood antecedent of "passive-aggressive" personality disorder in the adult (a conjecture offered by DSM-III-R). The CD child—in extreme "pure culture"—neglects societal requests, and if he believes he can "get away with it," he may simply carry on with the cruelty, callousness, or other antisocial behavior in which he was previously engaged, without guilt or remorse. The point is that all noncompliance is not created equal.

Temperamentally, many ADHD children act as if they were locked into the chronological stage of the "terrible twos." Parents of hyperactive children report that most disciplinary measures seem unsuccessful: rewards, deprivation of privileges, physical punishment. "He wants his own way . . . he never learns by his own mistakes . . . you can't reach him . . . he's almost immune to punishment."

The parents describe their hyperactive children as "obstinate," "forgetful," "stubborn," "negativistic," "indifferent," "not minding." The parents' reactions to their difficult children are understandable, but more precise observations indicate that the children do respond to the effects of *immediate* positive reinforcement. However, the effects do not last—that is, the reinforced behaviors extinguish rapidly. Parental inefficacy in socializing such children is often interpreted psycho-genetically, so that the child's behavior may be interpreted as a re-sponse to inconsistency or unconscious encouragement. Of course, children influence parents and shape *their* behavior, and parents whose disciplining efforts are not reinforced by success may become lax about enforcing rules and consistently rewarding compliance or punishing noncompliance. There is a two-way directionality of effect (Bell, 1968). Thus, it is often difficult to determine how the child would have re-sponded to more consistent disciplining, and with that issue in doubt confusion may remain as to whether the child is ADHD, CD, ODD, or some combination.

Disobedience also has secondary consequences: the adult reaction can produce a "vicious circle" of further, reactive negativism and non-compliance in the child. In this frequently unrecognized pattern of "deviation amplifying feedback" or "positive feedback," the parents' criticism itself amplifies the maladaptive behavior (Wender, 1968).

ADULTHOOD

Adult ADHD patients may recall that they were frequently repri-manded for not carrying out requests, but often they do not remember the circumstances of noncompliance. Some adults will describe them-selves as having been noncompliant or disobedient but having been "brought back into line" by firm or rigid rules at home or school. One man whose mother had been very physically abusive remarked, "I probably would have been a discipline problem at school except that I knew that then my mother would have *really* beaten the shit out of me." Another ADHD patient reported, "I was so hyperactive in the first grade that I was tied to my seat."

Essentially, however, there are no data on noncompliance in adult-hood. In our own drug studies on adults, we did not include adults who may have been marked noncompliers in childhood; children who had been ODD or CD entered our samples as adults only if they had out-grown those characteristics. Patients with a diagnosis of or several symptoms of Antisocial Personality Disorder (ASPD) were excluded. Many of the spouses of our drug-responsive patients report that the medication seemed to help the patients to "listen better" and take others' interests into consideration more. However, it is hard to deter-mine whether altered responsivity to implicit and explicit social de-mands plays a role or whether the changes are the consequence of improved attention and patience and decreased irritability and impulsivity.

ALTERED INTERPERSONAL RELATIONS

∎

CHILDHOOD

A number of interpersonal traits seem associated with ADHD. ADHD children are frequently characterized by parents and teachers as bossy, domineering, stubborn, and bullying. They want to play the game their way, by their rules. Since such traits are often combined with social immaturity, inability to stick with games, and athletic clumsiness, many ADHD children have few friends. They are not socially avoidant or beset by social anxiety, but others may reject them because of attributes that are seen as unattractive.

Some of these children—particularly when younger—*may* have an insatiable demand for attention. In part, such a demand might be seen as a response to frequent rejection, but in other children the quality is apparent to mothers even in early infancy. Many of the children do obtain attention later by acting as a class clown. Others may try to win friends by buying them with stolen goods. ADHD children are also frequently teased. Other children—excellent diagnosticians that they are—soon learn that the ADHD child has multiple incompetencies and deficits. They find that his threshold of response is low, he may be grossly overreactive, and he is a ripe target—a cinch to "get a rise out of."

Finally, one gets the impression that many ADHD children lack age-appropriate interpersonal sensitivity—that their awareness of others' feelings, behavior, and motivation is more like that of a child several years younger. Admittedly, this is a vague comment; nevertheless, my experience leads me to urge clinicians to keep it in mind.

ADULTHOOD

Although some ADHD adults are also described by spouses or others as stubborn and "bossy," there are no systematic data about such traits in the group as a whole. Certainly, ADHD adults affect others by failure to pay attention and by loss of temper (see next section), but it is difficult to think of the group of ADHD adults in overall interpersonal terms. Some subtle and complex problems are highlighted, however, when drug treatment is effective. The wife of the owner of a small business reported that "it was as if he *finally* saw the light . . . he saw what was obvious to everyone . . . mostly with his employees. . . ." "How?" "Several things . . . he listened to them, and found some were right . . . and one time admitted he was wrong . . . he stopped being angry and then going too far . . . he didn't feel everyone had to like him . . . he was finally able to fire people he should have fired a long time ago."

ALTERED EMOTIONALITY: TEMPER AND MOOD

■

CHILDHOOD

The ADHD child often has very labile mood—dysphoric at one time and overexcited another (one mother aptly described her son as "mercurial"). The excitement is not euphoric but is more that of being out of control and "unwinding." It is the way a young child is at the end of a long and tiring day, often described as "overtired." "Stimulus-rich" situations that most children regard as pleasurable often produce excessive excitement, while unpleasurable ones can produce temper outbursts. Many young children become excited at the supermarket or the circus; ADHD children tend to become overexcited and to lose control with only brief exposure to such situations. The lability is also noticeable as a spontaneous as well as a reactive phenomenon.

Such "affective instability" also produces excessive anger—and a hot temper. ADHD children are variously described as having a short fuse, a low flashpoint, and a low boiling point. As adolescents, they sometimes have a history of fighting although this is more typical of CD youngsters.

Some of these children *appear* to have a decreased ability to experience pleasure. They are, to coin a neologism, "hypohedonic"; the term "anhedonia," used in connection with major depression to indicate the inability to experience interest or pleasure, seems too severe (extreme). In their classic article, "Hyperkinetic Behavior Syndrome in Children," Laufer and Denhoff (1957) described the concern of many mothers that from infancy on they had not been able to make their "hyperkinetic" children "really" happy. The mothers attributed their failure to maternal ineptitude, but Laufer and Denhoff saw the condition as a congenital attribute of the child and suggested the importance of conveying to the mothers that the difficulty was not their fault. This decreased ability to experience pleasure that seems characteristic of some ADHD children now is understood as possibly the product of co-existing early major depression and ADHD. At the time Laufer and Denhoff wrote their paper, major depression was thought to be extremely rare in pre-adolescent children, but it is now recognized as not uncommon. Furthermore, it apparently has a greater than chance association with childhood ADHD: Carlson and Cantwell (1980) found that one-quarter of their outpatient sample of children with a diagnosis of major depression had a diagnosis of ADHD or conduct disorder as well.

Even when they do not have symptoms of major depression, many ADHD adolescents frequently seem demoralized—that is, they feel that they are helpless, ineffectual, and unable to solve their problems (Klein, 1974). Their schoolwork is too hard and too boring, they are disorganized, they lack stick-to-it-tiveness. The defeats and failures they experience are real, and demoralization is an understandable psychological consequence.

One final "emotional" characteristic of ADHD children is low self-esteem, which can be explained in two ways. First, the psychological basis is clear. The ADHD child receives a steady diet of negative feedback from parents, teachers, and peers. He is frequently punished, while his siblings are not. His teachers tell him that he could do better if he tried or ask him why he does not work as hard as his brother. Peers tease him, laugh at him when he plays the class clown, and do not invite him to parties or sleepovers. If his parents are also afflicted with ADHD, they may even physically abuse him. With such constant negative input, it is rational for the ADHD child to think of himself as bad, stupid, and unlikable.

Second, there may also be physiological components to the ADHD child's low self-esteem. The hypohedonia and boredom are clues, for the level of self-esteem is related to mood. Manics think they are terrific; major depressives think they are no good. Thus, the biological factors that are believed to have important links with mood may also play a role in the normal regulation of self-esteem. The biological correlates of self-esteem are reflected in the precarious psychological status of substance abusers: they are grandiose when "high" on cocaine or amphetamines, and they feel helpless and worthless when they "crash." Both psychological and pharmacological factors apparently play a role in the increase in self-esteem produced in medication-responsive ADHD children. The change in feedback and in self-esteem produced by successful stimulant treatment was illustrated by a seven-year-old informant who described his medication as turning him into a "good boy" who received praise rather than criticism from teachers, invitations to birthday parties, and compliments from his parents, and who now had fewer fights with his siblings.

ADULTHOOD

Affective lability is usually present in the ADHD adult in a form similar to that in the child. Patients report that it antedates adolescence, and when they can remember their childhood, they may relate that it extends back as far as they can remember. The mood shifts are characterized by "ups" and "downs" that occur both autonomously and in reaction to readily identifiable life experiences. Their duration is often short—minutes to hours—and several shifts per day are not uncommon. Patients may describe their moods as roller-coaster-like and nod affirmatively when the interviewer makes a sine-wave gesture with his hand. The "ups" of the ADHD adult are more like the excitement of the overstimulated child in the supermarket or circus than like the elation of the euphoric or hypomanic. The patients report that as they became older the spontaneous ups tended to disappear while the downs persisted. The downs are usually not accompanied by anhedonia, and even when prolonged, they are usually not accompanied by the neuro-vegetative alterations seen in major depression. The "downs" are often described as discontentment or boredom. Unlike the major depressive, the ADHD patient maintains the ability to experience pleasure; good news, a party, or an encounter with an attractive member of the opposite sex can quickly raise his mood.

Some patients, particularly when younger, seek excitement as an antidote for "boredom." The ADHD adolescent may engage in dangerous activities such as motorcycle racing, rock climbing, and playing "chicken." Such "sensation seeking" probably puts the ADHD adolescent at increased risk for accidents (Zuckerman, 1985). Lastly, there is the powerful association between alcoholic intoxication, automobile accidents, and fatalities in the young. To the extent that ADHD increases the risk for early alcohol and other substance abuse, ADHD adolescents and adults would be expected to constitute a disproportionately large fraction of drivers in serious accidents.

Although the ADHD patient's spontaneous depressions are generally shortlived, the ADHD patient's propensity to get himself into realistic life difficulties is constant and may produce prolonged "depressions" or demoralization. The combination of academic, vocational, and interpersonal difficulties often causes the ADHD patient to construct and fall into a deep morass from which he cannot extricate himself readily. However, such "depressions" respond well to simple supportive therapy of various kinds.

Explosive temper often also persists well into adult life. In general, ADHD adults calm down quickly between explosions, but some are chronically irritable. Some are frightened when they lose control, but others fail to appreciate the connection between their angry outbursts and the destruction of personal relationships. For example, a husband who is abusive in the morning sometimes cannot understand the decline in his wife's interest in sexual relations that evening.

ADHD anger is generally very different from the brooding, continuous anger seen in borderline patients and from the chronic anger and irritability seen in some patients with major depression. In many borderlines and some depressives one sees a constant anger that periodically breaks through, while in the ADHD patient the anger often seems provoked by a stimulus rather than released from a persisting source.

The amount of abusiveness in the samples we have studied is spuriously low because our samples have been skewed. Nonetheless, our patients have reported many instances of loss of control: fists through walls; destruction of hundreds of dollars worth of hi-fi equipment, china, and car interiors; and verbal and physical spouse abuse. This tended to decrease with age, but early episodes often left lasting scars on relationships.

STRESS INTOLERANCE

■

Stress intolerance is common in ADHD adults, but I do not know of any systematic data about stress sensitivity in ADHD children. Their "low frustration tolerance" and lack of "stick-to-it-tiveness" both denote an inability to handle difficulty and a tendency to "give up" under pressure, but in general stress is an area of adult rather than childhood concern.

Many ADHD adults relate that they are overreactive to the ordinary stresses of daily life, that they lack resilience and are unable to persevere. They respond excessively or inappropriately to ordinary demands, particularly if unanticipated. They describe themselves as easily confused, "discombobulated," "stressed out," and "hassled." These anxious feelings often induce a vicious circle: the ADHD adult under stress becomes more impulsive, more disorganized and less competent, generates further difficulties and becomes increasingly overwhelmed and demoralized.

As with their related feelings of depression, ADHD patients often respond exceedingly well to reality-based or supportive psychotherapy, or to concrete social intervention (helping the family with realistic goods such as food, clothing and shelter or enabling the children to get medical care)—that is, extricating them from their self-dug hole. Any kind of stress reduction is likely to mitigate impulsive and disorganized attempts to solve problems. Because the therapeutic response to a sensible, concrete approach is often rapid, it is important for the therapist to realize that the risk of relapse remains high.

RESPONSE TO MEDICATION

■

CHILDHOOD

In addition to the signs and symptoms, the response of ADHD children to stimulant medication is so striking that it can almost serve as a confirmation of the diagnosis. In medicine in general and psychiatry in particular response to treatment often is a weak diagnostic indicator. In this instance, the behavioral changes seen in highly drug-responsive ADHD children are almost qualitatively different from the response to somatic treatments in other psychiatric disorders. In some respects, the response is often more dramatic than the best response of a severe melancholic to electroconvulsive therapy (ECT). The major difference is that effective stimulant treatment does more than return the ADHD child to the *status quo ante:* It often allows him to function better than he has in his entire life. The dramatic response of some ADHD children to stimulant medication has led this author to comment that it almost seems as if some ADHD children had been born with congenital atrophy of the amphetamine gland and that stimulant drug treatment is replacement therapy. I will briefly describe the effects of stimulant medication, but most of my discussion of this subject will be presented in Chapter 6 on treatment. These remarks apply to the 60 to 80 percent of ADHD children who have been demonstrated in controlled studies to manifest a "moderate to marked" response to stimulant medication, as summarized in Barkley (1990).

In drug-responsive ADHD children, "inappropriate" hyperactivity is diminished. Stimulants do not slow down the child on the playground, but they do decrease his restlessness in the classroom or at the dinner table. Attention, concentration, and memory all appear to be improved. Impulsivity is decreased in the classroom and elsewhere. Lability is decreased, and temper outbursts are reduced in frequency and degree. In sum, the drugs enable the children to move through life more successfully and thus to be more comfortable with themselves, their parents, their teachers, and their peers.

ADULTHOOD

Drug-response effects appear to be identical in adults. They report that they are able to sit still and relax, remaining at the table after dinner and sitting through whole television programs, movies, and sermons. Not only can they sit still but they can concentrate for the first time in their lives. College students report that, when necessary, they can study for hours and that for the *first time in their lives* they enjoy learning. Several of the patients in our long-term study who had dropped out or flunked out of school, have returned and gotten A's and B's rather than C's and D's. One patient who had "read two or three books in my whole life" developed a passion for reading and consumed nonfiction as well as fiction at the rate of a book per week. Patients also report decreased distractibility, and perseverance is improved. Patients who formerly made impulsive stabs at things but dropped them when unsuccessful now complete their tasks. They are able to persist on a "thin schedule of reinforcement."[4] The decreased impulsivity in adults has multiple effects. Conversational interruption lessens, and a typical response is, "I used to interrupt a lot . . . wait impatiently for the other person to finish . . . and didn't listen . . . just waiting my turn . . . now I listen." Patients also report that they think more before talking. One subject reported after treatment with stimulants that he had stopped drawing technical fouls for cursing during basketball games. The decrease in impatience and impulsive anger is particularly noticeable in driving, where tailgating, honking, and cursing diminish. One patient had become so angry that he had forced other cars (three in one year) off the road in order to make citizen's arrests. Medication helped him to practice tolerance toward other drivers. Impulse buying is also curtailed, a change that literally can save patients from bankruptcy. Furthermore, stimulant-responsive adult patients describe several changes in their mood: decreased mood lability and boredom, and increased initiative and pleasure of accomplishment. As a result of all these changes, relations with others clearly improve. If a patient slows down, listens, becomes reflective, stabilizes in mood, is not explosive or irascible, functions more efficiently around the house and at work, and does not impulsively squander money, his spouse may feel greatly relieved.

SYNDROMES AND CONDITIONS ASSOCIATED WITH ADHD

■

Three additional sets of symptoms are not always found but are sufficiently frequent in ADHD children to be described: Minor Physical Anomalies, Learning Disorders, and Conduct Disorder. In different forms their presence can also be detected in adults.

MINOR PHYSICAL ANOMALIES

Childhood

The biological abnormality most frequently associated with ADHD is minor physical anomalies (MPAs; see review in Krouse and Kauffman, 1982). An association between minor physical anomalies and motor hyperactivity in normal preschool boys was reported by Waldrop et al. in 1968. The anomalies assessed included widely spaced eyes (hyperteleorism); epicanthal folds (in Europeans); malformed, low set, and asymmetrical ears; a high (arched) palate; furrowed tongue; small curving fifth finger; abnormalities in length, spacing, and webbing of toes. High stigmata scores have been described in clinical samples of hyperactive children (Quinn et al., 1974; Firestone et al., 1976; Firestone et al., 1978; Lerer et al., 1979), as newborn predictors of attentional problems and impulsivity in three-year-olds (Waldrop et al., 1978), and in children with "minimal brain dysfunction" (Gillberg and Rasmussen, 1982). Since ADHD appears to have important genetic contributions (see Chapter 4 on etiology), it is important to note that these anomalies have also been interpreted as markers of abnormal development in the first trimester of pregnancy (Smith, 1982; Lindahl and Michelsson, 1986), and have been found to be associated with maternal alcohol use (Jones et al., 1973). The latter two associations suggest that some children and adults with ADHD might have a nongenetic phenocopy of the disorder related to toxic fetal environment. However, the association with maternal alcohol use is ambiguous because hyperactivity in children is also associated genetically with alcoholism in the parents. Thus, an alcoholic mother might transmit ADHD to her child by virtue of both her genes and the biological environment to which her fetus is exposed.

Adulthood

There are several studies of MPAs in adults. Firestone et al. (1978) examined MPAs in the parents and siblings of "hyperactive children," retarded children, and controls; the siblings and parents of the hyperactive children and the retarded children had equal numbers of MPAs, and they were significantly higher than in the siblings and parents of normal controls.

Deutsch et al. (1990) examined the first-degree relatives (parents and siblings) of (1) 24 ADD children; (2) 24 adopted ADD children (their adoptive parents and siblings); and (3) 28 normal children. There were two principal findings. First, the number of MPAs was increased only in the biological parents and siblings of the nonadopted ADD children, a finding compatible with genetic transmission of both ADD and the associated MPAs. Second, ADD probands who were not dysmorphic had an increased number of first-degree relatives who were dysmorphic but not ADD.

LEARNING DISORDERS

Childhood

Learning Disorders have a greater than chance association with ADHD in childhood. Particularly relevant disorders are Reading Disorder, Disorder of Written Expression, and Mathematics Disorder. These terms replace older terms such as "learning disability" (the catch-all phrase) and "dyslexia" and "dyscalculia." In childhood, they refer to the discrepancy between expected performance (based on age and IQ) and the measured level of performance (achievement). They are characterized by inadequate development of specific academic, language, speech, and motor skills and are not due to demonstrable physical or neurologic disorders, childhood psychosis, mental retardation, or deficient educational opportunities. The guideline used to determine such disorders is arbitrary and is usually the number of months the child is behind in some skill, typically 18, 24, or 28 months. For example, a 10-year-old child with an IQ of 100 has expected reading and spelling levels of an average 10-year-old. If 24 months is the arbitrary maximum discrepancy considered normal, and if this child is reading at below the level of a normal 8-year-old, he will be said to have a Reading Disorder. If at the same age he had an IQ of 180 and was reading at the 10-year level, he would be more than 24 months behind his expected level of performance and would in this instance too be said to have a Reading Disorder.

The child with a Reading Disorder in most cases is slow in learning to read. When he does learn, he has more difficulty in reading aloud than he does silently, and in absorbing and remembering written material (as opposed to verbal material that is *heard*).

Of the various malfunctions that characterize Disorder of Written Expression, poor spelling is the most identifiable. As with reading, the diagnosis is made on the basis of spelling performance predicted from the subject's age and intelligence. The various spelling abnormalities of such children include reversal of letters (e.g., "b" for "d"), substitution of wrong letters, reversal of letters in words (e.g., "teh" for "the"), reversal of words ("was" for "saw"), phonetic substitutions (e.g., "f" for "ph"), and deletion or addition of letters or syllables (e.g., "didtt" for "didn't"). (See Miles, 1983, for additional examples.)

In Mathematics Disorder, common errors include reversals of numbers that are being dictated—for example, writing "16" for "61"; difficulty in remembering the mechanical rules of arithmetic—for example, that one multiplies from right to left rather than left to right; difficulty in remembering the multiplication table. Children with this disorder also tend to forget arithmetic skills easily after learning them.

Children with Learning Disorders also can have several associated problems, such as difficulty in learning to tell time on nondigital clocks or watches; difficulty in remembering directions, telling right from left and east from west; difficulty in learning sequences, such as the days of the week and the months of the year.

Learning Disorders seem to occur with increased frequency among both ADHD and conduct-disordered children. The strength of the association—the fraction of ADHD children who have "learning disabilities"—has not been well established. Children with Learning Disorders or CD almost always have academic difficulties and become "underachievers." Children with both deficits have an even greater handicap and likelihood of school failure.

Adulthood

Manifestations of Learning Disorders often continue to characterize the functioning of the ADHD adult. The most prominent (and not surprising) clinical manifestation of "dyslexia" in a subject's history is never having enjoyed reading, even in areas of interest to him. For example, not only may he have avoided reading geography as a child but also he may not have read about cars as an adult although he was an automobile addict.

A Reading Disorder is compatible with a high IQ and high vocational achievement. One man who had acquired both an M.D. and Ph.D. confided that his reading rate was only 70 words per minute. The question was, then, how he had obtained his degrees. His answer was simple. He rarely forgot what he heard and taped the lectures he attended. He was painfully slow finishing long reading assignments, but he was able to absorb them more rapidly and thoroughly by having his wife read the material to him—she could read out loud more rapidly than he could silently. Rutter points out (1978, p. 26) that in Learning Disorders the spelling disability is often more severe than the reading retardation. Thus, adults who may have made up lost ground in reading may retain some spelling impairment. We have not studied academic skill disorders in adults, but in a study of treatment with pemoline (Wender et al., 1981) we administered the Wechsler Adult Intelligence Scale and the Wide-Range Achievement Test (WRAT). The WRAT levels for men were below those that would be anticipated on the basis of their IQ and education. Their mean IQ was 110—the 75th percentile—while their spelling was in the 25th percentile.

Interestingly, in Mathematics Disorder, the arithmetic difficulties do not affect mathematical abstraction, and a "hard" scientist who suffers from ADHD may make frequent arithmetic errors but be at ease with calculus and higher mathematics. Although he was facile with differential equations, the productive M.D., Ph.D. already mentioned could not balance his checkbook or tabulate and calculate the figures from his experiments, because he reversed numbers in columns just as he reversed letters in words. His wife managed the household finances, and his laboratory technician took care of tabulating research measurements. In another example, an extremely bright and very "dys-lexic" 40-year-old could play chess well but had not mastered arithme-tic. Working as a surveyor (in precalculator days), he would master the multiplication table only to have to relearn it each summer. That kind of knowledge did not seem to be lodged in his long-term memory.

The associated abnormality involving problems in right-left discrim-ination may also persist well into adult life (into the forties and fifties) despite normal or superior intelligence. Many adults with this problem develop compensatory tricks. One woman placed her wristwatch on her left hand where there was a barely visible mole. She then had only to remember to place her wristwatch on the wrist with the mole.

CONDUCT DISORDER

Childhood

In diagnostic reappraisal of the concepts of "Minimal Brain Dysfunc-tion" and the "hyperactive child syndrome," investigators increasingly began to feel that these syndromes were composed of two partially distinct and partially overlapping syndromes— Attention Deficit Dis-order (now Attention-deficit Hyperactivity Disorder) and Conduct Dis-order. Nonetheless, it is important to emphasize that the now sep-arately defined disorders (no symptoms are rated on both) do in fact frequently overlap. Reviewing many studies, DSM-III-R states: "The symptoms of these disorders covary to a high degree" (Sandberg et al., 1978, 1980; Satterfield and Schell, 1984). Deciding which attributes should be used as criteria for each syndrome remains a familiar prob-lem.

One difficulty with the DSM-III-R diagnostic criteria for ADHD and CD is that they are applicable to two different age groups. Those for ADHD are for young children—for example, "has difficulty playing quietly"; but those for Conduct Disorder are applicable to an older age group—for example, "has stolen without confrontation of a victim on more than one occasion (including forgery)," "has forced someone into sexual activity with him or her," "has used a weapon in more than one fight." Obviously, these are not behaviors that even a future Jack-the-Ripper will usually engage in at age 7, so that a diagnosis of Conduct Disorder or mixed Attention-deficit Hyperactivity Disorder/Conduct Disorder in young children may be difficult or impossible to make.

Perhaps because psychiatrists have found the attributes associated with Conduct Disorder difficult to rate, DSM-III-R elected to establish criteria that were behavioral, clear-cut, and more likely to produce high interrater reliability. Unfortunately, these new behavioral criteria are given precedence over what seems to me a core psychological feature of CD: "no concern for the feelings, wishes, and well-being of others, as shown by callous behavior, and . . . lack [of] appropriate feelings of guilt or remorse" (DSM-III-R, p. 53; Cleckley, 1976). Similarly, Antisocial Personality Disorder, the adult version of CD, includes irresponsibility; lack of empathy, conscience, and remorse; failure to conform to social norms; and a "markedly impaired capacity to sustain lasting, close, warm and responsible relationships" (DSM-III-R, p. 343). Although DSM-III-R focuses on behaviors such as physical aggression, cruelty, stealing, lying, and cheating, there have been efforts to specify other, less age-dependent, age-specific but also less socially transgressive signs and symptoms. August and Stewart (1983) felt they could associate Conduct Disorder with attributes such as an increased frequency of "egocentricity," an excessive need for attention, blame projection, problems sharing with others, insensitivity to others' feelings, a lack of repentance, and (relevant because symptomatic of ADHD) "noncompliance," which is characterized by ignoring directions, resenting discipline, acting oppositional, and lacking respect for adults. Characteristics such as these may be better for discriminating Conduct Disorder in young children, whose antisocial potential is still compromised by their small size and their undeveloped capacities for serious transgression. Whether these alternative criteria prove useful is dependent on whether they can be evaluated reliably.

DSM-III-R also makes distinctions between Conduct Disorder, Group Type, and Conduct Disorder, Solitary Aggressive Type. There may be very great differences genetically, in natural history, in response to drugs, and in overlap with ADHD between the child with conduct disorder who lacks empathy and conscience and the child or adolescent who has these to an age-appropriate degree and engages in conduct disorder activities with his peer group. It is important to consider the transgressions that would qualify a child for a diagnosis of Conduct Disorder, Group Type; three of the following would suffice: stealing without confrontation; often truant; often lies; fire setting; vandalism; often initiates physical fights. These symptoms should be contrasted with more serious ones: has broken into someone else's house, building, or car; has deliberately destroyed others' property (other than by fire setting); physical cruelty to animals; has used weapons in more than one fight; has forced someone into sexual activity; stolen with confrontation (mugging, extortion, armed robbery); has been physically cruel to people. These distinctions have not yet been reported in epidemiological studies, so that we have no data about their frequency in conduct-disordered children or the association of the two types with ADHD.

DSM-III-R further refined diagnosis in this area by introducing Oppositional Defiant Disorder, which it placed together with ADHD and Conduct Disorder under the designation of Disruptive Behavior Disorders. DSM-III-R states: "The essential feature of this disorder is a pattern of negativistic, hostile, and defiant behavior without the more serious violations of the basic rights of others that are seen in Conduct Disorder" (p. 56). ODD children are described as angry, resentful, deliberately annoying, lacking in insight, and blame projecting. DSM-III-R further states that in Conduct Disorder all of the features of ODD are likely to be present, so that "Conduct Disorder preempts the diagnosis of Oppositional Defiant Disorder" (p. 57). ODD "in childhood or adolescence apparently predisposes to the development of [Passive Aggressive Personality Disorder]" (DSM-III-R, p. 357).

The interrelatedness of ADHD, CD, and ODD are discussed in two excellent reviews, "On the Distinction Between Attentional Deficits/ Hyperactivity and Conduct Problems/Aggression in Child Psychopathology" (Hinshaw, 1987) and "Diagnostic Conundrum of Oppositional Defiant Disorder and Conduct Disorder" (Loeber et al., 1991).

Adulthood

Studies of adults are not dependent on the solutions to these nosological problems. Clinicians will find themselves examining some ADHD adults who do and some who do not have histories of CD and ODD. In turn, some of these ADHD adults may also fall into the diagnostic categories of Antisocial Personality Disorder or Passive Aggressive Personality Disorder, while others do not.

It is not surprising that ADHD and Conduct Disorder commonly used to be "lumped together" by clinicians. One observes every degree of combination between ADHD and CD, but "pure" Conduct Disorder is uncommon. Developmentally, some children appear to begin as "pure" ADHD and then go on to develop Conduct Disorder—that is, antisocial behavior—as they become older (Huessy, 1973; Gittelman et al., 1985; Mannuzza et al., 1991). The central issue in deciding which criteria to employ in *defining* ADHD and Conduct Disorder is the empirical one of whether there are additional nonsymptomatic validating measures. For the clinician evaluating the adult with ADHD, the presence of antisocial traits or "soft" symptoms of Antisocial Personality Disorder is suggestive. Since CD responds much less well than ADHD to stimulant drugs, the drug responses of ADHD adults with a history of conduct disorder or of "soft" ASPD characteristics need to be studied.

An atheoretical and practical way of summarizing the association and overlap of ADHD, CD and Learning Disorders is illustrated in the accompanying Venn diagram (Figure 2.1).

THE COMORBIDITIES OF ATTENTION-DEFICIT HYPERACTIVITY DISORDER

■

Figure 2.1 is qualitative, not quantitative. It is based on studies of children, but it has implications for work with adults. It calls attention to the frequent comorbidity but does not indicate the degree of overlap—that is, the sizes of the symbols are not meant to indicate the fraction of subjects who are pure ADHD, pure CD, mixed ADHD/CD, and so on. Available data evaluating the degree of overlap among these syndromes will be discussed in Chapter 3 on prevalence. The various intersects identify the combinations of the three syndromes that are frequently seen. In pure form, the syndromes seem to have different family and natural histories, and different responses to medication and education. In regard to treatment, ADHD children manifest a good response to stimulant medication in approximately 60 to 80 percent of instances (Barkley, 1990); children with Learning Disorders but without ADHD receive no benefit from stimulant medication with their reading or spelling difficulties. The child with both ADHD *and* "dyslexia" who responds well to medication benefits from increased attentiveness, which may produce greater response to special teaching efforts. The response of conduct-disordered children to stimulant medication remains to be evaluated. Another problem is that even "dramatically" stimulant-responsive ADHD/CD children have been reported to become tolerant to medication after several years (Klein et al., 1980, p. 702).

An awareness of these various "subtypes" is indispensable to both the therapist and the student of ADHD in children and in adults. In Chapter

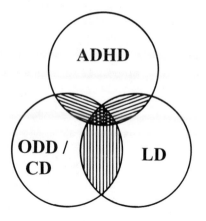

ADHD - Attention Deficit Hyperactivity Disorder

ODD - Oppositional Defiant Disorder

CD - Conduct Disorder

LD - Learning Disorders

Figure 2.1 The comorbidities of attention-deficit hyperactivity disorder.

6 on treatment, I will explore further the responses of these different forms of psychopathology to pharmacological and nonpharmacological treatment.

NOTES

1. Since ADHD is much more common in boys (at least in childhood), I will employ the male pronoun "he" most frequently and intermittently use "her" to remind the reader that the diagnosis of ADHD is not another exclusively male prerogative.

2. From *Animal Farm:* "All pigs are equal, but some pigs are more equal than others."

3. Since restless feet are readily observed—in cafeterias, waiting rooms, and group meetings—the diagnostic sensitivity and specificity of this and related hypotheses theoretically could be rapidly tested in such areas by inquiring about individual and family histories of, say, alcoholism, academic achievement, and imprisonment in a random sample of those with jiggling and stationary feet. The design is straightforward, but its execution poses practical ethical problems.

4. This phrase comes from operant psychology. For example, a pigeon continues to peck a key even though pellets—the reinforcement—appear at every fiftieth rather than every tenth peck.

3

The Prevalence of ADHD in Adults

■

The prevalence[1] of Attention-deficit Hyperactivity Disorder in adults is unknown because no epidemiological studies have been conducted that evaluate "residual ADHD." However, it is possible to obtain a rough estimate of the prevalence of ADHD. If it is true, as we suspect, that ADHD does not appear *de novo* in adults,[2] we can crudely estimate its prevalence in adults by: (1) examining the data on its prevalence in childhood, and (2) examining the natural history of ADHD in childhood—that is, its prognosis. The prevalence in childhood multiplied by the percentage of ADHD children in whom ADHD symptoms persist approximates the prevalence in age-specified adults.

Assessing the prevalence of a psychiatric disorder may seem like a straightforward task, since textbook descriptions of medical disorders always discuss prevalence (and incidence). It is trivially true that the prevalence of ADHD—both in children and in adults, and like any other psychiatric disorders—depends on the diagnostic criteria employed. Before proceeding, I would like to make one frequently overlooked point: the use of the word "diagnosis" in psychiatry carries an implicit and misleading connotation that stems from the use of the word in other areas of medicine, where diagnostic tests and diagnostic signs and symptoms are *validated against an independent criterion* for determining the presence or absence of the disorder.

This was not always true. Until the advent of gross and microscopic pathology at the end of the nineteenth century, diagnosis in medicine, like current diagnosis in psychiatry, was based solely on signs and symptoms. With the development of the sciences of pathology and microbiology, and later of physiological and biochemical measures, it became possible to understand the etiology of medical disorders. Physicians were then able to diagnose underlying disorders far more accurately because the relationship had been determined between manifest signs and symptoms and the underlying biochemical, anatomical, or tissue pathology. One could use a "gold standard" of whether the disease was present or not.[3] For example, defining active tuberculosis by the presence of tuberculous bacillae in the sputum, one could determine the accuracy of physical examination, chest X-rays, or tuberculin skin tests in diagnosing the disorder. *No such etiological diagnoses are available for "functional" psychiatric disorders in general or ADHD in particular.* Accordingly, there is no way of determining the accuracy—the "sensitivity" and "specificity," to use modern parlance—of current diagnostic techniques because there are no methods, biological or otherwise, for independently determining the presence or absence of etiological factors.

In estimating prevalence, there are two approaches to diagnosis. The first technique is categorical. Diagnosis is based on whether an individual has certain necessary symptoms. In the case of ADHD the number has varied in the successive DSM editions—eight of sixteen in DSM-III, eight of fourteen in DSM-III-R, and now twelve of eighteen for ADHD, Combined Type in DSM-IV (or between six and eleven for one of the other subtypes). With any of these schemes, the required number equals the syndrome, and one less means absence of the syndrome.[4]

The second technique for diagnosing ADHD is dimensional. It is based on standardized rating scales (or questionnaires) administered to parents and teachers. The prevalence of ADHD is then determined by examining the percentage of children with scores above a particular cutoff point. The resemblance to medicine is again misleading. It is similar to measuring blood pressure and designating values greater than 140/90 mm Hg as hypertensive and those between 139/89 and 90/60 as normotensive, but in that case the "cut" is made on the basis of systematic *data* detailing the medical histories of large numbers of people with different blood pressures. There is a correlation between blood pressures greater than 139/89 and an increased risk for developing cardiovascular disease.[5]

But using such a procedure to determine the prevalence of ADHD in the population constitutes a prejudgment. The investigator has tacitly assumed that ADHD simply represents an extreme position on the

distribution curve and has already decided what percent of the childhood population will be designated as ADHD. The approach of arbitrarily setting a cutoff point is dignified by precedent but not by logic. If
the distribution were normal—that is, Gaussian—approximately 6.7
percent of children would be expected to have a score greater than 1.5
standard deviations above the mean and 2.3 percent would have a score
greater than 2 standard deviations above the mean. For example, Trites
et al. (1979) examined prevalence as a function of cutoff scores in his
own and others' studies from four different countries and obtained the
following results. With a standard deviation of 1.5, the percentage of
hyperactive boys varied from 9 to 22 percent, and of hyperactive girls
from 2 to 9 percent. With a standard deviation of 2.1, the percentage of
hyperactive boys was 5 to 7 percent, and of hyperactive girls 2 to 4
percent.

Thus the predecided cutoff scores arbitrarily determine what prevalence will be found. There are no solid independent validating measures; these are pseudo measures. In consequence, the "cutoff problem" cannot be resolved by studying the diagnostic behavior
of clinicians because what is being measured is reliability (agreement) rather than validity ("truth").

What can be said for the scientific merits of the categorical and
dimensional approaches? Robins (1985, p. 921) makes an important
point when she says that the variability of estimates "is implicit in the
fact that psychiatric disorders lack definitive tests for their existence.
The presence or absence of disorder is decided on the basis of degree of
resemblance of a particular patient's self-report and the physician's
observations of the patient to the ideal type of the diagnosis." She
continues,

> Whether one thinks dimensionally or categorically, in fact the operations
> by which such psychiatric disorders are defined are dimensional. The cate-
> gorical hypothesis that there is a qualitative discontinuity between every
> psychiatric disorder and normal reactions to adverse experiences cannot be
> proved without definitive biological tests. It is the current lack of such
> tests that allows arguments about dimensional versus categorical diag-
> nosis and about whether many diagnoses are "real." Lacking a definitive
> test, whether one takes a dimensional or categorical approach to diagnosis
> is simply a matter of whether or not one finds it advantageous to choose a
> single cutting point on that accumulation of characteristics used to define
> a disorder beyond which disorders are defined as present.

The dimensional approach jibes with the finding of psychopathologi-
cal continua in other psychiatric disorders. Bleuler described "latent

schizophrenia" in the relatives of schizophrenics, and Kretschmer wrote of a "spectrum" moving from the "healthy schizothyme" to the sicker "schizoid" and then to the schizophrenic. He extended this approach to manic depression with the notion of the cycloid temperament (Kretschmer, 1936). The notion of genetically mediated continua in psychiatry was also demonstrated in the adoption studies of schizophrenia (Kety et al., 1975), which found that "mild cases of schizophrenia" were much more common than severe forms and were seen with increased frequency among the biological relatives of adopted schizophrenics. The notion of a spectrum of severity has been extended for other disorders, including the major mood disorders and antisocial personality.

Thus, one must recognize that with current techniques, various diagnostic approaches can only provide approximate measures, and even those can be adversely affected by the techniques employed. Bearing all these caveats in mind, what aspects of a prevalence study should be examined? (1) The population surveyed. In a community study, what fraction of those contacted agreed to participate? If a substantial number did not, was there a sampling bias (e.g., were families of children with ADHD more or less likely to participate)? (2) What was the age range of the sample? (3) Sex proportions of the sample? (4) Measuring device? Categorical (diagnostic) or dimensional (rating scale) or both? Is it measuring what you want to measure?[6] (5) If category-based, what is the interrater reliability?[7] This is usually reported as satisfactory (as the result of the use of structured interviews, such as the Diagnostic Interview Schedule for Children [DISC], the Kiddie SADS, etc.), but a cautionary note should be sounded on the basis of the findings in the NIMH Epidemiologic Catchment Area Project (ECA). Many years of effort have been spent in formulating diagnostic criteria and structured interviews for the major psychiatric disorders—many more than for ADHD. In the ECA study, rates of psychiatric disorders were assessed with structured interviews. In one part of the study prevalences in St. Louis were compared with those in Baltimore, with the following result: "Overall, estimates based on psychiatrists' interviews at one site differed an average of threefold from their estimates at the other site" (Robins, 1985, p. 920). In contrast, trained lay interviewers at the two sites differed very little, indicating that the two groups of psychiatrists were interpreting interviews differently rather than dealing with populations with different regional characteristics.

Before proceeding, I would like to use Table 3.1 to review how prevalence changes when diagnostic criteria change.

Table 3.1. Sensitivity, Specificity, and Prevalence

Test Result*	Disease State	
	Present	Absent
Positive	a (true positive)	b (false positive)
Negative	c (false negative)	d (true negative)

Sensitivity $= \dfrac{a}{a + c}$, the fraction of true positives detected by the test.

Specificity $= \dfrac{d}{b + d}$, the fraction of true negatives detected by the test.

Prevalence $=$ the fraction of true positives in the population evaluated,

or $\dfrac{a + c}{a + b + c + d}$

*Remember that this is hypothetical. There is no method for determining true positives and negatives.

What happens if you alter the number of diagnostic criteria? If you lower the number of symptoms necessary for diagnosis—for example, if you use a six-symptom rather than an eight-symptom cutoff for ADHD—you increase the sensitivity because the number of true positives detected increases (as, obviously, does the prevalence). But the price that must be paid is a decrease in specificity because the number of false positives increases and true negatives decrease; thus you overdiagnose.

As an excellent discussion by Robins (1985) points out, we may want to adjust the sensitivity and specificity of our criteria, depending on our *purposes* (since there is no method for determining "real" or "true" prevalence). Two examples follow.

1. *To determine the magnitude of a health problem.* If one is interested in determining the need for treatment, one is interested not only in diagnosing the presence of a condition but also in determining the degree to which it interferes with functioning. The issue then becomes one of deciding what fraction of individuals meeting diagnostic criteria should receive treatment. This, in turn, is dependent on available resources *and* the costs and effectiveness of treatment. One may wish either to increase the sensitivity of a test or to decrease the number of requisite diagnostic signs on the basis of this information. If the disorder impairs functioning and is treatable, one must examine the risks and benefits of treatment and nontreatment (perform a "decision analysis"). This issue is discussed in Chapter 6 on treatment, where it is argued that ADHD in adults is common and readily treatable, that the

risks of treatment are low, and that it pays to increase sensitivity even at the expense of decreased specificity.

2. *To identify possible risk factors associated with a disorder.* To do this, one wants to increase the specificity because false positive instances (cases without the disorder who are misclassified as positives rather than negatives) may cloud the relationship between the disorder and the supposed risk factors. This is likely to happen in genetic linkage studies, where a few false positive diagnoses can obscure linkage.

In the light of the current studies of the prevalence of ADHD in children, what is a reasonable estimate? On the basis of the brief descriptions of the main studies that I provide below, I believe that one can make only an order of magnitude approximation and would accept, tentatively, a figure of 6 to 10 percent. Looking at the same data, the reader may disagree. The important point that I want to emphasize in this discussion is that one cannot decide beforehand that only six percent of the population can be called pathological. When investigators report prevalence values of ten percent and greater, critics of the concept of ADHD are apt to say that these figures are artifacts of the criteria and that ADHD is being overdiagnosed. This is related to a semantic confusion arising from the ambiguous usages of the word "normal": normal *as average* and normal *as optimal*. Unfortunately, pathology of all kinds is very common. A National Institutes of Health Consensus Development Panel (1985) on obesity agreed that a 20 percent excess in weight over desirable weight was associated with an increased health risk, and that by this criterion 20 to 30 percent of men and 30 to 40 percent of women were obese. In the white suburban population of the Framingham Study, almost 20 percent had blood pressures greater than 160/95 and 50 percent had pressures greater than the maximal "normal" blood pressure, 140/90 (Dannenberg et al., 1988). The lifetime morbidity risk for major depression has been estimated to be as high as 10 percent for men and 20 percent for women. Nonoptimal conditions can be very common.

A related question that has been asked is whether or not the incidence of ADHD is increasing. There are no data that support this proposition, but it is possible. Analogously, examination of the incidence and prevalence of the mood disorders suggests that not only are these conditions common but their incidence may be *increasing*. This has been shown in a prospective study by Hagnell (Hagnell et al., 1982) that employed the same diagnostic criteria throughout and reported the prevalence of depression in a Swedish sample followed since 1947. Hagnell judged the cumulative probability of contracting severe and medium depression to be 18.4 percent for men and 32.6 percent for women. Between 1947 and 1972, the risk for "medium" and "severe" depression increased by a factor of 1.8. However, for men between 20 and 39, the risk of medium and severe depression increased *tenfold* during the same time period. A similar finding was reported by Klerman et al. (1985) in an examination of the rates of depression in the relatives of depressives as a function of "birth cohort" (the decade of birth). The risk was approximately three times as great for those born in 1920 as for those born between 1910 and 1920. However, this study was retrospective, and the older subsamples' report of a lower incidence could be an artifact of inaccurate memory and possibly an age-associated reluctance to acknowledge psychiatric illness.

By analogy, it is *possible* that ADHD, like depression, affects a large fraction of the population and that its prevalence *might* be increasing.

MAJOR PREVALENCE STUDIES (CHRONOLOGICAL)

■

In this section, I review studies of the prevalence of externalizing behavior (pre-DSM-III studies), ADD, and ADHD. The pre-DSM-III studies employ variable diagnostic criteria. A summary table that allows for easier comparison appears at the end of this chapter (Table 3.3).

LAPOUSE AND MONK (1958)

Epidemiologic study of behavior characteristics in children.

Sample   482 boys and girls, ages 6 to 12, randomly selected from population.

Evaluative measure   Structured interview with mothers or "mother substitutes."

Findings   "Externalizing" (ADHD-relevant) symptoms: overactivity, 49 percent; temper loss 2 to 3 times a week or more, 48 percent.

Comment   This study tells us something about the informants' expectations and, perhaps, that about half of school-age children are more active and prone to "temper loss" than adults would like.

HUESSY AND GENDRON (1970)

Prevalence of "hyperkinetic" syndrome in public school children in Vermont.

Sample   The entire second grade in several public schools: 501 boys and girls, and 430 of same group 2 1/2 years later.

Evaluative measures   Teacher questionnaire rating "hyperkinesis": hyperactivity, short attention span, emotional overreactivity, temper tantrums, coordination, and learning problems. Completed by second-grade teachers and by teachers of same group 2 1/2 years later.

Findings   "The children in the highest ten percentiles [43 children initially] were the ones the schools clearly identified as problems" (p. 246). Only one-third of those children remained in the upper decile two and a half years later (in the fifth grade), but about 7 percent of the originally "normal" children moved into the upper decile at the same time. Thus, "hyperkinetic" problems existed in 8 to 9 percent of the children at both time spans (boys:girls, 4:1).

WERRY AND QUAY (1971)

Prevalence of behavior symptoms in younger elementary school children.

Sample   951 boys (926 rated) and 864 girls (827 rated); grades kindergarten, first and second, including children in special classes, in mid-size Midwestern city.

Evaluative measure   Quay-Peterson Problem Checklist completed by teachers.

Findings   Representative "ADHD" behaviors (percent boys, percent girls): restlessness, 50, 28; hyperactivity, always on the go, 30, 14; temper tantrums, 9, 5; disruptiveness, annoying others, 46, 22; short attention span, 44, 26; "laziness in school," 31, 16; distractibility, 48, 28. Mean number of symptoms per child decreased with age, in both sexes.

Comment   Individual ADHD symptoms are common in school-age children (cf. Lapouse and Monk, 1958).

TRITES ET AL. (1979)

Prevalence of hyperactivity in Ottawa.

Sample   14,083 children, junior kindergarten (age 4) to grade 6, inclusive, from all school boards in Ottawa region of Canada, stratified sample.

Evaluative measure   Conners Teacher Rating Scale (CTRS): factors for inattentive-passive, conduct problems, and hyperactivity. Cutoff mid-point for each factor, that is, average between "just a little" and "pretty much."

Findings   Using a cutoff score of 1.5 standard deviations above the mean, the percents of the sample (boys, girls) classified as having the following symptoms were: hyperactivity, 20.6, 7.5; conduct problems, 4.0, 1.7; inattentive-passive, 17.9, 9.4. The authors emphasize that the prevalence of "hyperactivity" is an "arbitrary" function of the cutoff scores employed.

Comment   The authors call attention to the fact that there is no a priori method of selecting a cutoff score. With the same instrument (the CTRS), the percent of children categorized as hyperactive varies not only as a function of the cutoff but also among countries, which may, the authors reflect, be due to cultural differences in the children or their teachers. Assembling data from different countries, they point out that with a 1.5 cutoff, the prevalence of hyperactive children ranged from 9 percent for boys and 2 percent for girls in the United States, through 12 percent and 5 percent in Germany, 21 percent and 8 percent in Canada, to 22 percent and 9 percent in New Zealand. Each increase in the cutoff score decreases the percentages, so that a 2.1 cutoff yields 5 percent for boys and 4 percent for girls in New Zealand, and 7 percent for boys and 2 percent for girls in Canada.

SANDBERG, WIESELBERG, AND SHAFFER (1980)

Hyperkinetic and conduct problem children in a primary school population.

Sample   226 boys, ages 5 to 9, selected from primary schools in the inner London area; the children were from very disadvantaged backgrounds.

Evaluative measures Conners teacher questionnaire (1969, 1973), Rutter (1967) teacher questionnaire, Conners parent questionnaire (1970).

Variable analyzed Overlap between boys in the upper 10 percent of hyperactivity scores and the upper 10 percent of conduct disorder scores, that is, the 90th percentile of both; on most measures these children were 1.5 standard deviations above the mean.

Findings Approximately half of the children in the 90th percentile of hyperactivity on teachers' ratings on the Conners questionnaire were in the 90th percentile of conduct disorder as well. Teachers and *parents* identified *different* children as disturbed. Teacher questionnaires failed to distinguish well between hyperactivity and CD; the parent questionnaire distinguished between them better.

SCHACHAR, RUTTER, AND SMITH (1981)

Characteristics of situationally and pervasively hyperactive children.

Sample 1536 boys and girls, ages 10 to 11, evaluated in a total population study on the Isle of Wight (Rutter et al., 1970).

Evaluative measures Rutter teacher and parent rating scales, with hyperactivity factor cutoff.

Findings Situationally hyperactive (hyperactive on *only* teacher *or* parent questionnaire), 14.3 percent; pervasively hyperactive (judged hyperactive on *both* teacher and parent questionnaire), 2.0 percent. (Pervasively hyperactive children showed greater behavioral disturbance and cognitive impairment and their problems had shown greater persistence.) In situationally hyperactive children, the ratio of boy to girl was 1.9:1; in pervasively hyperactive, it was 2.9:1. Comorbidity for conduct disorder was 30 percent.

Comment A large N, numerical cutoff, and a subcategorization.

SHEN, WANG, AND YANG (1985)

Epidemiological investigation of minimal brain dysfunction in six elementary schools in Beijing.

Sample 2770 children from urban, suburban, and "mountain" areas.

Evaluative measure Combination of Rutters (1967) and Conners (1967) rating scales, completed by teachers.

Findings With a score 2 standard deviations above the mean, 160 were "identified as cases of MBD" (5.8 %). The rate was lower in the urban (3.1 %) than in the suburban (7.8 %) and mountain (7.0 %) areas. Rates were 40 percent lower in children from the highest as compared to the lowest socioeducational groups.

O'LEARY, VIVIAN, AND NISI (1985)

Hyperactivity in Italy.

Sample 344 rural and urban children (186 boys, 158 girls) from northern Italy in the second through fourth grades.

Evaluative measure 39-item Conners Teacher Rating Scale filled out by teachers; used with a "traditional" cutoff of mean + 2 standard deviations.

Findings 7.5 percent of the boys and 1.3 percent of the girls classified as hyperactive.

SHEKIM, KASHANI, BECK, CANTWELL, MARTIN, ROSENBERG, AND COSTELLO (1985)

Prevalence of attention deficit disorders in nine-year-olds in rural midwest.

Sample 114 nine-year-old boys and girls, 3 percent of all nine-year-olds in the community.

Evaluative measures The Diagnostic Interview Schedules for Children (DISC) and for Parents (DISC-P).

Findings Nine boys and five girls (12 %) were diagnosed as ADD-H by the DISC-P, four boys (4 percent) were diagnosed ADD-H by DISC, but only two children were diagnosed as ADD-H by both DISC and DISC-P.

Comment The discrepancy between reports on the DISC-P and the DISC is typical; ADD-H children appear to deny or minimize symptoms.

SATIN, WINSBERG, MONETTI, SVERD, AND FOSS (1985)

General population screen for attention deficit disorder with hyperactivity.

  Sample   Stratified population survey in a semi-urban area; 94 six- to nine-year-old boys (one-third of the 294 that had initially been identified).

  Evaluative measures   Rating scales by parents and teachers, and unstructured interview by psychiatrist using DSM-III criteria. Diagnosis was made only if the "symptoms were sufficiently severe to warrant treatment or careful followup" (p. 758).

  Findings   The purpose of the study was to determine the sensitivity of rating scales, but the investigators obtained prevalence figures of 24 percent for ADD-H; 8 percent of the sample met ADD-H criteria from both teachers and parents, that is, were "pervasively hyperactive."

  Comment   The obtained prevalence is exceptionally high.

SHAPIRO AND GARFINKEL (1986)

Occurrence of behavior disorders in children: interdependence of Attention Deficit Disorder and Conduct Disorder.

  Sample   All children in grades 2 to 6 at a rural Minnesota public school, 315; mean age: 9 years 10 months.

  Evaluative measure   Interview with the child (Diagnostic Interview for Children and Adolescents [DICA]); and questionnaire completed by the teacher (Conners Teacher Rating Scale).

  Findings   DSM-III-R criteria were not employed, and the prevalences were categorized as "suggestive": inattentive/overactive symptoms suggestive of Attention Deficit Disorder, 2.3 percent; aggressive/oppositional symptoms suggestive of Conduct Disorder, 3.6 percent; ADD and CD symptoms, 3.0 percent.

  Comment   This study highlights the frequently found overlap between ADHD and CD. Diagnosis based on cutoff.

BOYLE, OFFORD, HOFMANN, CATLIN, BYLES, CADMAN, CRAWFORD, LINKS, RAE-GRANT, AND SZATMARI (1987); OFFORD, BOYLE, SZATMARI, RAE-GRANT, LINKS, CADMAN, BYLES, CRAWFORD, BLUM, BYRNE, THOMAS, AND WOODWARD (1987); AND OFFORD, BOYLE, FLEMING, BLUM, AND RAE-GRANT (1989)

Ontario Child Health Study: Methodology, six-month prevalence of disorder, and rates of service utilization (all cases found in a six-month interval).

Sample A subsample of 1981 census: 4- to 16-year-old children in the province of Ontario. N = 3289 (large urban, 2018; small urban, 402; rural, 869).

Evaluative measures Child Behavior Checklist with items chosen to operationalize DSM-III criteria for ADD, CD, and somatization. Checklist used with parents, teachers, and adolescents 12 to 16. Interviews with mother (or guardian) and child were based on the same items. To receive a diagnosis, a child had to manifest symptoms that should "Be associated with impairment specifically to the child and/or distress to the child, family, or community." Sophisticated discussion of cutoff scores in terms of sensitivity and specificity, using psychiatrists' DSM-III diagnoses as the criterion.

Findings Ages 4 to 16, hyperactivity, 8.9 percent of boys and 3.3 percent of girls, conduct disorder, 8.1 percent of boys and 2.7 percent of girls (conduct disorder increased between ages 4 to 11 and 12 to 16 in both boys and girls; hyperactivity decreased slightly among the older boys). For ages 12 to 16, 4.5 percent of the boys and 10.7 percent of the girls received a diagnosis of somatization (relation of somatization and ADHD is discussed in Chapter 4 on etiology). In further analysis of these data (Offord et al., 1986), the overlap of conduct disorder with hyperactivity was considerable: approximately 57 percent of conduct-disordered boys and girls ages 4 to 11 and 34 percent of those ages 12 to 16 were diagnosed as hyperactive.

An additional refinement (Szatmari et al., 1989) showed that although prevalence of ADD-H in boys decreases between ages 4 to 11 and 12 to 16, ADD without hyperactivity seems to remain constant.

ANDERSON, WILLIAMS, MCGEE, AND SILVA (1987)

Prevalence of DSM-III disorders in preadolescent children; large sample from the general population in New Zealand.

Sample   792 eleven-year-old children (416 boys, 376 girls) in a longitudinal study.

Evaluative measures   Structured interview of the child (Diagnostic Interview Schedule for Children, Child Version); Rutter questionnaires for parents and teacher; earlier questionnaires for behavioral history. Diagnostic criteria: DSM-III.

Findings   ADD, 6.7 percent (boy to girl ratio, 5.1:1); oppositional disorder, 5.7 percent (boy to girl ratio, 2.2:1); conduct disorder (aggressive), 3.4 percent (boy to girl ratio, 3.2:1).

Overlap between diagnoses: Of 53 ADD children, 25 (47 %) were CD or ODD; of 72 CD or ODD children, 25 (34 %) were ADD.

Comment   Representative population sample has been followed since birth and has been evaluated with multiple instruments. A very valuable sample for learning about the natural history of childhood psychiatric disorders. ADD and ADD-H not distinguished. Note later study of 15-year-olds from same sample, described below (McGee et al., 1990).

YAO, SOLANTO, AND WENDER (1988)

Prevalence of hyperactivity among newly immigrated Chinese-American children.

Sample   250 boys and girls, grades 1 to 6, elementary schools, New York Chinatown. Bilingual and English-language classes, both regular and remedial classes. Of 36 teachers, 15 declined to cooperate.

Evaluative measures   Conners 28-item Teacher Rating Scale and CATRS.

Findings   2 standard deviations above mean. On CATRS: boys, 8.8, girls 1.7. On 28-item scale: boys, 12.7; girls, 1.7.

Comment   Higher rate than many other samples using a cutoff of 2 or more standard deviations above mean.

COSTELLO (1989)

Child psychiatric disorders and correlates.

Sample Consecutive children, ages 7 to 11, attending primary-care pediatric clinics. First-stage screening sample, 789; psychiatric interviews with subsample of 300 parents and children.

Evaluative measures Child Behavior Checklist completed by parents plus structured interviews of child and parent (DISC-C and DISC-P). Teacher Report Form. Global Assessment Scale for children, completed by interviewers.

Findings ADD with hyperactivity, 2 percent (males, 3.0%; females, 1.1%); ADD without hyperactivity, 0.2 percent (all boys); oppositional disorder, 6.6 percent (males, 7.3%; females, 6.0%); conduct disorder, 5.2 percent (males, 8.8%; females, 1.4%).

GOODMAN AND STEVENSON (1989)

Examination of hyperactivity scores in monozygotic and dizygotic twins (see Chapter 4 on etiology).

Sample 285 twin pairs obtained from two sources in London; 76 percent of the potential sample of 374 twin pairs.

Evaluative measures Rutter parent (mother and father) and teacher questionnaire.

Findings As in the Isle of Wight study (Schachar et al., 1981), the children were characterized as hyperactive at home *or* at school, *or* hyperactive in both settings ("pervasively hyperactive"); 4.6 percent were pervasively hyperactive, 12.7 percent were hyperactive at home only, and 7.2 percent at school only. The ratio of boys to girls was 1.4:1 overall and 2.3:1 for the pervasively hyperactive. The prevalence of pervasive hyperactivity in children of low socioeconomic status was 6.1 percent, as compared with 1.9 percent in children of higher SES.

Comment 4.6 percent constitutes a minimum figure for clinically relevant ADHD rather than situational hyperactivity (at home *or* at school), which British clinicians have asserted is the hallmark of the hyperactivity syndrome.

VELEZ, JOHNSON, AND COHEN (1989)

Longitudinal analysis of selected risk factors for childhood psycho-pathology.

Sample Random selection of 776 children from census tract in up-state New York, examined longitudinally. First wave in 1975; second wave in 1983 and again in 1985. Ages 9 to 20.

Evaluative measures Structured interviews (DISC-C and DISC-P), with mothers in 1975, and with both children and mothers in 1983 and 1985. Diagnosis based on DSM-III-R criteria.

Findings Of particular interest are the longitudinal data. Values reported were for "severe" instances of the disorder. The following figures are averages of the 1983 and 1985 findings. ADD, age 9 to 14, 15 percent; ages 13 to 20, 8.3 percent. Conduct disorder, ages 9 to 14, 11 percent; ages 13 to 20, 11 percent. Oppositional disorder, 9 to 14, 19 percent; ages 13 to 20, 16 percent.

Comment Note the 45 percent decrease in the prevalence of ADD between the two age periods, while the prevalence of conduct disorder is unchanged.

BIRD, GOULD, YAGER, STAGHEZZA, AND CANINO (1989)

Risk factors for maladjustment in Puerto Rican children.

Sample A population-based subsample, 777 boys and girls, ages 4 to 16 (92.2% of targeted households).

Evaluative measures Child Behavior Checklist from parents and teacher, followed by interviews by child psychiatrists with one parent and child. Interview included DISC. Diagnosis based on DSM-III criteria and the Children's Global Assessment Scale, but two ratings are given: *definite* maladjustment, and *some* maladjustment regardless of severity.

Findings Definite ADD, 9.5 percent; apparent ADD regardless of severity, 16.2 percent. Definite oppositional disorder, 9.9 percent; apparent oppositional disorder, 19.4 percent.

MCGEE, FEEHAN, WILLIAMS, PARTRIDGE, SILVA, AND KELLY (1990)

DSM-III disorders in large sample of New Zealand adolescents (see Anderson et al., 1987, described earlier).

Sample   943 adolescents from a longitudinal population study. Age 15, boys and girls.

Evaluative measures   Structured interviews of adolescents, parent questionnaire. Diagnostic criteria: DSM-III.

Findings   With 95 percent confidence limits: ADD, 2.1 percent (sex ratio, 2.3:1); ADD and CD/ODD, 0.4 percent of population (20 percent of ADD subjects). The authors state that 5.4 percent (51) of the children had been diagnosed with ADD at age 7 and 11, and that it had persisted in about 40 percent. ADD and anxiety disorder, 0.4 percent. Conduct and oppositional disorder, 9 percent.

Comment   The lack of parent interviews or teacher questionnaires undoubtedly underestimated the prevalence of ADD in this older group.

BHATIA, NIGAM, BOHRA, AND MALIK (1991)

Attention deficit disorder with hyperactivity among pediatric outpatients in India.

Sample   1000 boys and girls, ages 3 to 12, at pediatric outpatient clinic; all screened for ADD-H.

Evaluative measures   Conners parent rating scale, interview with parents, Wechsler tests of intelligence, and other psychological tests. Diagnosis based on integration of data; DSM-III criteria used for ADD-H.

Findings   Prevalence of ADD-H: boys, 15.7 percent; girls, 4.1 percent.

Comment   A clinical sample rather than a population (e.g., school) sample. Documents probable similarity and identifiability of ADHD in other cultures.

PELHAM, GNAGY, GREENSLADE, AND MILICH (1992)

Teacher ratings of DSM-III-R symptoms for disruptive behavior disorders.

Sample 931 boys, ages 5 to 14, in regular classrooms from schools in 48 states and several Canadian provinces.

Evaluative measures Teachers filled out rating scales, including one composed of DSM-III-R diagnostic criteria for ADHD, CD, and ODD, defined by the number of symptoms rated "very much." No structured interviews.

Findings There is some confusion about the findings because their total prevalence figure of 8.3 percent for disruptive disorders (78 of 931) does not match the figure shown in an illustrative diagram (63 of 931), 6.8 percent. The ADHD prevalence is 6.5 percent.

Comment A sophisticated study. It reports sensitivity, specificity, positive and negative predictive power of *individual symptoms*, using diagnosis as the criterion. However, the recurrent cutoff question here depends on the validity of DSM-III-R criteria.

SUMMARY: CHILDHOOD PREVALENCE STUDIES

I conclude that with all the differences in methodology, the variation among the studies is not surprising. Even with structured interviews and well-established diagnostic criteria, the variability in rates can be substantial. The picture is further clouded by uncertainty about some of the diagnostic criteria—for example, the popular Conners Abbreviated Teacher Rating Scale (CATRS). Normative data on the 1973 CATRS compiled by Sprague et al. (1974) led them to recommend a cutoff score of 15 or greater (2 standard deviations above the mean) to distinguish "hyperactive" from normal children. Ullmann et al. (1985) reexamined the old data and collected rating scale scores from a new large sample of children. Their conclusions were that with a cutoff of 15 the Abbreviated Teacher Rating Scale was insensitive to inattention—that is, children with difficulties in attention but not in hyperactivity would falsely be diagnosed as not having ADD. Their data further revealed that an overall cutoff of 15 was too low (despite the insensitivity to inattention), and that the basic 39-item scale from which the 10-item CATRS was derived also had major problems.

Recognizing problems of this kind, what can be concluded?

1. ADHD and conduct disorders are common in childhood.

2. Determining their prevalence on the basis of distribution/percentile is unjustifiable.

3. The lower prevalences of hyperactivity are obtained by the British for "pervasive hyperactivity": 2 percent (Schachar et al., 1981) on the Isle of Wight; 4.6 percent in London (Goodman and Stevenson, 1989). The most meaningful figures are based on the criterion of Boyle et al. (1987): to receive a diagnosis, a child must manifest symptoms that are associated with impairment specifically to the child and/or distress to the child, family, or community (Boyle et al., 1987; Offord et al., 1987; Offord et al., 1989). With that criterion 8.9 percent of the boys and 3.3 percent of the girls received a diagnosis of "hyperactivity," and 8.1 percent of the boys and 2.7 percent of the girls received a diagnosis of conduct disorder.

4. ADHD is more common in boys than in girls.

5. The prevalence of ADHD may be increased in children of lower socioeconomic status.[8]

6. ADHD is associated with CD on a much greater than chance basis. In most epidemiological studies, about half of the ADHD children also have conduct disorder, and the percent increases with the severity of "hyperactivity." Using the figures from the Ontario Child Health Study, 8.9 percent of the boys were hyperactive and 8.1 percent were conduct disordered. Almost half (44.1%) of the hyperactive boys had both diagnoses, substantially more than the number expected if the two conditions were uncorrelated.

As with hyperactivity, conduct disorder is less common in girls, although what may be manifestations of the CD/ASPD/alcohol/somatization disorder spectrum—perhaps a "CD equivalent"—increased in adolescent girls to 10.7 percent, which compares with 10.4 percent for conduct disorder in boys.

7. ADHD and CD decrease with age, as will be discussed in the next section on natural history.

This discussion of ADHD in children focuses on their behavior, not their feelings. Our adults with ADHD not only have behavioral abnormalities (signs) that are visible to others but have symptoms that cause them pain. Such symptoms are related to lability and overreactivity (mood and temper), and include their responses to their functional debility, to their disorganization, impulsivity, etc. We are able to assess these characteristics readily in adults because some are articulate introspectors. We do not know their frequency in the childhood population.

Finally, we should not expect DSM-IV to resolve our difficulties in determining the true prevalence of ADHD since it does not give us an independent measure to validate the diagnosis. That depends on scientific advancement and not redefinition.

THE NATURAL HISTORY OF ATTENTION-DEFICIT HYPERACTIVITY DISORDER

■

With some idea now of the various estimates that have been made of the prevalence of "hyperactivity" in childhood, we can proceed to examine the natural history of the syndrome. Twenty years ago when I wrote my monograph, on minimal brain dysfunction in children, the common wisdom was that "hyperactivity" diminished in adolescence and disappeared by adulthood. That assumption began to be invalidated by the systematic accumulation of data from three types of studies: (1) Cross-sectional studies that investigated the childhood psychiatric status of adults with certain psychiatric syndromes, specifically alcohol and substance abuse or dependence; (2) retrospective or follow-back studies that used clinic records to identify children who would now be diagnosed as ADHD or "hyperactive" and then investigated their current psychiatric status; (3) prospective studies in which the investigators identified a sample with a diagnosis of "hyperactivity" or ADD (ADHD) and followed that sample over time. As always, the pre-DSM-III children called "hyperactive" manifested varying mixtures of "externalizing disorders": ADHD, CD, and ODD.

CROSS-SECTIONAL STUDIES

The cross-sectional studies begin with a sample of adults with specified adult psychiatric disorders and then determine what fraction could retrospectively be diagnosed as hyperactive.

These studies cannot provide information about the natural history of ADHD unless one knows the prevalence of the syndrome being studied. For example, one might find that one-quarter of patients with syndrome X have a history of "hyperactivity," but one cannot calculate the fraction of ADHD children who develop this syndrome unless one knows the prevalence of ADHD in childhood, the prevalence of syndrome X, and whether the sample being studied is a representative one. Thus all these studies can do is to inform us that ADHD children may develop syndrome X when they become adults and that, perhaps, treatments that are effective for the children may be effective in the treatment of adults. Once again, if or when we have a biological correlate or a genetic marker for ADHD, these studies may identify forms of adult psychopathology in which we should evaluate such attributes.

A number of studies have reported an increased frequency of a history of "hyperactivity" in adult alcoholics or distinct personality characteristics in "hyperactive" alcoholics. Tarter et al. (1977) subdivided 66 outpatients and inpatients into "primary" and "secondary" alcoholics. Primary alcoholics had an early onset, tolerance, increased withdrawal symptoms and personal and interpersonal problems before age 40. The primary alcoholics were found to have higher scores than the secondary alcoholics on a rating scale of childhood "MBD" symptoms (Tarter et al., 1982). DeObaldia et al. (1983) and DeObaldia and Parsons (1984) replicated Tarter's findings that primary alcoholics had a greater number of MBD characteristics than did secondary alcoholics, and that the primary alcoholics had a trend toward poorer neuropsychological functioning.

Alterman et al. (1985) studied 99 inpatient alcoholics and separated them by the median of a rating scale previously used. The minimal brain *damaged* subgroup had more interpersonal problems and more use of nonalcoholic illicit drugs.

Wood et al. (1983) investigated alcoholics in a partial hospitalization program and found that one-third qualified for a diagnosis of ADD, Residual Type, using the Utah Criteria. The childhood diagnosis was partially based on the Parents' Rating Scale and may not discriminate between ADHD and CD children.

Goodwin et al. (1975) reported that in their Danish study of alcoholism those adoptees who were alcoholics were more likely than the nonalcoholics to have had symptoms of "hyperactivity" (ADHD, CD, or both) as children.

These studies examined the prevalence of ADHD-like syndromes in a non-ADHD population. In another study, Shekim et al. (1990) examined the prevalence of other psychiatric disorders in 56 adults referred for evaluation and treatment for "adult hyperactivity"; they met DSM-III-R criteria for ADHD, and 91 percent of them met the Utah Criteria for ADD,RT. The other diagnoses reported included dysthymic and cyclothymic disorders and hypomania, 54 percent; drug or alcohol abuse, 34 percent and 30 percent; generalized anxiety disorder, 53 percent. The high frequency of the nonmajor mood disorders may be the result of confusing the affective lability we have described in ADHD with subthreshold major mood disorders—dysthymia and cyclothymia.

It is difficult to explain the high rate of anxiety reported in this sample. Two possibilities are that the patients had generalized anxiety disorder (GAD) in childhood, which was misdiagnosed as ADHD, or that individuals with ADHD were more likely to seek treatment if they suffered from GAD as well. This is a problem with all clinical samples: people with multiple ailments are more likely to seek help than those with single ailments of the same severity. Thus, people seeking help are more likely to be comorbid.

There are also a few case reports of ADHD in patients with different psychiatric diagnoses. Case reports of associations between possible ADHD and other syndromes prove nothing—they can only *suggest* the utility of systematic investigation. Cocaine abuse may or may not be associated with a history of or persisting ADHD, but Khantzian (1983) reported the usefulness of methylphenidate in reducing craving in four cocaine addicts with persisting ADHD. Others have not found methylphenidate useful in non-ADHD cocaine-dependent individuals. Bromocryptine (Cocores et al., 1987) and pemoline (Weiss and Mirin, 1985)—both dopamine agonists—have also been reported to be dramatically effective in this subgroup of cocaine abusers.

FOLLOW-BACK STUDIES

In this design, one attempts through records to identify individuals who were or could be retrospectively diagnosed as "hyperactive" and then examines their current psychiatric status. These studies have utilized available data to dispel the notion that hyperactivity is outgrown at adolescence. Seven studies reviewed by Thorley (1984) have also shown that "childhood hyperactivity is not associated nonspecifically with psychiatric disturbance but only with certain types of psychopathology" (p. 128)—such as sociopathy and alcoholism. However, they suffer from a number of methodological difficulties (see Thorley)—for example, the problem of making an accurate retrospective diagnosis (particularly in regard to the separation of ADHD and CD) and the question of determining normal, nonpsychiatric controls.

PROSPECTIVE STUDIES

As in the rest of medicine, prospective studies provide the most useful information about natural history. Mannuzza et al. (1991) have summarized the most important methodological features of studies to determine the natural history of childhood hyperactivity (or any psychiatric disorder) as follows: "Ideally, follow-up studies should be prospective, include appropriate controls, employ specific selection criteria, have adequate sample size and follow-up duration, show low attrition, obtain data from multiple sources, and rely on assessments that are conducted blind to group membership" (p. 77). I will focus on two longitudinal studies of ADHD from childhood to adulthood, the studies by Weiss, Hechtman et al. (Hechtman et al., 1984; Weiss and Hechtman, 1993) and Mannuzza, Klein [Gittelman], et al. (1990, 1993), both of which have followed cohorts of "hyperactive" children past the age of 25 and have also studied control groups.

Before proceeding, however, I would like to summarize two studies that followed "hyperactive" children through adolescence. Although other such studies have been done, these two used more rigorous research criteria.

Satterfield et al. (1982) obtained student official arrest records for serious offenses in Los Angeles in 110 ADD-H and 88 normal boys for an average of five years. The ages ranged from 13 to 21, with a mean age of 17 years. Rates of single and multiple arrests, and institutionalization for delinquency, were significantly higher in the hyperactives—for example, the percentage of hyperactive adolescents arrested at least once was 58 percent in the lower class, 36 percent in the middle class, and 52 percent in the upper class, compared to 11 percent, 9 percent, and 2 percent for the controls. This more recent study differs significantly from other prospective studies in both the number of arrests and their seriousness. Weiss and Hechtman (1993) point out that in several somewhat earlier studies repeated antisocial behavior varied from 10 percent to 25 percent (p. 57). They add, however, that serious crime committed by youth is increasing, especially in the Los Angeles area.

Barkley and his colleagues (Barkley et al., 1990, 1991; Fischer et al., 1990) followed prospectively a large sample of ADHD and normal children for eight years after their initial evaluation. The follow-up sample comprised 123 hyperactive children (111 male) and 66 normal children (62 male), between 4 and 12 years of age, which represented 78 and 81 percent, respectively, of the original sample pool. At follow-up (average

age of hyperactives, 15; of controls, 14), 71.5 percent of the hyperactives met the DSM-III-R criteria for ADHD, versus 1.5 percent in the control group. About 43 percent of the hyperactive group qualified for a diagnosis of CD, versus only 1.6 percent of the control group. For both ADHD and CD, when the cutoff score was changed to 2 standard deviations above the normal mean, a larger percentage of the hyperactive sample could be diagnosed as ADHD (83.3 percent) and CD (60 percent).

A number of critical variables affect the validity of longitudinal studies, whether they are of adolescent or adult outcome. Before examining the results of the two adult outcome studies, I will list major research factors that must be considered.

CRITIQUE OF PROSPECTIVE STUDIES

1. *Diagnostic criteria.* Throughout I have discussed the confusion earlier studies caused by their failure to distinguish between ADHD and CD. This is an issue that is critically related to outcome since approximately one-half of conduct-disordered children develop Antisocial Personality Disorder.

The major studies reviewed chose their probands prior to the introduction of DSM-III. Inclusion in these samples was based on the category of the "hyperactive child" and, in varying and unknown proportions, included children who would now be diagnosed with concurrent oppositional defiant disorder, conduct disorder, or learning disorders. The inclusion of multiple subtypes would be more realistic—it is what one sees clinically. However, studying samples subdivided into any combination of the foregoing diagnoses means that a larger total sample (N) is necessary if each of the subgroups is to be sufficiently large.

An additional diagnostic consideration is how to interpret any change in the symptom picture, because the diagnosis of ADHD is not made on the basis of pathognomonic features but on the presence of more than a certain *number* of symptoms. If a "hyperactive" child entered a sample with eight DSM-III-R symptoms and five years later had only seven, should one say that he was no longer "hyperactive" or that his hyperactivity had diminished by about 12 percent?

2. *The age at which probands are evaluated.* The younger the age at first evaluation, the more likely children destined to develop CD will not have the defining symptoms, which are clearly age-related. CD may not be evident at age 5 or 8 but may be very evident at 10 or 12.

ODD may be identifiable earlier and in some instances is a precursor to CD (Loeber et al., 1991).

3. *Sample attrition*. Sample attrition is due to both lack of cooperation and loss to follow-up. Noncompliers are nonrandom. They are at increased risk for psychopathology in general and probably "acting out" psychopathology in particular. Their loss is likely to decrease the difference between the probands and the comparison group (Cox et al., 1977). Those who disappear may have died from suicide, homicide, or accident, may be lost through institutionalization, or, maintaining no social ties, may have left no forwarding address. All are likely to be associated with Antisocial Personality Disorder. Loss of subjects will therefore probably *decrease* the difference between the ADHD (and probably ODD and CD) probands and the comparison group. The Weiss et al. study was particularly susceptible to this criticism; they lost nearly 30 percent of the original sample (104 "hyperactive" children aged 6 to 12) at 10-year follow-up and more than a third by the 15-year follow-up.

4. *The sex of the sample*. There are no studies of girls with sufficient sample sizes to study their natural history as compared to boys. The only systematic study (Mannuzza and Gittelman, 1984) has an *N* of 12 girls (compared with 24 hyperactive boys and 24 male controls) and found no difference. There is obviously a risk of failing to find a difference which indeed exists—a Type II error.[9] An additional complication is the interesting possibility—raised by Huessy—that "minimal brain dysfunction" in girls may not be manifest until after adolescence (defining MBD on the basis of lability, overreactivity, and impulsivity).

5. *The choice of comparison groups*. Studies of the natural history of ADHD have used a number of different comparison groups. The one most methodologically suspect is patients' siblings. Since the disorder is probably genetic, one anticipates an increased frequency of ADHD-like behavior in the siblings, even if they are included because they do not meet criteria for ADHD. To the extent that ADHD has genetic components, their inclusion will diminish the difference between ADHD and non-ADHD subjects as adults (i.e., increase the likelihood of a Type II error).

Other options for comparison groups include "average" children—for example, a sample getting routine immunizations (psychologically screened and without any psychiatric disorder)—or children with another psychiatric diagnosis. The choice depends on which questions one wants answered. The first asks whether or not the developmental course of "hyperactivity" differs from that of normal or average (they are not synonymous) children. The second comparison group asks whether the developmental course of "hyperactive" children differs from that of children with other psychiatric disorders.

Comparisons are also affected by the nature of the ADHD group. Although it is generally tacitly assumed that a clinical sample is a random sample of ADHD children in the community, it may constitute a biased subsample of ADHD children with more severe symptoms. If the children were referred by social agencies, their parents could be incompetent, neglectful, or abusive. Conceivably the problems of such children might have been exacerbated by their parents, and the children may have been less severely ill if raised in an average "good-enough" environment.

6. *Follow-up techniques.* In follow-ups—as in initial evaluations—interviews are better than paper-and-pencil tests, structured interviews are better than unstructured interviews, and blinded interviews are better than nonblinded interviews.

With such factors in mind, let us return to the comparison of the Mannuzza et al. and Weiss et al. longitudinal studies. The Mannuzza and Klein study (Mannuzza et al., 1993) began between 1970 and 1975 with 103 white boys, ages 6 to 12 years, who had been referred by their teachers to a no-cost research psychiatric clinic for treatment of behavior problems. The boys were diagnosed as having hyperactivity, which at that time was called hyperkinetic reaction of childhood, and were treated largely by pharmacotherapy. The controls, 100 white males who were recruited about ten years later at the time of the adolescent follow-up, were provided by an adolescent medicine outpatient clinic. They were matched to the probands (the experimental subjects) for age and social class and were admitted to the study if they had had no behavior problems before age 13.

At the adolescent follow-up, mean age 18, information was obtained on 98 percent of the original sample. Full or partial ADD-H was diagnosed in 40 percent of the probands versus 3 percent of the controls. Further, 27 percent of the probands versus 8 percent of the controls were diagnosed as having either Conduct Disorder or Antisocial Personality Disorder. In addition, 16 percent of the probands versus 3 percent of the controls had an ongoing alcohol substance use disorder. These findings were replicated on an independent sample of 94 hyperactive boys and 78 controls.

The adult follow-up was conducted with 91 of the original cohort (88%) at an average age of 26 years. Of the 100 controls, 95 were interviewed at adult follow-up.

One-third of the probands versus 16 percent of the controls were diagnosed as having an ongoing mental disorder at adult follow-up. Antisocial Personality Disorder (18 percent versus 2 percent in controls) and nonalcohol substance use disorders (16 percent versus 4 percent) were both significantly more prevalent in probands than controls ($p<.01$). Substance abuse of any kind in the probands was higher among those with ASPD (40%) than among those without (13%). For ADHD, however, the difference between probands and controls (8 percent versus 1 percent) yielded only a trend ($p<.10$). An additional 3 percent of probands reported clinically impairing ADHD symptoms, bringing the total of affected cases to 11 percent versus 1 percent in controls, a significant difference ($p<.05$).

The changes between ages 18 and 26 are summarized in Table 3.2. The studies by Weiss and Hechtman and their colleagues (Weiss and Hechtman, 1993) began in 1962-65 with 104 children, ages 6 to 12, who were suffering from pervasive restlessness and poor concentration at home and at school and were taking part in a series of drug studies. Retrospectively the authors believe that all of the subjects had ADD-H and that the majority had some degree of associated conduct problems.

At a five-year follow-up in 1968, mean age 13.4, the 91 subjects interviewed scored worse on ADD-H symptoms than a matched group of 35 normal controls. The authors comment that a shortcoming of the study was the use of "normal" rather than patient controls.

At ten-year follow-up (1974), mean age 19, Weiss et al. were able to interview only 75 of the original sample. The control group at that time was enlarged to 45. About half of the original group continued to have

Table 3.2. Changes at Follow-up Periods: Mannuzza and Klein Study

| | Average Age at Follow-up | | | |
| | 18 | | 26 | |
Mental Disorder	Probands (%)	Controls (%)	Probands (%)	Controls (%)
ADD-H or ADHD, full or partial	40	3	11	1
Conduct Disorder or Antisocial Personality Disorder	27	8	18	2
Nonalcohol substance abuse disorder	16	3	16	4

significant problems of the original syndrome, particularly impulsivity and hyperactivity.

The study was completed with a fifteen-year follow-up, at which time 61 subjects and 41 controls were included in the analysis (90 percent of each group were male). Two-thirds of the 61 subjects (39) complained about at least one symptom of restlessness, distractibility, or impulsivity, versus 7 percent of the controls. About 22 of the 39 continued to have moderate or severe problems, while the other 17 had mild problems. Antisocial Personality Disorder was found in 23 percent of the original hyperactives and 2 percent of the controls. Unlike the Mannuzza study, nonalcohol substance abuse did not differ significantly between the two groups.

Thus, the percent of Antisocial Personality Disorders in the adult samples was similar for both studies (18 percent versus 2 percent in the Mannuzza study and 23 percent versus 2 percent in the Weiss study), but the two groups differed greatly in regard to the presence of symptoms of hyperactivity. The Mannuzza group found that 8 percent of the subjects continued to meet diagnostic criteria for hyperactivity (i.e., continuing attentional problems, impulsivity, and hyperactivity) and that an additional 3 percent had one or two symptoms of the disorder. The Weiss group found that two-thirds of the subjects had at least one disabling core symptom (restlessness, distractibility, or impulsivity), and that in about a third of their probands combinations of problems were moderately to severely troublesome.

How can we explain these very discrepant findings about continued presence of hyperactivity? Possibly they are related to the experimental designs, specifically interviewers' knowledge of the subjects and of their parents' judgment in the two studies. In the Mannuzza et al. study the interviewers did not know the subjects, and in their most recent follow-up they did not query the parents (parents of adults know less about their behavior than do the parents of adolescents) because a much smaller number of the subjects lived at home. In their earlier, adolescent follow-up study, in which 31 percent of the probands still manifested the full ADD-H syndrome (40 percent showed full or partial ADD-H), Mannuzza and Klein found that the prevalence of reported symptoms differed greatly between parents' reports about the subjects and subjects' reports about themselves: attentional problems, parents = 36 percent, subjects = 19 percent; impulsivity, 41 percent versus 16 percent; hyperactivity, 32 percent versus 21 percent. Weiss and Hechtman, on the other hand, were not blind to their sample. They did know their subjects, had to varying degrees seen them every five years, and had spoken to many of the parents throughout the time of follow-up. The difference between childhood patient-reported and parent-reported prevalence of symptoms jibes with our finding with adults—namely, that the adult ADHD's "other" reports many more symptoms than does the patient.

This finding of inaccurate self-perception has also been reported by Satterfield (1994, personal communication). He administered the Wender Utah Rating Scale (WURS) in two forms to ADHD adolescents and controls. In one form of the WURS, the published version, the subject evaluates his own behavior between the ages of 6 and 10; in the second form, the subject rates his current behavior on the same descriptors. The ADHD subjects rated their childhood as significantly more "hyperactive" than did the controls, but they rated their current behavior as normal, i.e., their ratings did not differ from those of the normal controls.

Conceivably, as Mannuzza and Klein both have said (personal communication), the Mannuzza adult rate (8% + 3%) should be doubled (22%) because of the absence of reports by "others" on the adult behavior. However, Weiss and Hechtman may have been oversensitive to psychopathology and thus vulnerable to overdiagnosis. In regard to impairment, Mannuzza et al. based their decisions on responses to standardized questions. Weiss et al. knew their patients' current academic or vocational level and had evaluated their intelligence in the past. Thus they could assess the discrepancy between potential and actual accomplishment—that is, the extent to which symptoms were impairing. Unquestionably, however, such discrepant results in part depend on the definition of "disabling."

A final important comparative feature is that the Mannuzza group was able to interview 88 percent of its original 103 hyperactive males after a mean of 16 years but that the Weiss group lost over a third of its original hyperactive subjects to follow-up. Researchers assume that these subjects are likely to have had more psychopathology than their locatable cohort members. Although the Weiss group found higher percentages of ADHD and ASPD than Mannuzza and Klein, the prevalence of continuing psychiatric disorders may have been underestimated.

Finally, what figure do I think we should employ as the best estimate of continuing ADHD symptoms in hyperactive children grown up? I would suggest as a minimum the Weiss group's figure of one-third. I say as a minimum because even their contact with the families is limited, and differential loss of subjects to follow-up has probably reduced that

Table 3.3. Prevalence of Hyperactivity in Childhood: Summary

Study	Study Focus	Sample b = boys g = girls	Ages or Grades	Evaluative Measures	Findings	Comment
Lapouse & Monk (1958)	Behavior characteristics	482 b & g	Ages 6–12	Structured interviews, mothers, or "mother substitutes"	Overactivity and temper loss, 48–49%	Half of school-age children are more active than adults would like
Huessy & Gendron (1970)	Hyperkinetic syndrome	430 b & g	Grade 2	Teacher questionnaire	Hyperkinetic problems, 8–9%	
Werry & Quay (1971)	Behavior symptoms	1815 (951 b, 864 g)	Grades Kg, 1, 2	Quay-Peterson Problem Checklist, by teachers	ADHD-type behaviors from 5% (girls temper) to 50% (boys restlessness), and everywhere in between (e.g., boys hyperactivity, 30%)	ADHD-type symptoms common in school-age children
Trites et al. (1979)	Hyperactivity	14,083 b & g	Grades Jr. Kg (age 4) to 6 incl.	CTRS[1]	Cutoff 1.5 SD, boys, girls: hyperactivity 20.6, 7.5%; conduct problems, 4.0, 1.7%	Authors emphasize relationship of prevalence to cutoff
Sandberg et al. (1980)	Hyperkinetic and conduct problem children in Inner London primary school	226 b	Ages 5–9	CTRS; Rutter teacher questionnaire; Conners parent questionnaire	On CTRS, about half of children in 90th percentile of hyperactivity were in 90th percentile of conduct disorder; different ratings from parent questionnaires	

Study	Focus	N	Age	Measures	Results	Comments
Schachar et al. (1981)	Situationally & pervasively hyperactive children on Isle of Wight	1536 b & g	Ages 10–11	Teacher and parent rating scales	Situationally hyperactive, 14.3%; pervasively hyperactive, 2.0%	
Shen et al. (1985)	Minimal brain dysfunction in elementary schools in Beijing	2770 b & g	—	Rutter and Conners rating scales	MBD at 2 SD = 5.8%	
O'Leary, Vivian, & Nisi (1985)	Hyperactivity in northern Italy	334 (186 b, 158 g)	Grades 2–4	CTRS	Hyperactivity at 2 SD: boys 7.5%, girls 1.3%	
Shekim et al. (1985)	ADD and ADHD	114 b & g	Age 9	DISC & DISC-P[2]	ADDH: by DISC-P, boys and girls, 12%; by DISC, boys 4%	Typical discrepancy (denial) between DISC & DISC-P scores
Satin et al. (1985)	ADDH	94 b	Ages 6–9	Rating scales by parents & teachers; diagnoses by psychiatrists on DSM-III	ADDH: situationally 24%; pervasively 8%	Exceptionally high
Shapiro & Garfinkel (1986)	Interdependence of ADD & CD	315 b & g	Grades 2–6; Mean age 9 yrs 10 mos	Diagnostic interview for children & adolescents; CTRS	"Suggestive" prevalences: ADD 2.3%; CD 3.6%; an additional 3.0% had both	Highlights frequent overlap between ADD & CD; diagnosis based on cutoff
Ontario Child Health Study Boyle et al. (1987) Offord et al. (1987,1989)	Child disorders	3289 b & g	Ages 4–16	Child Behavior Checklist with parents, teachers, adolescents 12–16; interviews with mother & child	Ages 4–16: hyperactivity, boys 8–9%, girls 3.3%; conduct disorder, boys 8.1%, girls 2.7%	Considerable overlap of hyperactivity and conduct disorder

(Continued)

Table 3.3. (Continued)

Study	Study Focus	Sample b = boys g = girls	Ages or Grades	Evaluative Measures	Findings	Comment
Anderson et al. (1987)	DSM-III disorders in preadolescent children in New Zealand	792 (416 b, 376 g)	Age 11	Structured interview of child (DISC-C); Rutter questionnaires for parents & teacher; behavioral history	ADD, 6.7%; CD, 3.4%; 47% of ADD children with CD	ADD & ADDH not distinguished
Yao et al. (1988)	Hyperactivity in immigrant Chinese-American children in NYC Chinatown	250 b & g	Grades 1–6	Conners 28-item TRS; CATRS[3]	Hyperactivity 2 SD: CATRS, boys 8.8%, girls 1.7%; 28-item, boys 12.7%, girls 1.7%	Higher rates than many other samples
Costello (1988)	Child psychiatric disorders in pediatric clinics	789 b & g	—	Child Behavior Checklist by parents; DISC, DISC-P, others	ADD with hyperactivity, 2%; ADD without hyperactivity, .2%, all boys; ODD, 6.6%; CD, 5.2%	
Goodman & Stevenson (1989)	Hyperactivity in monozygotic and dizygotic twins in London	285 twin pairs	—	Rutter parent and teacher questionnaire	Pervasively hyperactive, 4.6%	
Velez et al. (1989)	Longitudinal study of selected risk factors for childhood psychopathology	776 b & g	Ages 9–20	DISC, DISC-P	ADD: 9–14, 15%, 13–20, 8.3%; CD: 9–14, 11%, 13–20, 11% ODD: 9–14, 19%, 13–20, 16%	45% decrease in ADD between two time periods; no change in CD

Bird et al. (1989)	Risk factors for maladjustment in Puerto Rican children	777 b & g	Ages 4–16	Child Behavior Checklist from parents and teachers; DISC, DISC-P	Definite ADD, 9.5%; apparent ADD, 16.2%
McGee et al. (1990)	DSM-III disorders in adolescents in New Zealand; longitudinal study	943 b & g	Age 15	Structured interviews of adolescents; parent questionnaire	ADD, 2.1%; ADD & CD/ODD, 20% of ADD subjects; persistence of ADD in about 40% of children diagnosed earlier (5.4% earlier)	Lack of parent interview or teacher questionnaire may mean under-estimated prevalence
Bhatia et al. (1991)	ADDH among pediatric outpatients in India	1000 b & g	Ages 3–12	Conners parent rating scale; interview with parents; others	ADDH: boys 15.7%; girls 4.1%	Clinical rather than population sample; documents probable similarity of ADHD in other cultures
Pelham et al. (1992)	Teacher ratings of DSM-III-R symptoms for disruptive disorders	931 b	Ages 5–14	Teachers' rating scales ADHD, 6.5%		

[1] CTRS = Conners Teachers Rating Scale.

[2] DISC = Diagnostic Interview Schedule for Children; DISC-P = Diagnostic Interview Schedule for Parents.

[3] CATRS = Conners Abbreviated Teachers Rating Scale.

estimate. An estimate of one-third matches my clinical impression of the persistence of ADHD in adulthood among ADHD patients' parents who had themselves had ADHD in childhood. In other words, one cannot predict that the childhood symptoms will go away.

Combining the ADHD prevalence in childhood of 6 to 10 percent in the entire population and the above follow-up data, I would therefore argue that one-third of 6 percent is a minimal figure, and that two-thirds of 10 percent is a high estimate. In sum, the best guess about the prevalence of persisting ADHD in the adult population is 2 to 6 or perhaps 7 percent.

NOTES

1. "Prevalence" refers to the frequency of a condition as assessed at a particular time; "incidence" is assessed by determining the number of *new cases that arise in a specific time interval.*

2. Hans Huessy thinks that what he believes to be the cardinal symptoms of ADHD—impulsivity, overreactivity, and lability—frequently do develop in adolescent girls who in grade school had not been "hyperactive" but who were "more involved in daydreaming than in the typical acting out" of their male counterparts (Huessy et al., 1979, p. 27).

3. But it is frequently not that simple. We often must use less accurate procedures—for example, we obtain ECGs and blood enzymes to diagnose a myocardial infarct, and do not do a biopsy.

4. The criteria are probably honored in the breach. I suspect that experienced clinicians often use a banned gestalt impression and may diagnose ADHD in the presence of a smaller-than-necessary number of solid signs and not diagnose it in the presence of the required number of signs that are rather weak.

5. With increasing knowledge about the natural history of hypertension, and the development of effective, less noxious antihypertensive drugs (e.g., the ACE inhibitors), the cutting point has been decreased to 135/85. This is a good example of how the definition of a disorder can be a function of more than a list of signs and symptoms or a quasi-arbitrary cutting point. But do people with blood pressures of 140/90 have a significantly greater risk of cerebrovascular accidents and cardiac disease than people with blood pressures of 139/89? It is extremely doubtful, but there may be a different outcome for people with blood pressures of 141/91 versus those with blood pressures of 135/85.

6. For example, in using DSM-III-R criteria, one might want to know how many patients had eight symptoms (and "have ADHD") as opposed to those who "only" have seven symptoms.

7. Even if employing identical criteria, one can expect variations in inter-rater reliability. A recurring problem is that the relevant behaviors are dimensional (e.g., hyperactivity) rather than qualitative (hallucinations).

8. Lower SES may be the result of a disorder and not the cause of it. The prevalence of schizophrenia is greater in individuals of lower SES, but this is

due to "downward drift" produced by their illness (Wender et al., 1976). In the case of ADHD, all other things being equal, afflicted individuals are at a disadvantage in learning—and thus education—and job performance, and can be expected to move downward in the social hierarchy. Since—as will be seen—ADHD is a genetic disorder, lower SES parents will have a greater likelihood of having ADHD children. Similarly, higher SES parents, who are less likely to have ADHD, are less likely to produce ADHD children.

9. A "Type II error"—failing to find a difference which really exists, because the sample size is too small.

4

Etiology

■

In 1971 and 1972, I wrote that one subgroup of Minimal Brain Dysfunction (MBD) might be genetic in origin and produced by decreased catecholaminergic functioning. My conjectures about genetic origin were based on (1) an *apparent* increased frequency of MBD among the siblings of MBD children; (2) an apparent increase of mixed (depressive, alcoholic, sociopathic) psychopathology among the parents of "MBD" patients and the absence of such psychopathology in parents who had adopted MBD children; (3) a few instances of the syndrome in foster children whose biological parents had psychiatric illnesses. The reasons for hypothesizing decreased catecholaminergic activity were:

1. "MBD-like" ("postencephalitic behavior disorder") behavior was produced in children who recovered from von Economo's encephalitis during an epidemic in the late teens and early 1920's (described below).
2. Adults who recovered from the acute symptoms of von Economo's encephalitis frequently manifested symptoms of Parkinson's syndrome, and adults who died from the illness had lesions of the basal ganglia.
3. "Idiopathic" Parkinson's Disorder is associated with dopamine depletion due to degeneration of dopaminergic neurons in the nigrostriatal system and is associated with decreased levels of the principal metabolite of dopamine, homovanillic acid (HVA), in cerebrospinal fluid.

4. Some drugs were often dramatically effective in reducing or eliminating the symptoms of MBD, often as if they were remediating a basic biological deficit (see Chapter 6 on treatment).
5. The drugs that were most effective were those which were dopaminergic—and not those which were ostensibly noradrenergic, such as the tricyclic antidepressants.
6. Dopaminergic drugs decrease MBD-like behavior in animals (see, e.g., Corson et al., 1976; Bareggi et al., 1979a).

Until recently, the only data concerning etiology dealt with ADHD in children, which might again raise the question of the relationship between the causes of ADHD in childhood and the causes of ADHD in adults. However, as previous chapters indicate, the question is probably not relevant because if the disorder is a lifelong one, then whatever plays a role in the etiology of ADHD in childhood probably plays the same role in the etiology of ADHD in adults.

A legitimate problem that does arise in the investigation of ADHD in adults involves diagnostic heterogeneity. How can one meaningfully examine the etiology or etiologies of a probably heterogeneous group of patients? Paradoxically, attempts to discover an etiology are dependent on a homogeneous sample, but obtaining such a sample may require a knowledge of etiology. If a clinician studies "the" infectious disease pneumonia but cannot distinguish between viral pneumonia, pneumococcal pneumonia, and pulmonary tuberculosis, he is going to have a difficult time finding the exact "cause." The corresponding problem in genetic disorders is even more complicated because of the phenomenon of "genetic heterogeneity," a term used to describe identical (or very similar) disorders produced by multiple genetic causes. A clear instance of this phenomenon occurs in the disorders of coagulation of the blood. The syndrome was first called "hemophilia" and was found to be transmitted by an X-linked recessive gene. Further study revealed that "hemophilia" was the result of two different deficiencies in protein factors involved in clotting, hemophilia A ("classical hemophilia"), a deficiency in Factor VIII, and hemophilia B (Christmas disease), a deficiency in Factor IX. Much rarer are defects in Factors V, VII, X, and XIII. A phenocopy—that is, an environmentally produced mimic—is produced by a vitamin K deficiency. Identification of the specific cause of the disorder in a hemophiliac is essential. The symptoms of classical hemophilia can be eliminated by transfusing a concentration of Factor VIII but will not be controlled by Factor IX or vitamin K. The molecular abnormalities of hemophilia A and B are now being elucidated by cloning and the complementary DNA mapped on the X-chromosome.

As mentioned in the Introduction, an even more elaborate example of genetic heterogeneity occurs in the hyperphenylalaninemias (HPAs, formerly phenylketonuria or PKU), abnormalities in the utilization of phenylalanine hydroxylase, which catalyzes the oxidation of phenylalanine to tyrosine in the liver. This genetic disorder was first recognized as a distinct form of severe mental retardation which was accompanied by seizures, hypopigmentation, and a particular "mousy" odor of the skin and urine. The classical form of the disorder was found to be transmitted as a recessively inherited deficiency of the hepatic enzyme phenylalanine hydroxylase. The increased plasma level of phenylalanine activates other metabolic pathways (one manifestation of which is increased phenylketone) and interferes with, among other things, tyrosine hydroxylase activity, amino acid transport, protein synthesis, and myelin synthesis. A therapeutic breakthrough was the discovery that the symptoms of classical PKU could be mitigated by placing the infant at risk on a very low phenylalanine diet. Currently, more than forty forms of the HPAs have now been identified, with enzyme activity ranging from undetectable to 25 percent (Medical Research Council, 1993). Further genetic heterogeneity exists because increased plasma phenylalanine (together with other metabolic abnormalities) can be produced by a deficiency in tetrahydrobiopterin, a necessary cofactor. This form is classified as "malignant," cannot be corrected by diet, and is usually rapidly fatal. Finally, there is a phenocopy. PKU women who had been treated successfully with a phenylalanine-deficient diet throughout childhood and adolescence had then been placed on a normal diet. Their increased blood levels of phenylalanine did not harm them, but when they became pregnant, their fetuses were exposed to elevated levels of phenylalanine and became severely retarded.

Still another etiological complication emerges because with the same genetic load and psychological experiences, different individuals may manifest symptoms to a greater or lesser degree. This is the phenomenon of "variable penetrance" or "variable expression." A good example of variable penetrance is neurofibromatosis, which is dominantly transmitted by non-allelic genes on chromosomes 17 and 22. The severity of the disease may vary from instances in which there are only café-au-lait spots, to peripheral neurofibromas with impaired neurological function, to malignant glioblastomas. Variable expression can also take the form of "incomplete penetrance," in which a dominant abnormality skips a generation. All of these variations can occur because of the effects of other genes or of environmental factors. If we think about ADHD in terms of these phenomena, we can postulate that "simple" genetic errors—such as one in an enzyme regulating the synthesis of a particular neurotransmitter—might produce hyperactivity in one person, impulsivity in a second, inattention in a third, and full ADHD in a fourth. One sometimes sees such diversity in the siblings of ADHD patients, or in their relatives of different generations.

A related phenomenon is "pleiotropism," in which at least one genetic abnormality produces multiple and different effects. A dramatic example is diabetes mellitus, in which insulin deficiency may lead to atherosclerosis, renal failure, heart disease, and blindness.

Ideally, one would hope to separate illnesses on the basis of pathophysiology. In the case of psychiatry, this would appear to be an attempt to solve a difficult problem by a harder one. However, one can attempt to construct homogeneous categories on the basis of symptom pattern, natural history, and response to treatments. Etiological data of this kind can point to diagnostic clarifications, and vice versa, although one might be pulling oneself up by one's conceptual bootstraps.

Before presenting the evidence for the possible role of genetic factors in the transmission of ADHD, I must add that there is evidence—of varying degrees of persuasiveness—that MBD has nongenetic phenocopies (environmental mimics of genetic conditions). They may be produced by: (1) maternal use of alcohol or cigarettes during pregnancy (Shaywitz et al., 1980; Streissguth et al., 1984; Bennett et al., 1988);[1] (2) environmental toxins such as lead; (3) viral infection, such as a specific viral infection that occurred over 70 years ago and has not occurred since. I shall provide a description of a phenocopy by describing below that specific infection.

The first widespread description of an ADHD-like disorder followed the pandemic of encephalitis lethargica (von Economo's encephalitis) that occurred during the late 1910s and early 1920s. Reports began to appear describing behavioral sequelae of the illness in children—for example, a report by Hohman (1922) saying that following recovery from the acute phase of the illness, some children underwent "profound changes in character and behavior" and became "irritable . . . restless . . . quarrelsome . . . teased other children unmercifully . . . [were] disobedient . . . no longer amenable to discipline . . . emotionally quite unstable . . . capriciously moody" (pp. 372–373). Phillips (1923), summarizing several case reports from the French literature about the "after effects of encephalitis" in children, stated that "change in the moral character was present in all the cases. Lying, outbursts of temper, turbulence, violence, thefts, distractibility of attention, backwardness in learning, were some of the symptoms which made their appearance for the first time in a subject previously normal" (p. 246). Hill (1928) reported that in "the mildest cases the patients have in common a liability to bouts of anger and fighting, and a general restlessness with [a] secondary inability to sit still for long or concentrate in school. . . . Attempts at mental concentration make their restlessness and behaviour worse, . . . the effect of discipline, etc., being quite superficial" (pp. 2-3).

Some of these children exhibited ego-dystonic[2] symptoms of conduct disorder: "They realize the atrociousness of their actions, often showing spontaneous regret for them and evidence of trying to control themselves, weeping or giving signs of the most genuine repentance and complaining that they 'could not help it'" (pp. 3–4). One boy said: "'I am a bad boy. I know I am a bad boy, but I can't help it'" (p. 4).

To these characteristics, Bond (1932) added "truancy, lying, stealing, fears and recklessness combined . . . returns to infantile habits . . . and mawkish affection" (p. 31). In his chapter on the sequelae of *Encephalitis lethargica*, Von Economo (1930) devoted an entire section to "pseudo-psychopathia." He stated, "We see here how organic encephalitic lesions may produce in previously normal individuals a strange alteration of personality which cannot be otherwise described than as a kind of *moral insanity*" ("moral insanity" was the phrase employed by Pritchard 100 years earlier [1835] to describe "psychopathy," which now is approximated by Antisocial Personality Disorder). Von Economo described these children as having "a state of slight maniacal excitation . . . with urge-like motor impetus . . . outbreaks of anger and fury also often occur. Generally, however, the clinical picture assumes milder forms. Formerly normal children who were not psychopathic become (according to Nonne) more talkative, importunate, impertinent, forward, and disrespectful; they lack inhibitions; they often become troublesome and antisocial and display a tendency to outbreaks of emotion. Full of pertness and chatter . . . they tramp, beg, lie, steal, write on walls, squander all the money they can lay hands on . . . cannot be controlled at school, run away from home" (pp. 128–129). As time passed these children were apparently forgotten, although some authors discussed the persistence of the symptoms (W. Holt, 1937; Levy, 1959).

In summary, postencephalitic children manifested symptoms of Attention-deficit Hyperactivity Disorder (distractibility of attention, impairments in learning, increased motor activity, and impulsivity) and of Conduct and Oppositional Disorders (impertinence, disrespectfulness, temper outbursts, lying, stealing, antisocial behavior, and sexual misbehavior), and some a mixture of the two. Thus, the behavioral changes apparently produced by viral infection may have mimicked the syndrome seen in the usual idiopathic forms of ADHD and CD.

Parenthetically, Still (1902; often cited but one thinks infrequently read), who was one of the first to describe hyperactivity, also characterized children who were predominantly conduct disordered. He stated that their predominant feature was "an abnormal defect of moral control" (p. 1008) but commented on "quite an abnormal capacity for sustained attention" (p. 1166). It is of interest that he mentioned the presence of minor physical anomalies, particularly a high arched palate and epicanthal folds.

An encephalitic phenocopy of idiopathic ADHD and CD would be of less interest were it not for the fact that the histopathology of *Encephalitis lethargica* was studied in both children and adults. While von Economo's encephalitis produced a postencephalitic syndrome in children similar to ADHD and Conduct Disorder, adults recovering from the acute phase of the illness developed a postencephalitic Parkinson's syndrome, including bradyphrenia, a slowing of movement. One might think of the children's hyperactivity as similar to akathisia, which, like bradyphrenia, is frequently produced by neuroleptics; both are attributed to dopaminergic blockade.

Von Economo and others who explored the histopathology of the brain in encephalitis lethargica in adults found damage to gray matter, "most considerable in the substantia nigra, less intense in the lenticular nucleus and hypothalamus, but still distinctly visible." With regard to children, von Economo stated that the changes "in juvenile patients have not yet been sufficiently elucidated by morbid anatomy . . . [but on the basis of the available data] we must [therefore] look not on merely [incidental cortical lesions] but on the apparently regularly occurring lesions of the brainstem as the primary anatomical cause of these psychopathias" (p. 148)—that is, the localization of the lesions appeared similar in children and adults. Leo Kanner (1962), the father of American child psychiatry, also reported that children who recovered from encephalitis had a mixture of restlessness, lability of affect, and antisocial tendencies. He suggested that organic damage destroyed ordinary inhibitions.

With an awareness that these major examples of ADHD-like phenotypes preceded the accumulated literature on ADHD, we now examine the evidence that the disorder is related to genetic factors. I conclude this chapter by presenting additional material on possible biochemical abnormalities in ADHD and by looking at directions for future research.

GENETIC STUDIES OF ADHD

■

Three types of studies have been used to evaluate the roles of genetic factors and psychosocial experience in the etiology of ADHD: (1) family studies; (2) twin studies; and (3) adoption studies. As might be expected, the earlier studies dealt with a heterogeneous group of children who would now be diagnosed as having various mixtures of ADHD, ODD and Conduct Disorder, and Learning Disorders.

All of these studies suffer from being clinical samples rather than random epidemiological samples. Clinical samples are subject to a number of sampling biases—for example, children referred to clinics may have more severe symptoms, be comorbid with different disorders, have more symptoms that are socially noxious, or have parents or caretakers who have a lower threshold for seeking help. Furthermore, the composition of clinical samples may be expected to vary depending on whether they came from a private setting, a teaching hospital, or an inner city hospital. Some of the investigators have been aware of these and other research problems—such as whether to use categorical diagnoses or a dimensional scale—but one must always keep in mind the difficulties of comparing the results in different studies.

1. *Family studies* are used to determine if there is an increased frequency in the amount and type of psychopathology in the biological relatives of children with ADHD. They are the simplest and most straightforward of the three types of studies. The studies to be reviewed examine the first-degree relatives (sibs and parents) of children with hyperactivity and Attention Deficit Disorder. The earlier studies investigated the mixed diagnostic category "hyperactivity," while later studies examined ADD children who did or did not have accompanying Conduct Disorder.

2. *Twin studies* can—given hypotheses which may not be fully acceptable—provide a rough measure of the etiological contributions of "nature and nurture."

3. *Adoption studies* provide a strategy that circumvents the limita-

tions of the twin method and permits a more accurate determination of genetic contributions to the disorder. They have also contributed to knowledge about the relationships between the adult psychiatric disorders that are seen with increased frequency among ADHD or CD children.

FAMILY STUDIES

As previously mentioned, the earlier family studies were of "hyperactive" children and did not discriminate between such disorders as ADHD and CD. These studies examined the frequency and nature of psychopathology in the biological relatives of "hyperactive" children. Morrison and Stewart (1971) evaluated the parents, aunts, and uncles of 59 hyperactive and 41 control children and found a statistically significant difference between the relatives of the hyperactive children and those of the control group. The Morrison and Stewart study is difficult to interpret because their text and illustrative tables do not fully agree, but according to the text: (1) about 20 percent of the "hyperactive" children versus about 5 percent of the controls had a parent hyperactive in childhood, and adding aunts and uncles produced a significant difference; (2) about one-third of the hyperactive children's parents versus one-sixth of the control group's parents received some psychiatric diagnosis, differing specifically in the prevalence of alcoholism, sociopathy, or hysteria; (3) finally, the data suggested that hyperactivity in childhood was a forerunner of these forms of adult psychopathology: about half of the parents who had been "hyperactive" in childhood received an adult diagnosis of alcoholism, sociopathy, or hysteria.

Similar findings were reported by Cantwell (1972), who studied the parents and other relatives of 50 "hyperactive" boys and 50 control boys. He found that about 35 percent of the hyperactive boys' parents versus about 10 percent of the controls' parents received a diagnosis of alcoholism, sociopathy, or hysteria (definite or probable). Ten percent of the parents of hyperactives had been "hyperactive" in childhood (versus 1 percent of control parents) and all of the formerly hyperactive parents received one of these three adult diagnoses, a finding which replicated that of Morrison and Stewart and suggested that these three disorders are genetically related and that childhood hyperactivity is frequently their precursor. Nearly half of the hyperactive children's parents versus less than one-fifth of the control children's parents had a psychiatric diagnosis.

Welner et al. (1977) conducted a study of the siblings of 43 "hyperactive" boys and a control group of 38 matched nonhyperactive boys. There was a statistically significant, threefold increase of hyperactivity in the brothers of the hyperactive probands (the experimental subjects) as compared to the brothers of the controls (26% versus 9%), and a sixfold increase in "depression" in the nonhyperactive brothers of the probands as compared to the nonhyperactive brothers of the controls (36% versus 6%). Neither diagnosis was more common in the sisters of the probands than in the sisters of the controls.

One problem in the studies discussed is whether the psychopathology seen in the relatives of hyperactive children is specific to that disorder or is nonspecifically related to any psychiatric illness in children sufficient to bring them for treatment. Morrison (1980) addressed this issue by investigating parental diagnoses for a large sample of "hyperactive" (N = 140) children and adolescents and for age- and sex-matched nonhyperactive, mixed psychiatrically ill patients (N = 91). He found a statistically significant increase of antisocial personality and Briquet's Syndrome (hysteria) but not of alcoholism in the parents of the "hyperactive" children as compared to those of the psychiatrically ill controls.

Stewart et al. (1980) called attention to two possible sources of error in previous family studies. First, the diagnosis of "hyperactivity" had been used in a broad sense and included children with antisocial and conduct problems; second, the comparison groups used in most previous studies were of the parents of normal children rather than of children with other psychiatric diagnoses (cf. Morrison above). They further reasoned that the increased frequency of psychopathology in the hyperactive children's parents might be nonspecific and related to any kind of psychiatric pathology in children; thus, they argued, one should compare the relatives of hyperactive children with those of children with other psychiatric diagnoses. Stewart et al. therefore investigated parental psychopathology in a group of 126 boys consecutively admitted to a child psychiatric clinic or ward. They separated them into the following diagnostic groups: unsocialized aggressive (N = 25); mixed unsocialized aggressive and hyperactive (N = 33); probable mixed unsocialized aggressive and hyperactive (N = 16); hyperactive (N = 20); and a comparison group of boys with phobic neurosis, depression, enuresis or encopresis, and undiagnosed disorders (N = 32). The authors found that primary alcoholism was significantly higher among the fathers of the hyperactive boys than among the remainder (26% versus 11%)—although the rate was equal if fathers with secondary diagnoses of alcoholism (e.g., individuals in whom alcoholism was subsumed under antisocial personality) were counted in the comparison. Hysteria was three times as common among the mothers of the hyperactive boys as it was among the mothers of the remainder (13% versus 4%), but this result did not reach a conventional level of statistical significance ($p < .06$). Lastly, antisocial personality was significantly greater among the fathers of the unsocialized aggressive boys than it was among the fathers of the hyperactives and others, taken together, but this finding is difficult to interpret because of an interaction between social class, antisocial personality, and proband diagnosis. The major thrust of the study was to suggest the importance of separating hyperactive children into homogeneous subgroups and, in particular, of separating them into subgroups of ADD alone, CD alone, and mixed ADD/CD. However, despite this design, the study failed to find an association between parental disorder and hyperactivity.

Another study designed to evaluate familial psychopathology as a function of homogeneous diagnostic subgroups was reported by August and Stewart (1983). They reanalyzed a subset of a previously studied sample (August and Stewart, 1982) by separating "hyperkinetic" boys into those with a positive family history of antisocial personality (FH+, $N = 36$) and those with a negative family history (FH−, $N = 31$). They then numerically rated the boys on eight dimensions of psychological and behavioral functioning as assessed by a structured interview with the children's mothers. The authors found that the two groups did not differ on inattentiveness, hyperactivity, anxiety, or depression, but that the FH+ manifested more aggression, noncompliance, antisocial behavior, and egocentricity. On the basis of these findings, they again suggested the utility of increasing diagnostic homogeneity by subdividing hyperactive children into those with and without a biological parent in the "antisocial spectrum." A normal or a nonhyperactive group with no family history of Antisocial Personality Disorder was not provided, so we cannot determine if the FH+, while less compliant than the children from FH− backgrounds, were less compliant than normal children or children with other psychiatric disorders (such as children with separation anxiety disorder or major depression). The variable that distinguished the two groups most was noncompliance, but an analysis of the data shows that the effect of family history was not strong.

Additional support for the utility of separating "hyperactive" children into aggressive and nonaggressive subgroups comes from the work of Loney and associates (Loney et al., 1978, 1981; Paternite and Loney, 1980; Loney and Milich, 1982). They assessed "a variety of psychiatric chart material" with independent judges and found they could identify two largely separate dimensions, an aggression-conduct disorder dimension and a hyperactivity (impulsivity, inattentiveness) dimension. The factor scores associated with these attributes had differential prognostic implications: aggression was correlated with adolescent delinquency, while hyperactivity predicted academic achievement problems in adolescents.

Biederman et al. (1986, 1990, 1991a, 1991b, 1992; Faraone et al., 1991) have published six family studies on ADD children and their families. The studies published in 1990 and 1991 have the same probands, but the separate studies consider different ADD subgroups (with Oppositional Disorders, Conduct Disorders, affective disorders, and anxiety disorders). A major problem in interpreting these studies is that the same probands must have multiple diagnoses (there are more diagnoses than subjects), and we do not know the relationship between the varying and combined psychopathologies in the probands and the psychiatric disorders in their relatives. The methodology is, in general, sophisticated and utilized blind structured interviews (Diagnostic Interview for Children and Adolescents—Parent Version [DICA-P]). In the first study three-quarters of the interviewers were trained research assistants with undergraduate degrees in psychology. The remaining quarter had more advanced training, comparable to the doctoral-level interviewers of the Mannuzza-Klein outcome studies described in the chapter on prevalence and natural history.

Biederman et al. (1986) reported an increased frequency of ADD, Oppositional Disorder (OD; a DSM-III category), and major depression in the first-degree relatives of 22 ADD probands (psychiatric referrals from an outpatient clinic in a teaching hospital, not broken down into comorbid diagnostic subgroups) as compared to those of a *normal* control group. The rates of these disorders in the relatives of the ADD probands hovered around 27 to 33 percent, as opposed to 5 or 6 percent in the normal controls. The diagnosis of ADD in childhood in the parents of the ADD children was based on the Diagnostic Interview Schedule for Children, Parent Version (DISC-P) and the DICA-P. Biederman et al. did not find an increase in ASPD or substance abuse in the relatives, although this has been a recurrent finding in the relatives of hyperactive (and variably CD) patients. Because comorbidity in the probands is not provided, one cannot determine whether the increase in OD in the relatives was mediated by ADD/OD or ADD/CD probands.

In 1990 Biederman et al. published an analysis of an enlargement of the earlier sample, now including 73 subjects. Again, the ADD probands were not separated into those with OD or CD. These probands' relatives were compared to those of a group with mixed psychiatric diagnoses and those of a "normal" group. The significant differences in diagnoses in the first-degree relatives of the probands, of a mixed psychiatric comparison group, and of the normal controls was for ADD, 25 percent versus 5 percent versus 5 percent; for antisocial disorders (now, but not in 1986), 25 percent (with slight discrepancy in accompanying table) versus 7 percent versus 4 percent; for affective disorders, 27 percent versus 14 percent versus 4 percent; for anxiety disorders, 19 percent versus 14 percent versus 5 percent. Most of the affective disorders were major depression. This is the second report documenting an increase in major depression in the first-degree relatives of ADD probands and raises a question about the composition of their sample. The retroactive diagnoses of ADD in the parents were based on answers to a structured interview, but the authors did not discuss the problem that must be directly addressed—how to determine whether the interviewed adult would in fact have merited such a diagnosis in childhood.

In 1991 the same group (Faraone et al., 1991) reported the blind, interview-based diagnoses of the parents and siblings of 73 ADD probands, now broken down into three groups: ADD, ADD/OPD and ADD/CD. (OPD, Oppositional Personality Disorder, is different terminology for OD, Oppositional Disorder, the term they had used earlier.) These diagnoses were compared with those of the relatives of the psychiatric patients and normal controls. The results were as follows:

1. There was an increased frequency in ADD among all first-degree relatives of the three groups of ADD probands versus psychiatric and normal controls: relatives of ADD/CD, 38 percent; of ADD/OPD, 17 percent; of ADD, 24 percent; of psychiatric and normal controls, 5 percent for both.

2. The risk for antisocial disorder was highest among relatives of ADD/CD (34%) and ADD/OPD (24%), which was significantly greater than the risk to relatives of ADD probands (11%) and psychiatric (7%) and normal controls (4%).

3. Both ADD and antisocial disorders occurred in the same relatives on a greater than chance basis. The authors conclude that ADD with and without antisocial disorders may be distinct disorders, but they may also be explained by a multifactorial hypothesis in which ADD, ADD/OPD, and ADD/CD occur along a continuum of familial etiology.

In two additional 1991 studies (Biederman, 1991a, 1991b), the Biederman group examined the familial association between ADD and anxiety disorders, and between ADD and major affective disorders. In both instances, the risk for ADD and for the disorders under investigation was greater among the relatives of the ADD probands than among the relatives of the normal controls.

Biederman et al.'s subsequent report (1992) extended previous findings by using both pediatrically and psychiatrically referred proband samples.

Another study of the familial associations of ADD and CD was reported by Lahey et al. (1988), who investigated the parents of an outpatient population of children with CD ($N = 14$), ADD-H ($N = 18$), ADD-H + CD ($N = 23$), and other diagnoses (clinic control group, $N = 30$). Assessment was made in most instances by obtaining information from one parent (usually the mother). The significant findings were an increased frequency of major depression, dysthymia, Antisocial Personality Disorder, history of fighting, arrests, and prison sentences among the mothers of the CD and ADD-H + CD probands versus the mothers of the "pure" ADD-H probands, and an increased frequency of Antisocial Personality Disorder, alcohol and substance abuse, history of fighting, arrests, and prison sentences among the fathers of the CD and ADD-H + CD probands versus the fathers of the "pure" ADD-H probands and controls. However, the characteristics of the sample make interpretation difficult. The parents of the ADD-H + CD probands had the lowest SES and the most psychopathology; the parents of the ADD-H probands and controls had the highest SES and the least psychopathology. Since CD has been previously reported to be associated with low SES (Robins, 1966; Stewart et al., 1981), the relationship between CD in the children and antisocial behavior in the parents may be affected by SES.

The high rate (33%) of major affective disorder in ADD probands and their relatives in Biederman's studies (1991b, p. 635) raises the question of whether those major depressions in probands and relatives are all alike or can be distinguished as melancholic or endogenomorphic depressions (in ICD-10, identified by biological concomitants such as a failure to suppress on the dexamethasone suppression test and tricyclic antidepressant responsivity) rather than reactive, depression spectrum "neurotic" or "atypical" depressions (hyperphagic, hypersomnic, lethargic and, perhaps, rejection sensitive).

What can be inferred from the family studies reviewed? First, there is an increased frequency of ADHD and ASPD characteristics among the relatives of "hyperactive" children. Second, when the probands are separated into those with "pure" ADHD and those with ADHD and CD, the study results differ, but there clearly is an increase of ASPD and related syndromes among the biological relatives of ADHD/CD probands and a suggested increase of such disorders among the biological relatives of "pure ADHD" probands. Thus, these family studies give evidence for the familial transmission of ADHD and provide some additional information regarding the relationship between Conduct Disorder and ADHD. ADHD and CD can be separated, but CD occurs with a much greater than chance association with ADHD. Abikoff (1987) reports that 89 percent of the CD children they studied were currently comorbid for ADHD and that most of the remaining 11 percent had ADHD in the past. Some "hyperactive" children develop CD as they become older (Mannuzza and Klein, 1993, as seen in the longitudinal follow-up studies). These findings may be only a result of the diagnostic techniques employed: it may have been ADHD children with CD attributes that were not above diagnostic thresholds who subsequently developed CD. Goodman and Stevenson (1989a, 1989b), whose twin study will be discussed below, found that comorbidity for CD was a function of the severity of "hyperactivity"; they found that 96 percent of children with pervasive hyperactivity (at home and school) were conduct disordered. Obviously, the overlap between ADHD and CD cannot be ignored.

Family studies cannot determine the contributions of genetic and nongenetic (usually assumed to be psychological) factors in the production of a psychiatric disease. Psychological abnormalities in the parents of ADHD children could be either an indication of the same disorder in them, which they have transmitted genetically to their children, or a possible source of deviant childrearing techniques, which led to the psychological development of ADHD in their children. Abnormalities in ADHD children's siblings may likewise be either a manifestation of the putative genetic abnormalities that they share with the proband or a reflection of their similar exposure to abnormal parenting.

Psychopathology might be psychologically transmitted by a variety of mechanisms, including identification with deviant parents; reaction to neglect, or physical or sexual abuse; "training" in a haphazard manner, with inconsistent reinforcement; or the systematic reinforcement of deviant behaviors, attitudes, and values.

One issue that the family and twin studies do not address because they employ categorical diagnoses rather than dimensional ratings is the frequency of mild, subsyndromal ADHD in the relatives of probands. As I mentioned in discussing prevalence, studies of schizophrenia and affective disorders have found it useful to examine less severe forms of these disorders (Kety et al., 1968, 1975), a "schizophrenic spectrum" and an "affective spectrum." Such examinations are based on the hypothesis that the major disorders occur along a continuum of severity and that there is an increased frequency of milder manifestations in the relatives of individuals with clear-cut instances of the disorder in question. Since the diagnoses of ADHD and Conduct Disorder are really quantitative (based on a certain number of symptoms above some threshold), it would be useful to investigate less severe forms of these psychopathologies in the close relatives of ADHD and CD probands. Appendix F illustrates the kinds of ADHD symptoms that occur in families of representative ADHD patients.

TWIN STUDIES

The strategy of studying monozygotic (MZ) and dizygotic (DZ) twins is based on both fact and hypothesis: the fact is that MZ twins are genetically identical and that DZ twins, on the average, share only half their genetic constitution; the hypothesis is that MZ and DZ twins share exactly the same psychological environment. Accordingly, it is reasoned that the increased "concordance" (the fraction of pairs in which both have the attribute—here psychiatric disorder) in MZ versus DZ twin pairs is due solely to genetic factors. Another issue is the rate of the disorder in question in twin populations compared to the non-twin general population. The rates seem to be the same for hyperactivity (see Goodman and Stevenson, 1989a), so that the disorder is not affected by biological factors associated with twins.

Appropriately designed twin studies require all the features discussed in the family studies. In addition, they require a systematically acquired sample. A clinical sample will not do, because in the study of any condition, unusual instances (such as concordant MZ twins) are more likely to receive clinical attention; there is the hazard that the sample will be biased in the direction of concordant pairs referred by clinicians struck by such concordance. Appropriate populations should be obtained from population registers or, in the case of children, from a complete survey of twins in a school system (although this, too, can be slightly biased through exclusion of severely disturbed children in institutions). Another, absolutely critical feature of twin studies is the precise determination of zygosity. Differentiation between monozygotic and dizygotic twins is the crux of the method. Earlier studies were based on such measures as appearance, fingerprints, and multiple blood types in each member of the twin pair. The current approach is to use DNA typing.

Lopez (1965) reported on MZ and DZ twins that were nonsystematically obtained from a variety of clinical sources and found that all of the four MZ sets and only one of the six sets of DZ twins were concordant for "hyperactivity." The MZ twins were all male, while two-thirds of the DZ twins were female. Since girls are less likely than boys to have ADHD, the sex differences of the MZ and DZ sets, along with the nonsystematic sample, make interpretation impossible.

Willerman (1973) investigated 93 pairs of twins obtained through a mothers' organization and evaluated activity level rated by the mothers on a behavior questionnaire used at that time. The author then used differences in scores between twin pairs (intraclass correlation) to determine the "heritability" of activity level, which was loosely defined as identifying hyperactivity. The heritability is the degree to which a trait, attribute, or disorder is due to genetic factors or the degree to which a phenotype is "caused" by a genotype. Willerman found a high heritability for *activity level*. Since this study evaluated motor activity alone in an ostensibly normal population of children, no inferences can be drawn about the genetics of the "hyperactivity" disorder. Similar twin studies that found genetic contributions to normal activity levels were also done by Scarr (1966) and Vandenberg et al. (1986).

Because Learning Disorders occur with increased frequency among ADHD children (see Semrud-Clikeman et al., 1992, for a review of the literature), the possibility of a shared genetic etiology for the two disorders is of interest. Gilger et al. (1992) used a twin study to investigate the etiology of that comorbidity and found data suggesting that reading disabilities and ADHD may be primarily genetically independent. However, trends and subtype analyses suggest that a genetically mediated comorbid subtype may exist. Here, as in other instances of comorbidity, it is difficult to separate disparate disorders from disorders that may be manifestations of a common cause or a causal relationship (Kendall and Clarkin, 1992; Clarkin and Kendall, 1992).

Goodman and Stevenson (1989a) investigated a sample of 13-year-old twins obtained from a birth register and school rolls. Of a potential sample of 374 pairs of twins, 285 pairs participated. Zygosity was evaluated with hierarchical measures, employing blood group typing in ambiguous instances. The hyperactivity measures that were employed included behavior questionnaires administered to parents and teachers as well as IQ and performance tests. The dependent variables studied were the *heritability* of inattentiveness and hyperactivity scores and diagnostic concordance in MZ and DZ pairs. The authors also analyzed *heritability* for those same-sex twin pairs in which at least one twin was hyperactive at home, at school, or in both settings—that is, "pervasive."

The pairwise concordance for the broad category of hyperactivity (including all three types) was 51 percent for MZ twins and 33 percent for same-sex DZ twins, with a ratio of MZ/DZ of 1.5. The derived heritability for broadly defined hyperactivity was 64 percent. Family factors such as marital discord, low parental warmth, or high parental malaise accounted for less than 10 percent of the variance. In a subsequent refinement of the data the authors found that pervasive hyperactivity was generally associated with high antisocial scores (1989b, p. 687).

A problem in this study is the recurrent issue of cooperation—for example, only 67 percent of the parents in one of the two original sources for the sample were willing to participate. Lack of cooperation may be associated with greater psychopathology in parents (and therefore in their children), and the sample will be biased toward less severely disturbed children. The second point that should be emphasized is that the variance not associated with genetic factors, the "heritability," is technically the "residual squares"—that is, that which is not genetic—but this need not necessarily be psychosocial. Monozygotic twins are not 100 percent concordant for a number of medical conditions. Many of these conditions show concordance rates in MZ twins similar to those found for psychiatric disorders, as seen in the examples in Table 4.1, some of which (e.g., TB) have clear-cut environ-

Table 4.1. Concordance for Various Medical Conditions in Monozygotic Twins

	Concordance (%)	
Condition	*MZ*	*DZ*
Diabetes mellitus	56	11
Atopic diseases	50	4
Hyperthyroidism	47	3
Psoriasis	61	13
Tuberculosis	52	22
Cholelithiasis	27	7
Mood disorders		
Bipolar	58	17
Unipolar	74	29

mental contributions (Vogel and Motulsky, 1986, p. 213; Tsuang and Faraone, 1990, p. 74).

The roles of "heredity" (nature) and "environment" (nurture) in the etiology of ADHD (as with other psychiatric disorders) cannot be determined by adding data from twin studies to the data from family studies. They can, however, be more conclusively separated by adoption studies, in which the parents providing the genetic constitution (the biological parents) and those who provide the psychological environment (the adoptive parents) are different people.

ADOPTION STUDIES

The most powerful clinical method for separating the effects of nature and nurture consists of adoption studies. Adoption constitutes a scientifically well-designed (but unintended) social experiment by which one can determine whether an individual adoptee's psychopathology is correlated with his nature or nurture: with his biological parents, who supplied his genes (and those of his siblings); or with his adopting parents, who provided him (and his siblings in his adoptive home) with his psychological environment. The adoption studies of "hyperactivity" and the CD-associated adult disorders, alcohol abuse and antisocial personality disorder, have employed the three strategies designed and carried out in the Danish adoption studies of schizophrenia: the family method (Kety et al., 1968, 1971, 1975); the adoptee and cross-fostering methods (Rosenthal et al., 1968, 1971; Wender et al., 1974; also used in the U.S. by Heston et al., 1966); and the adoptive parents method (Wender et al., 1968, 1971, 1976). These experimental designs will be discussed in context.

Critical features of the adoptive studies of ADHD are the following: (1) The specific diagnoses that were used to select the probands were "minimal brain dysfunction" or "hyperactivity" (with varying mixtures of ADHD and CD). Another aspect of diagnosis to watch for in the studies discussed below is the method by which diagnoses were made. When diagnoses of index and control cases are based on institutional records (hospital and legal) rather than interviews, there is a bias toward underdiagnosis. (2) In the case of the offspring from a psychiatrically disordered, *putative* biological father, verification of paternity is crucial. (3) The data are likely to be richer if an attempt (usually very difficult) was made to diagnose the biological parents of offspring given up for adoption using interviews rather than records. (4) Age at separation from the biological mother and time of transfer to the rearing home should be indicated. (Some children are placed in foster homes before their final transfer to the adopting home.) It is *possible* that disruption of early bonds may be pathogenic. (5) The fraction of identified subjects who participate should be indicated: as in all studies, the greater the better. Those lost to follow-up or unwilling to be interviewed are nonrandom and probably have greater psychopathology. (6) Adequate studies require a suitable comparison (control) group and examination of its members to ascertain that they are free of psychiatric disorder. (7) The results are more dependable if blind interviewing was employed—that is, the interviewer did not know if a given individual was the biological or adoptive relative of an index case or a control.

The first adoptive (actually foster) study was reported by Safer (1973), who used the family strategy. Safer investigated the psychological status of the full and maternal half-siblings of 17 MBD (19 full and 22 half) children, all of whom had been placed in different *foster* homes. The probands were a mixed group medically and psychiatrically: approximately one-half to one-third had abnormal EEGs, seizure disorders, or "gross motor incoordination"; one-fifth had congenital anomalies; and about 80 percent had "repeated childhood antisocial behavior" and were presumably conduct disordered. Diagnosis was made on the basis of chart review, coding the number and severity of symptoms and using a cutoff score. Approximately 50 percent of the full siblings versus about 10 percent of the half-siblings of the MBD probands were diagnosed as having "minimal brain dysfunction." This difference is statistically significant and consonant with the hypothesis of genetic transmission: If the disorder were transmitted as a simple dominant gene with full penetrance, one would expect one-half of the full siblings and one-quarter of the half-siblings to manifest the same illness.

There are several problems in interpreting the data: First, there was an increased frequency of biological abnormalities, low birth weight, seizures, and congenital anomalies in the full sibs, raising the possibility that the increased frequency of "minimal brain dysfunction" was being produced by biological but not genetic factors. As an answer to this first objection, when the biologically deviant children were deleted from the analysis, the differences between the full and half-sibs remained statistically significant. Second, the age of transfer to the foster parents was comparatively late, raising the possibility that the syndrome was the result of separation from the parents and that the observed concordance was produced by this shared psychological trauma. The half-sibs were transferred almost two years later than the full sibs.

This factor might be expected to increase their risk of MBD if MBD is produced or aggravated by late separation and so decrease the differences in concordance between the full and half-siblings. However, Heston et al. (1966) found no relationship between age of transfer to foster or adoptive home and psychopathology. David Rosenthal and I found a similar absence of a relationship between age of transfer and psychopathology in a group of Danish adoptees (unpublished). Finally, all of the children in this study were exposed to abnormal parenting, and such abnormal experience might be a *necessary* factor, even if not a *sufficient* one, to produce "MBD"—that is, the genetic disposition might be expressed only if such individuals were exposed to a psychologically pathological environment, a situation that here pertained to *all* of the children.

The next studies addressed the last problem by employing the "adoptive parent" strategy to separate the effects of "nature" and "nurture." In this technique, one compares parents who have adopted "hyperactive" children with biological parents who have raised their own "hyperactive" children (*not* the biological parents of the adoptees). One problem with the adoptive parents method is that the prospective adoptive parents have usually been screened by adoption agencies and excluded if they had significant psychopathology. In the first such study, Morrison and Stewart (1973) interviewed the adoptive parents of 35 "hyperactive" children and compared their rates of psychopathology with those of biological parents (again, who had raised their own children!) of 59 hyperactive children and those of the biological parents of 41 controls who had been admitted to the hospital for operations such as appendectomies and herniorrhaphies. They found a statistically significant, threefold increase in the frequency of alcoholism in the biological as compared to the adoptive parents (25% versus 8%) of hyperactive children, and a diagnosis of "sociopathy" or "hysteria" in 15 percent of the biological parents of hyperactive children but in none of the other parents.

In a similar study, Cantwell (1975) evaluated the adoptive parents of 39 "hyperactive" boys, the biological parents of 50 "hyperactive" children, and the parents of a group of 50 screened (and presumably normal) children. He found that 33 percent of the biological parents of hyperactive children received a diagnosis of alcoholism, "sociopathy" or "hysteria" versus 5 percent in the adoptive parents and about 10 percent in the controls. A history of childhood hyperactivity was twelve times as common in the first-degree and second-degree relatives of the index group as contrasted with the two comparison groups (12% versus 1%).

Cantwell's study replicated the findings of Morrison and Stewart (and, as will be discussed later, is subject to the same problems in interpretation).

Deutsch (1983) conducted an adoptive parents study of pure ADD, excluding children with ADD/CD. Subjects were 24 adopted children with ADD, 24 children with ADD living with their own biological parents and 24 normal control children. The diagnostic criteria were those of DSM-III. All the subjects were male and between the ages of 6 and 14. Psychiatric diagnoses were based on the "Hyperkinesis Index" from the Conners parent questionnaire and an infrequently used childhood depression rating scale. The parents rated themselves, the probands, and the probands' siblings on these scales, using adolescent norms for cutoffs. Using a Conners score in the 97th or higher percentile as diagnostic of ADD, 5 of the 24 biological fathers and 3 of the 24 biological mothers of ADD children were ADD, versus none of the adoptive parents of ADD children and none of the parents of normal children. The differences were statistically significant for the biological fathers ($p<.02$) or either parent ($p<.01$) but not for the biological mothers. A similar pattern emerged with the siblings of the ADD children raised by their biological parents: 7 of the 35 had ADD, versus none of the adoptive parents' biological children. This, too, was a significant difference ($p<.05$).

The adoptive parents method has also been used to study psychological test performance in the biological and adoptive parents of "hyperactive" children and the biological parents of "normal" children (Alberts-Corush et al., 1986). The findings are compatible with the genetic transmission of attentional problems as measured by these particular tests.

Two further adoption studies serendipitously found a relationship between parental psychopathology and "hyperactivity" in children. Both used the adoptee method. In this design one examines the psychiatric status of the "probands" (or "index cases") born to a biological parent with psychiatric syndrome "X" and adopted in infancy, and compares them with "controls," whose biological parents did not have syndrome "X" and who were likewise adopted in infancy. The controls are matched with the probands on relevant variables such as age, sex, social class, and the age at which they were transferred to their adopting parents.

Goodwin et al. (1973), focusing on alcoholism, conducted an adoptee study utilizing the NIMH Copenhagen adoption register and other records (Kety et al., 1968). They identified 55 male adoptees, each of whom had one biological parent (85 percent were fathers) with a history of hospitalization for alcoholism. The 55 adoptees were matched with a group of adoptees (N = 78) whose biological parents were considered non-alcoholic although they had not been *officially* screened by interview and found to be non-alcoholic. All the probands and matched controls were given blind interviews. An unexpected finding (1975) was that half of the men who were alcoholics (regardless of the alcoholism of their parents) versus about 15 percent of the non-alcoholics could be retrospectively diagnosed as "hyperactive." Similarly, 20–30 percent of the alcoholics versus 2–4 percent of the non-alcoholics were diagnosed as having often been truant or "antisocial" or "often disobedient" in childhood. In other words, Goodwin et al. obtained a history of ADD/CD-type behavior that was associated with current alcoholism—that is, the relationship was with the phenotype (being an alcoholic) and *not* with the genotype (being the son of an alcoholic). Goodwin et al. (1977a) also studied the adopted and non-adopted daughters of the same sample of alcoholic biological parents and a matched control group, adopted women of non-alcoholic parentage. Only one difference in childhood psychopathology emerged between the groups: women who had been raised by their alcoholic parents were two to three times as likely to describe themselves as having had few friends or having been shy. There were no differences between the adopted and non-adopted daughters in hyperactivity, school performance or truancy. However, the adopted-away daughters of the alcoholics did significantly less well in school than the daughters of the controls, a characteristic associated with ADD.

The second adoptee study relevant to hyperactivity was performed by Cunningham and Cadoret and their colleagues (Cunningham et al., 1975; Cadoret et al., 1975) in the United States. Employing adoption agency records, they located 88 adoptees who were 18 years old or older and whose biological parents had a psychiatric disorder, and 87 matched adopted controls whose biological parents were not *recorded* as having a psychiatric diagnosis (i.e., they were not screened with a psychiatric interview). About two-thirds of each group (59 index and 55 control adoptees) were willing to participate and were interviewed. Antisocial behavior items were significantly more common in the index cases than in the controls, while the difference in "hyperactive" behavioral items approached but did not reach a conventional level of statistical significance ($p < .08$). When the offspring whose biological parents were antisocial were compared with controls, there was a significant increase in the number of "hyperactive symptoms" in the index group. In a later report, Cadoret and Gath (1980) presented data on a larger sample of 143 index cases and 103 controls, which represented about two-thirds of the potential subjects. In this sample they found the diagnosis of "hyperactivity" to be two times as common among the offspring of antisocial biological parents as among those of the controls (which was not statistically significant) and five times as common among the offspring of alcoholic parents as among those of the controls (which was statistically significant).

Specific problems of these adoption studies include: (1) About one-third of the potential subjects refused to participate or could not be located. (2) The diagnosis employed was of "hyperactivity," so there is the familiar ADD/CD diagnostic problem of how the subjects would be diagnosed currently. (3) In some of them (e.g., Morrison and Stewart, 1973; Cantwell, 1975) the interviewers were not blind to the status of the relatives (that is, whether they were index or control cases) they were interviewing.

Another interesting finding related to adoption that suggests the action of genetic factors is the increased prevalence of adoptees in children referred for psychiatric treatment, which was reported by Schecter et al. thirty years ago (1964). A related phenomenon has been investigated systematically by Deutsch et al. (1982). They found that the rate of adoption among ADD patients in the clinical population was *8 to 16 times the prevalence of adopted children in the population at large* and the prevalence of adopted children with medical disorders. The rate of ADHD in adoptees is probably higher than that in nonadoptees. There are a number of possible explanations.

First, adoptive parents may have a lower threshold for seeking help than demographically similar biological parents of children. To investigate this possibility, Deutsch, Swanson and Leech (in preparation) solicited parents' questionnaire ratings on a total sample of adoptees (50% of whose parents complied). The adoptees were then compared with the biological children of the adopting parents in terms of categorical diagnoses of ADD made with varying criteria: for lax criteria, the proportions were 35 percent for the adoptees, 17 percent for their siblings who were the biological children of the adopting parents; for moderate criteria the rates were 11 percent versus 3 percent. Thus the high rate of adoption among ADD patients is not explicable by a systematic sampling bias. Another possible explanation is that the biological parents of children placed for adoption might have an increased frequency of genetically transmitted ADHD (see above).

In addition, mothers whose children are placed for adoption might receive inadequate antenatal care or might consume more substances noxious to fetuses than mothers not placing their children for adoption. Horn et al. (1975) examined the Minnesota Multiphasic Personality Inventory (MMPI) scores in 363 women admitted to homes for unwed mothers, a control sample of 28 married pregnant women, and over 2,000 twelfth-grade girls. The most marked differences were on the psychopathic deviation (Pd) scale: the mean scale score of the unwed mothers was higher than that of 84 percent of the controls, and about 18 percent of the unwed mothers had scores 2 standard deviations above that of the comparison group (i.e., in the upper 2.3 percent of the population). We do not know the diagnostic breakdown of the adopted-away offspring of mothers with high psychopathic deviation scores on the MMPI, but they are probably at increased risk of "hyperactivity." To the extent that there is an association between the Pd scores and ASPD, the mothers would probably be at increased risk for substance abuse during pregnancy. Furthermore, if there is assortative mating, their mates might have an increased frequency of "antisocial" traits. Finally, as mentioned earlier, psychological variables associated with placement for adoption—such as separation from the mother in a critical period—*might* increase the risk of ADHD (but we have no data to support psychological etiologic factors).

CONCLUSIONS BASED ON GENETIC STUDIES

What have these adoption studies added to the data on ADHD from the family and twin studies? First, they have provided more solid data showing that "hyperactivity" (broadly defined) has genetic contributions. Second, the adoptive parents studies have shown that psychopathology in the rearing parents does not necessarily accompany the development of ADHD. Third, they have shown that some psychiatric disorders associated with conduct disorder—"alcoholism," Antisocial Personality Disorder ("psychopathy," "sociopathy"), somatization disorder ("Briquet's syndrome," "hysteria")—are associated with hyperactivity and are also genetically transmitted.

A very interesting feature of this clustering of psychopathology is that a large number of studies from the Washington University group in St. Louis (Perley and Guze, 1962; Arkonac and Guze, 1963; Guze et al., 1969, 1971; Cloninger and Guze, 1970, 1973; Guze and Goodwin, 1972; Cloninger et al., 1975) have shown that alcoholism, sociopathy, and Briquet's syndrome—the "St. Louis triad"—not only run in families but also cluster in families. The close relatives of a person with one of these disorders are not only more likely than controls to have that disorder but are also more likely to have one of the other two disorders. Thus, the brothers and fathers of "hysterics" are at increased risk for alcoholism and antisocial personality; the sisters and mothers of male felons have an increased frequency of "hysteria"; females with anti-social personality have an increased frequency of hysteria in their mothers and sisters; male sociopaths have an increased frequency of sociopathy and alcoholism in their brothers and fathers. Some support for this picture occurs in Swedish reports (Bohman et al., 1984; Cloninger et al., 1984; Sigvardsson et al., 1984).

Parenthetically, some adoption studies of criminality, which is related to but not the same as Antisocial Personality Disorder, have also shown a genetic component (Crowe, 1972, 1974; Hutchings and Mednick, 1975). However, rearing does play a role in criminality (Hutchings and Mednick, 1975), and in the Swedish studies criminality does not show a genetic factor unless linked with alcoholism (Bohman, 1978; Bohman et al., 1982; Cloninger et al., 1982).

I have mentioned other data on alcoholism in reporting on the adoption studies, but the Swedish work mentioned above, which was a major adoption study of alcohol abuse (Bohman et al., 1981; Cloninger et al., 1981), deserves closer attention. Examining the influence of sex, three levels of severity of alcohol abuse, and postnatal environmental factors, the investigators obtained different results for men and women. Alcohol abuse in men could be broken down into two syndromes: Type I, "milieu limited," occurring in 13 percent of adoptive men, was usually mild, and required no treatment. Both genetic predisposition and postnatal factors (e.g., lower social class) were necessary for its development. Type II, "male-limited," occurring in 4 percent of adoptive men, was of moderate to marked severity, occurred only with a strong genetic disposition, and was unaffected by postnatal experience. Alcohol abuse in adopted women followed a complex genetic pattern, but the daughters of alcoholic women were at greater risk for alcoholism than the daughters of alcoholic men.

Other research that has contributed to the data on the relationships between ADHD and alcoholism or substance abuse includes the following: DeObaldia et al. (1983, 1984) found a significant association between primary alcoholism and scores on Tarter's minimal brain dysfunction questionnaire. Eyre et al. (1982) found that 22 percent of 157 patients (male, 76%; female, 24%) applying for treatment at a drug treatment unit could be diagnosed as having childhood hyperactivity.

In Rounsaville's (1991) evaluation of comorbidity in a sample of co-caine abusers seeking inpatient ($N = 149$) or outpatient ($N = 149$) treat-ment, none of the patients were diagnosed with current ADD, but 35 percent had a history of childhood ADD. Conduct Disorder was not assessed.

An examination of the similar symptomatic overlap that occurs with the schizophrenias and the affective disorders is of interest and may provide us with plausible hypotheses. The schizophrenias and affective disorders are generally considered distinct syndromes that in some instances overlap. Schizophrenics have an increased frequency of bipo-lar affective disorder in their relatives (Cloninger, 1985). A frequency plot of the specific symptoms of schizophrenia and the affective disor-ders should show a bimodal distribution, but Crow (1986) found that when cases were scored on the sums of the most characteristic features of schizophrenia and affective disorders, a unimodal rather than a bi-modal distribution resulted. As Crow observes, "such findings cast doubt on the common clinical assumption that most cases of psychosis can be relatively easily classified as either affective or schizophrenic" (p. 420). What about etiology? Do schizophrenia and the affective disor-ders "breed true"? The question is obviously rhetorical. Crow cites a number of earlier studies which found that parents with affective disor-ders have children with an increased (and expected) frequency of simi-lar affective disorders but also with an increased frequency of schizo-phrenic disorders. The same is true, to a lesser degree, among the offspring of schizophrenic parents, who show not only an (expected) increased risk for schizophrenia but may also show an increase of affec-tive disorders as well.

What about the frequency distribution of ADHD and CD symp-toms? In Chapter 3 on prevalence and in some of the studies here, I have discussed the high co-occurrence of these disorders (e.g., Good-man and Stevenson, 1989b). Many clinicians feel that although ADHD without CD is relatively common, pure CD without ADHD is uncom-mon. The genetic studies of ADHD that have been reviewed suggest that ADHD and CD may likewise not "breed true." What we need to examine is the frequency of ADHD and CD in the offspring of adults with a history of CD (with and without current ASPD) but without a history of ADHD, and of adults with ADHD but without a history of ODD or CD. There are no definitive studies. To answer the question with clinical methods would require a study of the type of psycho-pathology found in the adopted-away offspring of pure groups of ADHD and ASPD biological parents; such a study has not been performed. The analogy with schizophrenias and affective disorders is suggestive but of course insufficient. The analogy does illustrate that the overlap (continuum) problem exists with disorders (dementia praecox and manic-depressive psychosis) whose symptoms and natural history have been extensively studied for nearly a century, whose family patterns of transmission have been studied for nearly 70 years, and whose response to somatic treatments has been studied for over 50 years.

The slow progress of these studies in resolving the etiological problems of the functional psychoses warns us of the difficulty of the task of unraveling the etiological mysteries of ADHD. The difficulty is further compounded by the incomplete definitions of some of the overlapping symptoms. For example, with reference to CD and ASPD, in the past "psychopathy" and "sociopathy" were terms often used in a pejorative sense rather than as crisp diagnostic designations. The criteria for ASPD are now behavioral and clearly increase reliability. The symptoms of CD and ASPD are weighted toward behavioral *signs* of criminal behavior, and the behavioral criteria may miss the essential characteristics of the psychopath who is not grossly antisocial—the character type, in the extreme, described by Cleckley (1976). Cleckley's characteristics include unreliability, untruthfulness, lack of remorse (a weak superego), poor judgment, failure to learn by experience, egocentricity, absence of insight, and absence of a life plan.

In particular, the white-collar psychopath may have the personality characteristics of psychopathy without having committed the diagnostically necessary transgressions of DSM-III-R or DSM-IV. A Danish adoption study of psychopathy that used a definition similar to Cleckley's yielded results consistent with genetic transmission (Schulsinger, 1972). It would be useful to see if the relatives of ADHD probands have an increased frequency of the characteristics of Cleckley's psychopathic personality, without meeting the criteria of ASPD. Similarly, Tarter's study (1977) and the Swedish studies (Bohman et al., 1981; Cloninger et al., 1981) suggest the existence of at least two forms of alcohol abuse.

What the studies have clearly shown is, first, that there are major genetic contributions to ADHD: the concordance of ADHD in MZ twins is as high as that of several purely biological conditions; and second, that there appears to be little environmental contribution to ADHD, as shown by the finding that family factors account for only 10 percent of the variance. These findings have been confirmed by the adoption studies.

Despite their helpfulness, the adoption studies have not solved the pressing problem of separating the ADHD/CD spectrum disorders (formerly called "minimal brain dysfunction") into homogeneous subgroups. The adoption method is clearly not the best way of resolving the diagnostic problems. In the next section we take a look at evolving scientific methodologies that may help us to make progress in these difficult areas.

BIOLOGICAL STUDIES OF ADHD

■

The existence of ADHD in adults has resolved one problem in studying the biology of ADHD. When one studies biological variables in children, it is doubtful that they can give truly informed consent for invasive studies (such as lumbar puncture) or for studies of experimental interest but of doubtful therapeutic benefit (such as the administration of pharmacological doses of amino acids). The existence of ADHD adults resolved these dilemmas and allowed us at last to conduct several categories of studies (described in this section) which had been indefinitely postponed.

The techniques available to measure the activity of specific neurotransmitter systems in the brain have been very limited. They include (1) the measurement of transmitter metabolites in the cerebrospinal fluid, blood, and urine; (2) the psychological and physiological response to precursors of putative neurotransmitters and the administration of drugs that block the receptors of putative neurotransmitters; (3) the psychological and physiological response to drugs with ostensibly specific mechanisms of action—for example, MAO-B inhibitors; and (4) brain imaging techniques such as positron emission tomography (PET). With these techniques, at present we are testing only a minute segment of possibly relevant biological functioning.

From a methodological point of view additional complications are that reliabilities of measurement over time are not usually available, and low sample sizes limit the power of the statistical tests. That is, the risk of a Type II error—missing a biological difference that does exist— is high. Thus, one can anticipate a failure to detect real differences in specific subgroups. Furthermore, in evaluating biological correlates by nonbrain techniques—for example, by examining the blood or blood cells—one must keep in mind that the human genome contains fifty to one hundred thousand genes, half of which may be expressed only in the brain. This means that for biological abnormalities that may be expressed only in the brain, no specific abnormalities may be detected in the periphery (for example, in plasma levels of particular substances). Of the current methods, molecular genetic techniques appear to offer the best possible way around this problem. The entire genome (the total genetic information of the DNA of the organism) can be obtained from peripheral sources—for example, white cells—which will allow evaluation of those twenty-five to fifty thousand genes that are expressed only in the brain.

STUDIES OF AMINE METABOLITES IN CEREBROSPINAL FLUID

The results of a plethora of studies of the metabolites in urine and blood of ADHD children have been inconclusive, so researchers have turned to a direct method for assessing the activity of biogenic amines in the brain—measuring the concentration of their metabolites in cerebrospinal fluid (CSF). This approach has been based on the hypothesis (and hope) that such levels will reflect the activity of amine *systems* in the brain. Critical issues include (1) determining the relative amounts of these metabolites that are removed from the brain and transferred into the bloodstream versus those transferred to the cerebrospinal fluid;[3] (2) determining the source of the metabolite in question. Whereas 5-hydroxyindolecetic acid is derived from the spinal cord and brain, lumbar homovanillic acid (HVA) is believed to largely reflect brain dopamine turnover (Post and Goodwin, 1978). There are two tacit assumptions as well: First, that level reflects turnover; and second, that turnover is a measure of neuronal activity. One might also assume that high levels—already assumed to be manifestations of high turnover—are compensatory attempts to increase the activity of a downregulated or underactive system. The relationship between pathological functioning and low values or the absence of HVA in the CSF was discovered in a series of studies of Parkinson's syndrome (Hornykiewicz, 1973). There are some data suggesting that decreased central dopaminergic activity is associated with an ADD-like syndrome that responds to dopaminergic agents (Wender, 1978). I comment later on the contradictory nature of some of these data in comparison with data from other sources.

There have been two studies of biogenic amine metabolites in the CSF of children. Shetty and Chase (1976) investigated the levels of

HVA in the CSF of 23 "hyperkinetic" children and 6 controls. Baseline CSF HVA did not differ between the two groups. Ten of the hyperkinetic subjects were treated with D-amphetamine and 5 with placebo, and a second sample of CSF was obtained and analyzed. The authors found a strikingly high correlation between the degree of clinical improvement and the degree of HVA reduction in cerebrospinal fluid ($r=.91$, $p<.001$) with those receiving D-amphetamine but not those receiving placebo. However, despite random selection, the initial values of HVA happened to be twice as great in the 10 patients treated with D-amphetamine as in the placebo subgroup. A more conservative analysis would have employed an analysis of covariance since the greater decreases in the treated group might be an artifact of the initial difference.

Shaywitz et al. (1977) investigated monoamine metabolites in spinal fluid in 26 controls and 6 children with "minimal brain dysfunction" (MBD). The children had been pretreated with probenecid, which interferes with the active transport of acid metabolites and thereby increases their level within the spinal fluid.[4] The initial finding was that there were no differences in the concentration of HVA in the two groups. However, the children with MBD had higher values of probenecid than did the controls and it is possible to argue that this increased level spuriously increased the levels of HVA in the "MBD" children. When levels were calculated on the basis of concentrations of probenecid (i.e., the concentration of HVA divided by the concentration of probenecid), the children with MBD had decreased HVA as compared to controls ($p<.05$). Unfortunately, HVA levels in normal and "MBD" patients off and on probenecid have not been studied so that the procedure of dividing by probenecid levels cannot be justified.

There has been one study of CSF in adults with ADHD. Reimherr et al. (1984) examined biogenic amine metabolites in 15 adults meeting the Utah Criteria for DSM-III ADD with hyperactivity and 13 age- and sex-matched controls. An additional 21 controls were obtained from the National Institute of Mental Health. Following a brief hospitalization for the lumbar puncture, all subjects were entered in a double-blind random assignment crossover trial of methylphenidate and placebo. Eleven subjects experienced moderate-to-marked improvement and 4 subjects did not improve or had an accentuation of their symptoms. The levels of homovanillic acid (HVA) and 5-HIAA (5-hydroxy-indolectic acid) prior to drug treatment are shown in Table 4.2.

Responders had significantly lower levels of HVA than nonresponders and a trend for lower HVA than controls; nonresponders had

Table 4.2. Mean Values for Responsive, Nonresponsive,
and Control Subjects

Subjects	n	(HVA) (ng/ml)		(5-HIAA) (ng/ml)	
		Mean	SD	Mean	SD
Responders	11	31[a]	9	19[a]	9
Nonresponders	4	52[b]	10	36	12
Utah controls	13	37[c]	12	24[c]	14
NIMH controls	21	38	14	18[d]	5

Probabilities, one-tailed t-tests:

[a] Different from nonresponders, $p < .02$.

[b] Different from Utah controls, $p < .05$.

[c] Different from responders, $p < .10$.

[d] Different from Utah controls, $p < .10$.

significantly *higher* HVA than did the Utah controls. In the case of
5-HIAA, levels were significantly lower in responders than in nonresponders and there was a trend for responders to have lower levels than
the Utah controls. These findings are consistent with the hypothesis
that ADHD is associated with decreased dopaminergic function, but
they do not constitute robust support for it. The unexpected finding of
interest is that one subgroup of ADD patients—those whose symptoms
were unaffected or aggravated by methylphenidate—had *increased*
levels of HVA. This is consonant with two *mechanisms*: (1) that dopamine receptors are subsensitive and that, homeostatically, more dopamine is being produced; and (2) that excessively high dopamine produces an ADHD-like picture. The second instance might be
comparable to one in which normal individuals receive large doses of
stimulants and become agitated (hyperactive) and scattered (a short
attention span). Finally, the findings for a *trend* for HVA to be lower
in patients than controls could be a result of heterogeneity in the
syndrome; our sample is much too small to determine if there is an
underlying bimodal distribution with low HVA and normal HVA subjects.

Animal studies have also shown variations of amine metabolite
levels in responding and nonresponding "hyperactive" subgroups (Bareggi et al., 1979b; Ginsburg et al., 1984), suggesting a dopamine deficiency in responders. Both the human studies and the animal studies
point to possible explanations of variable responses to medication in
ADHD patients and in control subjects.

ADMINISTRATION OF AMINO ACIDS (PRECURSORS OF DOPAMINE) IN THE TREATMENT OF ADHD

Another test of the hypothesis that activity of dopaminergic function-ing is reduced in ADHD patients is the administration of pharma-cological doses of the amino acids that are the precursors of dopamine. As seen in Figure 4.1, phenylalanine is hydroxylated to tyrosine, which in turn is hydroxylated to L-dopa. L-dopa is decarboxylated to form dopamine. By the principal of chemical equilibrium, increasing the amount (concentration) of a precursor compound should drive the reac-tion and increase the amount of the products. Wurtman et al. (1980) have reviewed the evidence which indicates that pharmacological doses of the appropriate dietary amino acid lead to increased brain levels of a specific neurotransmitter.

Based on these findings, our research group decided to give phar-macological doses of precursor amino acids in order to try to increase levels of monoamines in the brain. All subjects in these studies met the Utah Criteria for adult ADHD and were in the 95th percentile of "hy-peractivity" on the Parents' Rating Scale. Clinical status was measured by means of the Clinical Global Impression and the seven ADHD target symptoms.

The first precursor amino acid that was studied was L-dopa (Reim-herr et al., 1980; Wood et al., 1982), which is decarboxylated to dopa-mine. We expected a reaction in ADHD adults similar to that in pa-

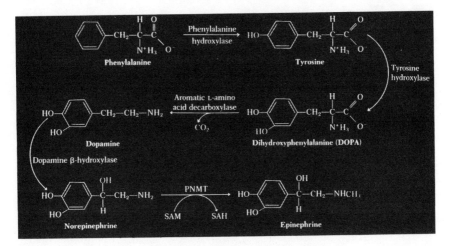

Figure 4.1 Biosynthesis of catecholamines.

tients with Parkinson's syndrome. In Parkinson's patients L-dopa is presumably taken up by dopamine-containing cells, decarboxylated to dopamine, and released by these dopaminergic cells. The design was open and L-dopa was administered with carbidopa.[5] Patients were begun on 100 milligrams of L-dopa and 10 milligrams of carbidopa per day in divided doses. Dosing was flexible: the dosage was to be gradually raised until substantial clinical improvement occurred or side effects prevented any further dosage increase; the maximum dose was to be 2000 milligrams per day of L-dopa. At the end of the first week of treatment, the physicians globally rated most of the patients as either moderately or slightly improved. At the end of the second week, the patients were rated as the same as before treatment, and all the patients experienced nausea. Interpretation of these results is complicated by the fact that L-dopa—a nonnaturally occurring amino acid—may be taken up by nondopaminergic neurons, where it may be converted to dopamine by ubiquitous decarboxylases and released when these nondopaminergic cells fire—that is, they act as "false" neurotransmitters and produce nonnaturally occurring effects. In particular, when levodopa is first administered, it seems to increase serotonergic activity by displacing serotonin. Later, it inhibits serotonergic activity, possibly by acting as a false transmitter in serotonergic systems (Bartholini et al., 1968; Barrett and Balch, 1971; Hutt et al., 1977; Nimitkitpaisan et al., 1977); this nonnatural effect may obscure the hypothesized increase in dopaminergic activity.

Because of L-dopa's possible function as a false neurotransmitter, we next elected to investigate the natural amino acid precursors of dopamine. We began with phenylalanine (Wood et al., 1985). The rationale for using phenylalanine is that the amino acid is not only the initial precursor of dopamine but is also the precursor of phenethylamine. Work by Borison et al. (1974, 1975) suggests that phenethylamine may be a neurotransmitter. Phenethylamine differs from amphetamine only in lacking the alpha-methyl group, which prevents oxidation of that molecule, and Borison's work also suggests that amphetamine may release phenethylamine. If underactivity of phenethylamine or dopamine does characterize ADHD, then dietary increases in phenylalanine would be expected to lead to increased functional amounts of phenethylamine and dopamine, producing amelioration or a reversal of the signs and symptoms of ADHD. The design was a random assignment, double-blind crossover with racemic phenylalanine and placebo. Dosing was flexible, beginning at 50 milligrams three times a day and rising to a maximum of 1,200 milligrams a day in three divided doses. The drug produced fatigue, and after the completion of the trial it was found that the average tolerated dose of phenylalanine was slightly less than 600 milligrams a day. There were statistically but not clinically significant improvements in mood and mood lability. All patients became tolerant to the therapeutic effects after two to three months on open trial.

The last amino acid trial was of L-tyrosine, the immediate amino acid precursor of dopamine (Reimherr et al., 1987). The admission criteria and outcome measures were the same as those in our previous study. The design was a single-blind, one-week placebo washout followed by an open trial of L-tyrosine, which was rapidly increased from 50 to 150 milligrams per kilogram per day in three divided doses. Fifteen subjects remained after the placebo washout; 12 completed the trial. Maximal clinical changes were seen at four weeks: marked improvement in 2 patients, moderate improvement in 6, slight or no improvement in 2, and slight worsening in 2. Medication was continued to eight weeks, at which time there was clinical regression to the pretreatment status. The condition of one subject was worsened after two weeks of treatment, and the amino acid was discontinued when he became progressively more angry and suspicious. His diagnosis was reconsidered and he was classified—after the fact—as having possible paranoid personality disorder. Although this study was not placebo-controlled, the effects of tyrosine should be compared to those of the other two amino acids, which seem to have behaved like placebos. Another finding that supports an active role for the tyrosine was that the substance was therapeutically effective only after two or more weeks. This delay is similar to that found by Gelenberg et al. (1980) in the tyrosine treatment of depression and to that encountered with the use of tricyclic antidepressants and monoamine oxidase inhibitors in the treatment of depression. The delay seen with antidepressants parallels the changes in receptor function and suggests that analogous changes may have to occur before L-tyrosine becomes therapeutically effective. In our previous studies of phenylalanine and L-dopa, the pharmacological response was immediate, so we did not predict a delay in L-tyrosine response, further decreasing the likelihood of a placebo response.

All the patients who responded to L-tyrosine became tolerant to its therapeutic effects. The clinical reports on the effects of L-tyrosine on depression (Gelenberg et al., 1980; Goldberg, 1980) do not discuss the length of time that the treatment remained effective nor whether tolerance developed. One incidental observation that suggests that do-paminergic activity may have increased was the development of para-noid ideation in the patient mentioned earlier; this is analogous to the effects produced by amphetamine in such patients. Arguing against the hypothesis that the action of L-tyrosine and of phenylalanine was medi-ated by increase in dopamine synthesis is the fact that tyrosine hydrox-ylase is the rate-limiting enzyme in the production of dopamine (at least in rats) and that increasing L-tyrosine or phenylalanine concentra-tions in the brain should not drive the reaction more rapidly.

From a practical standpoint, none of these amino acids appears to have any clinical utility in the treatment of the disorder.

THERAPEUTIC TRIALS OF MONOAMINE OXIDASE INHIBITORS

As a further test of the hypothesis that ADHD was associated with underactivity of dopaminergic or phenethylaminergic systems, we de-cided to conduct therapeutic trials with medication that would be ex-pected to increase phenethylaminergic and dopaminergic activity. One way of doing this is to decrease the catabolism of phenethylamine and dopamine. Both are broken down by monoamine oxidase (MAO). MAO occurs in at least two forms: MAO-A and MAO-B (Johnson, 1968). The preferred substrates for MAO-A are predominantly norepinephrine and serotonin, while those for MAO-B appear to be phenethylamine and dopamine (Murphy et al., 1976). If decreased synthesis or increased breakdown of dopamine or phenethylamine play a role in the genesis of ADHD, we would predict that an MAO-B inhibitor would be thera-peutically effective.

We tested two drugs that in small doses have been found to be rela-tively specific blockers of MAO-B, deprenyl and pargyline. (These studies are discussed in Chapter 6 on treatment.) The major point to make here is that pargyline was very effective—of practical relevance—and that it produced typical unpleasant MAO-inhibitor symptoms. Al-though L-deprenyl (now selegiline) produced moderate to marked bene-fit in 6 out of 11 patients, none opted to stay on the drug because of prominent side effects. This may very well have been a function of our unwitting overdosing: the average dose was 30 milligrams a day. The use of lower doses in children with Tourette's syndrome and ADHD has been reported by Jankovic (1993), who found that 5 to 15 milligrams a day controlled the ADHD symptoms and did not aggravate the patients' tics.

IMAGING

Both positron emission tomography (PET) and magnetic resonance imaging have been used to investigate ADHD etiology.

There have been two studies of cerebral glucose metabolism, as measured by the PET technique, in adults with a history of childhood and continuing Attention-deficit Hyperactivity Disorder. Zametkin et al. (1990) investigated glucose metabolism in 50 normal adults and 25 "hyperactive" adults. Their principal finding was that total cerebral glucose metabolism was 8 percent lower in the ADHD adults than in the normal comparison group: among the men metabolism was 6 percent lower in the ADHD patients; in the women it was 13 percent lower. The difference between the sexes is not statistically significant, but the fact that the percent of lowered metabolism was twice as great in women—the sex less frequently afflicted—is of interest. A comparison of sixty regions showed no significant difference, but this may have been due to the large number of statistical comparisons. Matochik et al. (1993) examined the effects of methylphenidate and D-amphetamine on cerebral glucose metabolism in 27 adults with "hyperactivity." The effects on glucose metabolism were complex and differed for the two drug conditions. Amphetamine produced no consistent change in glucose metabolism. Methylphenidate increased glucose metabolism in some areas and decreased it in others. In addition, the increases and decreases produced were not the same for the two stimulants.

Giedd et al. (1994) used the technique of magnetic resonance imaging to examine the areas of a midsagittal cross section of the corpus callosum in samples of ADHD and normal boys. They found that two anterior regions, the rostrum and rostral body, were significantly smaller in ADHD children. The authors interpret this finding as supporting the hypothesis that there are abnormal frontal lobe development and functioning in ADHD.

These studies represent only a beginning. Imaging techniques are expanding rapidly, and it is hoped that they will allow more direct measures (e.g., receptor number) of more direct neurophysiological relevance.

I comment on the implications of these four types of biological studies in the next section.

THE ADHD RESEARCH HORIZON

■

In examining possible directions for future research in ADHD, I first recapitulate the hypotheses that have been advanced about the genetic and biochemical transmission of the syndrome, and then look at promising new investigative techniques.

THE TRANSMISSION OF ADHD: FRAGMENTARY DATA

Despite indications of a genetic component in ADHD, the mechanism of genetic transmission of ADHD is unknown. Morrison and Stewart (1974) first proposed that the mechanism of transmission is polygenic, calling attention to the fact that in their sample relatives with hyperactivity and allied conditions were found on both sides of the family (although this could also be a result of assortative mating—like with like—for example, alcoholic with alcoholic). Another possibility is that ADHD is polygenetic and that girls require a greater "load" to be above the threshold for expressing ADHD (Omenn, 1973). If so, there should be a higher prevalence of ADHD among the relatives of ADHD girls than among those of ADHD boys. However, the evidence for this possibility is mixed. Kashani et al. (1979) and Pauls et al. (1983) found such a higher prevalence; Mannuzza and Gittelman (1984) found an insignificant trend, but their sample was small. Biederman et al. (1990) did not find a higher prevalence of ADHD among relatives of ADHD girls. Faraone et al. (1992) report that, taken together, family studies do not find a greater prevalence of ADHD in the relatives of ADHD girls versus ADHD boys; they argue that girls do not have a higher threshold for expressing ADHD and that ADHD may be transmitted as a single major gene. With a single gene the sex difference could result from the interaction of genetic and other biological factors, as in baldness. In baldness the autosomal (non-sex) gene takes effect only with the secretion of androgens, as at puberty in a normal male.

One nonadoption study that deals with the genetic transmission of alcohol suggests another genetic possibility for ADHD, since alcoholism in fathers seems associated with "hyperactivity" in sons. Kaij and Dock (1975) investigated the prevalence of alcoholism in the grandsons of alcoholics. The sample consisted of 136 sons of the sons of alcoholics and 134 sons of the daughters of alcoholics. The authors do not report the comparative risks for alcoholism in the sons and daughters of the alcoholic grandfathers, but we can assume the frequency was considerably higher in the sons. The finding of theoretical interest was that the risk of alcoholism in the sons of the sons and the sons of the daughters was approximately the same, 21 percent and 18 percent respectively. If women can transmit but not manifest alcoholism, perhaps they can transmit but not manifest ADHD. Similarly designed research focusing on the inheritance of ADHD would be worthwhile.

Regardless of the mechanism of genetic transmission in ADHD, current thought favors the idea that genetic abnormality alters catecholaminergic functioning. My own hypotheses have focused on dopamine depletion. However, many of the neurochemical hypotheses that have been advanced to explain the etiology of psychiatric disorders are simplistic, and my dopaminergic and related hypotheses (Wender, 1972; Wood et al., 1982, 1983, 1985; Wender et al., 1983; Reimherr et al., 1987) are no exceptions.

For example, neuroscientists have currently identified five different dopaminergic receptors, and more may be forthcoming (Waddington and O'Boyle, 1989; Strange, 1993). Earlier studies of the D_1 and D_2 receptors found qualitatively different effects in response (increased activity versus sedation) to dose and type of dopamine agonist (Carnoy et al., 1986). Creese (1987) found that low doses of dopamine agonists (apomorphine) and another direct agonist (3-PPP, a putative dopaminergic autoreceptor agonist) decreased response to rewarding stimuli, while larger doses increased motor activity. These observations have been interpreted to suggest that with low doses the agonists bind with the autoreceptors on the presynaptic cell and decrease the rate of dopamine release, producing sedation. Higher levels are presumed to induce the presynaptic cell to release greater amounts of dopamine, with a resultant increase in motor activity. Thus, if there is a relationship between dopamine depletion and ADHD, it is a highly complex one.

Even *if* underactivity of a particular (e.g., dopaminergic) system is demonstrated, one cannot infer that such underactivity is *the* primary "lesion." The neuronal systems that modulate the dopaminergic system may either fail to stimulate its activity or inhibit such activity. An analogy would be fluid retention in heart failure, which is a common secondary phenomenon, a result of decreased cardiac output. The fact that the administration of diuretics reduces fluid retention and improves symptomatic functioning does not demonstrate that fluid retention is the fundamental abnormality in "congestive heart failure." We now know that fluid retention is the product of the primary underlying abnormality, which is death of myocardial tissue and decreased cardiac output.

If one posits that catecholaminergic systems have decreased activity in ADHD, the related questions become: What does this predict with regard to levels of metabolites of catecholamines, and where will these be found? For example, is decreased dopaminergic activity accompanied by high or low levels of dopamine's principal metabolite, homovanillic acid (HVA)? If the receptors are too insensitive, one might anticipate the homeostatic response of increased dopamine production and *increased* levels of HVA. But on the other hand, receptors might be supersensitive in response to decreased levels of dopamine release, which would predict decreased HVA in metabolites (in blood, urine, cerebrospinal fluid, etc.). Such possibilities make the interpretation of the metabolite studies difficult.

The possibility that noradrenergic activity also plays an etiological role in ADHD has been raised by Zametkin and Rapoport (1987), who state that stimulant drugs have major central noradrenergic as well as dopaminergic effects. The occasional successful use of tricyclic antidepressants as a combination treatment for ADHD supports this hypothesis (Ratey et al., 1991), but reports that beta-adrenergic blockers augment the response to stimulant drugs argue against it (Mattes, 1986).

Another reason that a unitary neurochemical hypothesis seems unlikely is that biological systems, including homeostatic processes, are very complex. Those of us proposing explanatory hypotheses for the presence of ADHD sometimes seem to have suppressed our knowledge of physiology. Are homeostatic neurological systems—for example, those modulating concentration, motor activity, affective lability and all the rest—less complex than the homeostatic mechanisms controlling coagulation of the blood? As a reminder, the clotting of blood is produced when thrombin catalyzes the formation of fibrin (insoluble) from fibrinogen (soluble) as the final phase of a complex cascade in which more than a dozen proteins interact (see Figure 4.2; O'Reilly, 1987). Evolution has "produced" a system which keeps blood liquid "when it should be," on the one hand avoiding exsanguination with a shaving cut, and on the other preventing thrombosis of the entire vascular tree when we sustain a bruise.

Do we suspect that the mechanisms that oversee the sensitivity and

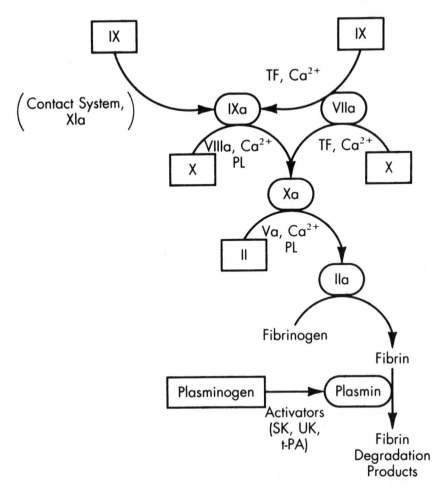

Figure 4.2 Major reactions of blood coagulation and fibrinolysis. Boxes enclose the coagulation factor zymogens and the ovals the active proteases. PL = platelets or phospholipids; TF = tissue factor; Va = activated factor V; VIIIa = activated factor VIII; SK = streptokinase; UK = urokinase; t-PA = tissue plasminogen activator. Majerus, P. W., Broze, G. J., Miletich, J. P., and Tollefsen, D. M. (1990). In A. G. Goodman, T. W. Rall, A. S. Nies, and P. Taylor, (Eds.), *Goodman and Gilman's the pharmacological basis of therapeutics. (eighth edition)*. New York: Pergamon Press.

reactivity of the brain are less complex? We would hope that the signs and symptoms of ADHD are produced by one mutation in one biochemical pathway. But it is prudent to consider how carefully important physiological processes are regulated by checks and balances. Clotting, for example, can be prevented by errors of lowered concentration or absence of an enzyme, or an ineffective mutant enzyme, at multiple points. Clotting malfunction can be corrected only by providing (if possible) the missing substance. Failure anywhere has a final common outcome: a failure to clot. It is not improbable that the systems regulating psychological functions—both general ones such as activation or inhibition and more specific ones such as mood or anger—are just as complex.

In attempting to refine the neurotransmitter hypotheses, we must remember that all the abnormalities discussed are biological *correlates*. Those of us who have had a traditional scientific education diligently teach students that correlation may have nothing to do with causation, and then we tend to forget it ourselves. Difficulties with the relevant studies are multiple, and many have not even been replicated. Among those that have been, the findings are often contradictory, and as in studies of ADHD treatment and family distribution, the findings are further confused by unclear diagnoses. As is always the case, the earlier studies are less sophisticated than the later ones.

Most of the biochemical studies remind one of the word Donald Klein invented to refer to high-level theoretical explanations of the mechanism of action of drugs—"metaneuropsychopharmacology." A parallel term would be "metaneuropsychophysiology." Both are relatives of "metapsychology": they cannot make precise—and hence refutable—predictions; they can retroactively explain anything; and they mask ignorance with air-filled logic. As Karl Popper holds, the best hypotheses must be potentially refutable. The hypotheses in these biochemical studies—particularly the metabolite ones—are not definite and refutable, and they cannot distinguish between primary and secondary abnormalities.

Further, we have two kinds of strong evidence in adults that ADHD is metabolically heterogeneous: (1) In our study of cerebrospinal fluid, described earlier, the ADHD adults who did not respond to methylphenidate had a significantly higher level of HVA than the responders (Reimherr et al., 1984). (2) The considerable variation in drug responsivity suggests heterogeneous metabolism. Some patients—indistinguishable clinically from the others—do not respond to stimulants. Others respond preferentially to either D-amphetamine or methylphenidate. Some patients have an arousal response to stimulants under certain conditions. A few have a robust response to tricyclic antidepressants; of those, a few do not develop tolerance. Reaction to bupropion is likewise variable, with some patients responding completely and some partially. Other patients respond to combinations of drugs, such as an antidepressant plus a stimulant. In fact, Murphy et al. (1987) have used differential drug responsivity to elucidate the etiology of depression.

Considering these highly unsatisfactory data, the most conservative hypothesis now is that the syndrome can be caused by several different biochemical abnormalities, and that some can be "corrected" by different medications. Although we suspect that most of these abnormalities are genetic in origin, we know that there has been at least one major phenocopy of ADHD—the syndrome of post-encephalitic behavior disorder.

Even a casual consideration of these genetic and biochemical complexities should be daunting to any clinical psychiatric researcher. If the regulation of attention, motor activity, impulsivity, anger and mood, and the other attributes of ADHD and related syndromes are as complex as the processes involved in, say, the physiology of hearing—which depends on the proper functioning of hundreds of genes and can also be affected by environmental factors—we should be extraordinarily cautious in interpreting the observations of all the relevant studies, from family, twin and adoption studies to monoamine analyses and PET scans. We know that genetic factors play a role in the etiology of ADHD, but we may reasonably expect phenocopies and a large amount of genetic heterogeneity. We can expect to see differences in symptom patterns, in penetrance, and severity, and therefore in familial association. If we wish to make further progress in our understanding of these disorders, it is essential that they be broken down into homogeneous subgroups. It is unlikely that we can expect much progress by refining our current techniques, observing more characteristics, attempting to group subjects on the basis of symptom patterns, obtaining better and larger samples, or using new statistical techniques.

One cannot discover genetic entities on the basis of signs and symptoms alone, because of the danger of circular reasoning. Even if one subdivides into apparently more homogeneous subgroups, he may be "splitting" a single pleiotropic disorder. "Differences in the phenotype are the most treacherous basis for decision on genetic heterogeneity. After all, similarity of phenotype is what leads to mistaken impressions of homogeneity (or unity) in the first place" (McKusick, p. 344).

As science progresses, molecular genetics may hold the solution. In the next section we will take a look at the possibilities in that developing field.

THE FUTURE: MOLECULAR GENETICS

What the techniques of molecular genetics might accomplish in the investigation of ADHD is analogous to what histopathology accomplished in internal medicine: correlation of specific tissue pathology with different syndromes led to definition of syndromes, which in turn led to the separation of seemingly identical disorders, which led to improved diagnosis, accurate epidemiology, study of natural history and evaluation of different treatments. With the techniques of molecular genetics one can ascertain the locations of genetic abnormalities and thus may begin to separate patients into genetically homogeneous groups. Having done that, one can explore the specific molecular abnormalities associated with each of the subtypes.

Techniques of this kind would vastly improve the possibility of threading one's way through the intricacies of genetic heterogeneity, pleiotropy, variable penetrance, phenocopies and the dangers of circular reasoning. They are also an improvement over current studies of possible biochemical correlates, which are limited not only by diagnostic uncertainty but by such factors as: (1) no peripheral correlates—i.e., extra-central nervous system manifestations—which means that some studies might have deceptively negative results; (2) the pertinent abnormality is structural rather than a biochemical abnormality in the brain; and (3) expression of the abnormality in the brain only at a certain level of development.

Modern techniques of molecular genetics provide two ways of determining whether a particular gene is abnormal: the first is the examination of "candidate genes"; the second is the exploitation of DNA polymorphisms. In the candidate gene method, one tries to examine the genes involved in the functioning of the suspected system. For example, the dopaminergic system is dependent on the synthesis of dopamine, its release, and its effect on dopamine receptors. If one knew the exact DNA structure of the normal dopamine receptors, one might hunt for a DNA sequence that seemed to code for a disorder of those receptors. Then one would attempt to determine if it was identical with the DNA coding for the same receptors in individuals with the disorder in question.

The second technique investigates linkages between the disorder in question and a particular site on a person's genome. This represents a powerful elaboration of the classic technique that linked genes on the gender-determining X chromosome, such as the genes for hemophilia and color blindness in males.[6] Study of the X genes was facilitated by the fact that men have only one X chromosome, which they receive from their mothers. Thus, one can easily identify which of the 46 chromosomes is the carrier of a sex-linked genetic malady. Recent investigation in molecular genetics has been attempting to expand such knowledge by establishing markers on the remaining 22 "autosomes" (the nonsexual chromosomes) inherited from each parent—that is, to map the human genome. The first relevant discovery was that almost 90 percent of the "genome" (the DNA in the chromosome) seems not to be expressed: it does not seem to initiate the sequence in which DNA "instructions" lead to particular forms of protein. Since it *apparently* conveys no information, it apparently is "free" to vary. If this is so, different individuals might have harmless variable DNA. But how could one determine such variability? The discovery of "restriction enzymes" now points to possible answers. "Restriction" enzymes cleave certain sequences in this "nonsense" part of the genome; thereby one can determine mutations in these regions that can be used as markers for an exact place on the chromosome. One then tries to see whether the disease being studied segregates with one of these markers.

Markers work best when there is one dominant gene. If several mutant genes are affecting different parts of the system being investigated (e.g., the dopaminergic), the genetic heterogeneity means that the impaired genes will probably be on different chromosomes. One could then locate a genetic factor only in large families in whom the same gene would be associated with all family members with the disorder. With current techniques it is thus much more difficult to analyze disorders that are genetically heterogeneous or polygenetic (multifactorial) in origin. Recent developments that will expedite the search for markers are: (1) a technique for rapidly synthesizing the amount of unknown DNA rapidly by the "polymerase chain reaction"; and (2) more and more genetic markers. The markers now reach all parts of the genome. As they become more finely distributed on the genome, the markers will allow more accurate measurement and establishment of more genetic linkages. An exciting example of such a linkage—and one that may be distantly related to ADHD—is the recent discovery of a "quantitative trait locus for reading disability on chromosome 6" (Cardon et al., 1994).

CONCLUSIONS

■

Taken together, what do these data tell us? First, that ADHD is transmitted genetically. Second, that the syndrome is etiologically heterogeneous. Third, that ADHD occurs with the "St. Louis triad" very much more frequently than would be expected on a chance basis, even though pure ADHD does not have such genetic relationships. Fourth, that ADHD is associated with (not necessarily caused by!) decreased dopaminergic activity. Lastly, that the most progress will occur if clinical research and molecular genetic research go hand in hand as a mutual bootstrap operation, each zeroing in on more homogeneous groups for the other to study. If we are lucky, we will discover that most or all forms of ADHD are due to a dominant major gene rather than to genetic heterogeneity or polygeneticism.

NOTES

1. Cause is confounded because ADHD is associated with alcohol abuse and the abnormalities in the offspring may be genetic, with the alcohol and nicotine abuse in the mother being markers of ADHD in her.

2. Egodystonic—refers to anything unacceptable to the ego and rejected by it. This contrasts with the experience of a psychotic who does not question reality of his hallucinations—he appears not to experience them as foreign.

3. Although if the percent released into the bloodstream does not vary appreciably between individuals and the percent transferred to the bloodstream is the same for individuals with and without the disorder, this factor is not critical.

4. A problem is that the degree of inhibition may be related both to levels of probenecid (which may or may not be corrected for) and to other factors. For these reasons the technique is no longer employed.

5. In the treatment of Parkinson's disorder, L-dopa is currently administered in combination with carbidopa. Many of the side effects of L-dopa are due to its decarboxylation outside of the brain, and originally L-dopa had to be begun at low doses and very gradually increased to allow patients to become tolerant to these peripheral side effects. This problem can be obviated by giving L-dopa in conjunction with carbidopa, which is a decarboxylase inhibitor that does not cross the blood-brain barrier. Thus, it prevents decarboxylation peripherally (and thus these peripheral side effects) but does not interfere with neuronal decarboxylation of L-dopa in the brain.

6. The reason that these abnormalities are much more common in males is that females have an almost always normal gene (allele) on one of their two X chromosomes that compensates for the abnormal allele on the other X chromosome.

5

Diagnosis of ADHD in Adults

■

In Chapter 2, "Signs and Symptoms," I described the characteristics of Attention-deficit Hyperactivity Disorder as seen in children and adults. In this chapter I elucidate how my colleagues and I have used such observational data to formulate diagnostic criteria for ADHD in adults.

Previously undiagnosed "minimal brain dysfunction" (MBD) can be identified in adult life, but the diagnosis is frequently missed because of the patients' "noisier" clinical characteristics: antisocial, histrionic, borderline, and explosive traits; alcohol and substance abuse; and chronic mood problems, which are sometimes diagnosed as an adult situational reaction or dysthymic disorder. When these signs and symptoms are causing the patient pain and destroying personal relationships, it is easy to overlook his fidgety hands and restless feet and his accounts of having had a "short attention span" in elementary school.

When we began our studies of "minimal brain dysfunction" in adults in 1973, the diagnostic criteria that we developed were based on my formulations of what was then a very loosely defined syndrome (Wender, 1971). As described in the Introduction, "minimal brain dysfunction" encompassed the whole cluster of externalizing disorders (DSM-III-R's Attention-deficit Hyperactivity Disorder, Conduct Disorder, and Oppositional Defiant Disorder) and the ill-defined group of "learning disorders," particularly the academic skill disorders. In this chapter I describe how we have refined both inclusionary and exclusionary criteria. I also include some specific approaches that we believe are helpful in diagnosing Attention-deficit Hyperactivity Disorder in adults.

INCLUSIONARY CRITERIA

■

Working with the clinic population at the University of Utah Medical Center, we began with adults who were symptomatic volunteers and thought they might have MBD symptoms, and with patients who were referred because their physicians thought the diagnosis possible. To ascertain the diagnosis, we had to determine what they had been like as children.[1] None of the patients we studied had been diagnosed or treated as children—which was not unexpected since they had been born in the 1950s and late 1940s, and during their childhood there was one child psychiatrist in Utah. All had to be diagnosed retroactively. Our patients' memories of their childhood were often sketchy. When possible, we asked them to contact their parents (usually mothers) and relay the family's accounts to us. Because we had no benchmarks for assessing the remembered childhood of adults with and without current psychiatric disorders, we decided to use a standardizable rating scale on which the patients' parents (or parent substitutes) could rate their offsprings' childhood characteristics. The scale we decided to use in the 1970s was the Conners Abbreviated Rating Scale, which was then the standard workhorse of pediatric psychopharmacology; it had been used both to select "hyperactive" children and as a measure of treatment response. We identified it as the Parents' Rating Scale (PRS) and requested that mothers (not teachers) rate their offsprings' behavior between the ages of 6 and 10; if a patient's mother was not available, his father or another older relative was asked to do the rating. The scale, its scoring, and the frequency distribution in a normal population are shown in Appendix B.[2]

Since we did not want to discard candidates whose parents were not available, we also constructed a rating scale on which the adult rated "MBD" behaviors in his childhood. Titled the Wender Utah Rating Scale (the WURS), it is shown in Appendix D, along with the scoring and the frequency distribution of the scores in normal adults, patients with unipolar depression, and ADHD adults.

Neither set of criteria derived from the scales is sufficient for retroactive diagnosis. The diagnosis must be based on the presence of certain highly specific behaviors, and not on the basis of generalized traits (inattentiveness, impulsivity). For the most part, the lower level descriptors in the scales provide only a sample of specific behaviors. Thus, the Utah Criteria for the diagnosis of ADHD in adults comprise two parts: (I) childhood history and (II) adult diagnostic criteria.

For the childhood history, the category of "Broad criteria" (I.B below) covers what patients can remember of their childhood with reasonable certainty. The category of "Narrow criteria" (I.A) is used when parents (or other adults who had been the patient's caretakers when he was a child) remember enough to fulfill DSM-III-R criteria.

Part I. A childhood history consistent with ADHD in childhood as defined by A or B.

A. *Narrow criteria:* The individual met DSM-III-R criteria for ADHD in childhood (8 of the 13 symptoms, or signs).

B. *Broad criteria:* Both characteristics 1 and 2, and one characteristic of 3 through 6.

1. Hyperactivity. More active than other children, unable to sit still, fidgety, restless, always on the go, talking excessively.

2. Attention deficits, sometimes described as a "short attention span," distractibility, daydreaming, failure to finish assignments in class or complete homework, was called lazy, was said not to remember, was told he could do better than he did. Underachievement not due primarily to learning disorders ("dyslexia")—or deficits in intelligence.

3. Behavior problems in school. Talking in class, disciplined more than classmates, called out for disrupting the class, stayed after school, etc. Disciplined by teachers, principal.

4. Impulsivity. Couldn't wait for turn, acted without thinking, blurted things out, got into accidents, reckless, etc.

5. Overexcitability or temper outbursts, got into a lot of fights.

6. Temper outbursts.

(As discussed, it is usually difficult to determine if the specific signs required by the DSMs were present, even with information obtained from parents or other adults who had been the patient's caretaker(s) when he was a child.)

The broad inclusion criteria reflect their heritage: they include characteristics of the conduct-disordered and oppositional child. The rationale for continuing to employ them is that there is considerable comorbidity of ADHD with CD and that about one-half of conduct-disordered children do not have continuing conduct disorder problems as they grow older—they do not develop Antisocial Personality Disorder (ASPD; Robins and Price, 1991). From a practical point of view the clinician can determine whether the adult patients they are evaluating manifest continuing symptoms as ASPD or as Passive Aggressive Personality Disorder (PAPD), which may be the later form of Oppositional Defiant Disorder (ODD). It will obviously be important to study and compare the natural history, familial association, and treatment responsiveness of ADHD and its common comorbid conditions (CD and ODD) in terms of whether CD and ODD disappear or continue in adulthood. For example, the etiological and treatment differences of the following combinations are not yet known:

	Adulthood	
Childhood	Outcome 1	Outcome 2
ADHD/CD	ADHD/ASPD	ADHD
ADHD/ODD	ADHD/PAPD	ADHD

Both the broad criteria for ADHD in childhood and the adult criteria for ADHD (which follow) specify the presence of hyperactivity, and in this respect these criteria are more restrictive than those of DSM-III and DSM-III-R. We elected to study the more typical "core" group. An analogy from adult psychiatry would be to study Kraepelinian dementia praecox rather than Bleulerian schizophrenia—that is, the narrow rather than the broad conceptualization of the syndrome.

DSM-III subdivided "Attention Deficit Disorder" into ADD with (ADD-H) and ADD without Hyperactivity. The latter was characterized by inattention and impulsivity. Some investigators have considered ADD without hyperactivity to be a more heterogeneous syndrome with less predictable stimulant response than ADD with hyperactivity, although some data suggest that many of these children do respond well to stimulant medication. Because the diagnosis of

ADHD in adults was controversial, we opted for underdiagnosis of a narrow category rather than a broader one for both scientific and legal reasons: (1) retrospective diagnosis of ADD without hyperactivity is difficult, and (2) it seems safer to introduce the use of controversial Schedule II drugs in a narrow and more definite form of the disorder rather than overprescribing and violating possible legal strictures of the Drug Enforcement Administration.

Ascertaining the presence of the adults' signs and symptoms is based on what the patient observes, what he relates others observe about him, *and,* whenever possible, the reports of a knowledgeable other. As with childhood ADHD, reports from an other—significant or not—are necessary. The patient himself will usually underestimate the extent of his symptoms and their change with treatment. I will discuss this in greater detail later. The adult section of the Utah Criteria is as follows:

Part II. The presence of (A.1) motor hyperactivity and (A.2) attentional difficulties, and at least two of the five characteristics listed in B.

A.1. HYPERACTIVITY

More or less continuous motor hyperactivity as manifested by restlessness, greater energy than most people, fidgetiness, playing with fingers (drumming) or twisting hair, rhythmic rapid flexing of the leg at the knee or of the foot on the floor or of alternating feet on the floor, inability to relax (sometimes labeled "nervousness"—in which case the clinician should determine if the patient means restlessness or anticipatory anxiety), inability to persist in sedentary activities (e.g., watching movies or TV, reading the newspaper), being always on the go, leaving the table immediately after finishing a meal, feeling dysphoric when inactive.

The ADHD adult may initially constrain his activity in the office—as may the hyperactive child in school—but as the interview continues his self-control decreases and, again like the child, hyperactivity rears its head. It is usually present in the waiting room, where the patient's diagnosis can often be made by the observant receptionist.

A.2. IMPAIRED CONCENTRATION

Attentional deficits as manifested by inability to keep mind on conversations, distractibility (being aware of other stimuli even though attempts are made to filter them out), inability to keep mind on current activity (e.g., on reading), difficulty keeping mind on job, frequent "forgetfulness," often losing or misplacing things (car keys, purse, wallet), forgetting plans, "mind frequently somewhere else."

As in childhood, inattentiveness may be overcome in areas of great interest. A few nondyslexic ADHD adults actually are "great readers," and some may refrain from continually changing the television channel. The problem is—as was true in elementary school—that some areas of less than riveting interest are important to the ADHD adult's functioning.

B.1. AFFECTIVE LABILITY

Usually described as antedating adolescence and in some instances beginning as far back as the patient can remember. Manifested by definite shifts from a normal mood to depression or mild euphoria or, more usually, a feeling of excitement or being "wired." The ups tend to decrease and disappear with age; the depression is described as being "down," "bored," or "discontented." Anhedonia is not present—the patient is capable of enjoyment, and his depression may be relieved by pleasurable events. He may have psychological inertia, having difficulty initiating activities that he knows will require effort. Mood shifts usually last hours to, at most, a few days and are present without significant physiological concomitants; mood shifts may occur spontaneously or be reactive. The depression may persist when life problems do. Usually this depression remits when the patient's life circumstances change for the better.

B.2. HOT TEMPER

Explosive, short-lived outbursts, transient loss of control, easily provoked or constant irritability, impatience. Overreactivity is variously described as "having a short fuse," a "low boiling point," or a "hair trigger." Loss of control can range from the verbal (yelling, being hurtful) to physical violence, which may be toward inanimate objects (throwing glasses or plates, or punching a fist through walls) or other people. Patients usually "cool off" quickly and do not brood; a frequently associated feature is their inability to understand why the other people involved can remain angry while they recover their composure so quickly. Our samples probably have a disproportionately low prevalence of physical violence because we have excluded patients with marked antisocial traits. Obviously temper tantrums can produce serious problems in all relationships.

B.3. INABILITY TO COMPLETE TASKS AND DISORGANIZATION

A lack of organization in running a household, performing school work, or in one's occupation; workspace, house, and office are sloppy and messy; tasks frequently not completed or completed after multiple delays and interruption; subject often switches from one task to another in haphazard fashion, beginning a new task before completing the previous one; disorganization in problem solving, organizing time, and planning expenditures; lack of perseverance and stick-to-it-tiveness, gives up easily.

B.4. STRESS INTOLERANCE

The patient cannot take ordinary stresses in stride and reacts excessively or inappropriately with depression, confusion, uncertainty, anxiety, or anger; low frustration tolerance—he is easily discouraged; emotional responses interfere with appropriate problem solving, and he is likely to become increasingly disorganized; he is easily "flustered" or "hassled," reacts to criticism and pressure by becoming "tense" or uptight; experiences repeated crises in dealing with routine life stresses.

B.5. IMPULSIVITY

Minor manifestations include talking before thinking things through, interrupting in conversations, impatience (e.g., while driving), frequently saying or doing something on the spur of the moment and without considering the consequences, and impulse buying. Major manifestations may be similar to those seen in mania and Antisocial Personality Disorder, including poorly thought-out decisions, often on the basis of insufficient information (e.g., quitting jobs, abrupt making or termination of relationships, foolish business investments); reckless driving; inability to delay acting without experiencing discomfort.

EXCLUSIONARY CRITERIA

■

We excluded an adult diagnosis of ADHD when the following symptoms were present:

1. Symptoms of the bipolar and depressive mood disorders and what are probably their *formes frustes* (Akiskal, 1983).
2. Signs and symptoms of schizophrenia, schizoaffective disorder, schizotypal personality disorder. The woolly (vague, meandering) thinking (speech) of schizophrenic spectrum disorder.
3. The following symptoms of Borderline Personality Disorder (BPD):
   a. A pattern of unstable and intense interpersonal relationships, characterized by alternating between extremes of overidealization and devaluation.
   b. Recurrent suicidal threats, gestures, or behavior, or any self-mutilating behavior.
   c. Prominent identity disturbances.
   d. Pronounced and chronic feelings of emptiness.
   e. Frantic efforts to avoid real or imagined abandonment, and intolerance of being alone.
4. Current criteria of Antisocial Personality Disorder, alcohol or drug abuse within the past year, or any history of stimulant drug abuse.

RATIONALE FOR INCLUSIONARY AND EXCLUSIONARY CRITERIA

■

The rationale for using both the inclusionary and exclusionary criteria was that we wished to study as homogeneous a group as possible. Such a "pure" group may be statistically atypical, but it is a useful one to employ in initial studies: it should decrease variance and improve the likelihood of detecting commonalities in family history, biological correlates, and response to treatment.

In addition, we excluded possible ADHD patients with these prominent symptoms for the following specific reasons. The mood disorders were excluded because they represent a different "family" of conditions: they tend to be episodic; their family histories are of mood disorders (rather than Antisocial Personality Disorder and alcoholism), and they respond to drugs (tricyclic antidepressants, lithium) that are generally ineffective in the treatment of ADHD. The schizophrenic spectrum disorders involve symptoms that might mask or be confounded with those of ADHD, and they are members of a family of disorders whose symptoms are generally aggravated by stimulants and mitigated by neuroleptics—whereas ADHD symptomatology in adults is generally mitigated by stimulants and unresponsive to the neuroleptics. Patients with Borderline Personality Disorder were excluded because the syndrome is heterogeneous and believed to be largely unresponsive to drugs. In addition, BPD patients may be at increased risk for abusing Schedule II drugs, including stimulants. Finally, we have excluded patients with antisocial characteristics because this population is unreliable and is at increased risk for alcohol and chemical substance abuse (whether acknowledged or not). In addition, conduct disorder, which is their childhood antecedent, is much less responsive to stimulant drug treatment than is childhood ADHD. Similarly, the unreliability of alcoholics rules against their inclusion in research of this kind, even though some *may* have a decreased urge to drink when treated with stimulants.

Although our research design required that we exclude many patients with probable ADHD who had "comorbid" diagnoses, these mixed clinical pictures are expectable, and the clinician must treat them. In addition, some "pure" ADHD patients develop new illnesses *after* initial diagnosis. Patients with mixed diagnoses usually need and respond to different, perhaps combined, treatments.

Biederman and colleagues (1986, 1987, 1990) have reported an increased prevalence of mood and anxiety disorders in the relatives of ADHD children. Mannuzza and Klein (1993) and Weiss et al. (1985) found no evidence that formerly hyperactive children were at increased risk for mood or affective disorder in adulthood. It is difficult to interpret this discrepancy. In addition to the nagging and persistent problems of sample differences, Mannuzza and Klein suggest that methodological differences may be playing a role because interviewers in the studies had different levels of training and different interview schedules.

DIFFERENTIAL DIAGNOSIS

Many of the symptoms and behaviors of ADHD in adults are similar to those seen in other psychiatric disorders and may lead to a false diagnosis of ADHD. Because Borderline Personality Disorder and mood disorders may sometimes be difficult to distinguish from ADHD, I list here their more important partial resemblances to ADHD and their identifiable differences.

Borderline Personality Disorder (BPD)

The similarities between Borderline Personality Disorder and ADHD are great enough so that in order to study homogeneous samples, the Utah Criteria exclude not only individuals who have BPD but also individuals who have unique BPD traits. The borderline attributes seemingly shared by the ADHD patient include impulsivity, angry outbursts, affective instability, and feelings of boredom. What are the differences in these signs and symptoms between patients with BPD and ADHD we have studied? They differ both qualitatively and in intensity. (1) The ADHD patient's impulsivity is short-lived: He buys impulsively, runs a traffic light, interrupts others, talks before thinking. The impulsivity is situational. It is milder and intermittent and appears to be thoughtless rather than compulsively "driven." This is different from the BPD's more severe and sometimes compulsive behavior, for example, shoplifting and bingeing. (2) Both the ADHD patient and the BPD may exhibit excessive or inappropriate anger. The DSM-III-R description of BPD anger is "inappropriate, intense anger or lack of control of anger, e.g., frequent displays of temper, *constant* anger, recurrent physical fights." The ADHD patients we have included in studies have had *episodic* anger, which is quick to rise and quick to cool, and ADHD patients do not maintain constant brooding anger. Recurrent physical fights are more likely to be seen in those ADHD patients with a history of conduct disorder in childhood and concurrent antisocial traits.

In addition to these distinctions, the major differences between BPD and ADHD patients are that the latter do not have the symptoms we specified in our exclusionary criteria: unstable, intense interpersonal relationships that alternate between idealizing and denigrating others; suicidal preoccupation (the ADHD patients we have studied have not intentionally injured or mutilated themselves or made repeated suicidal attempts); identity disturbances; feelings of emptiness; or fear of abandonment or of being alone.

Lastly, there are patterns of interpersonal behavior that many clinicians believe are strongly associated with BPD that we do not find in our ADHD study samples. Therapists working with ADHD adults do not feel manipulated by the patients and do not see "game-playing" in the patients' behavior; nor do they feel the frequently draining dependency demands (sometimes punctuated by periods of derogation or hostility) that BPD patients may manifest. As I pointed out earlier, clear signs and symptoms of ADHD and BPD can co-exist in the same patient. However, it is important to identify the two disorders clearly, not only for research purposes but in order to provide adequate treatment.

Mood Disorders

The mood abnormalities of ADHD differ from those of the major mood disorders in quality (including amplitude and duration), "typical" personality, age of onset and natural history, and family history.

The mood shifts of ADHD are described by ADHD patients as "roller-coaster-like," with changes from excitement to euthymia to depression typically occurring in minutes to hours, as contrasted with the episode duration of days to weeks for dysthymia and cyclothymia.

The excitement seen in ADHD is readily distinguishable from hypomania: the ADHD patient's motor is running too fast and his experience is one of excitement, not euphoria—it is the adult equivalent of the overstimulated five-year-old's "going into orbit" at the circus. It is very brief (usually no more than hours in length), is almost always triggered by readily identifiable events, and can be terminated by bad news, a rebuff, or a disappointment.

The ADHD's depression may persist if he falls into a self-dug hole in life—which occurs not infrequently. In these circumstances he may feel miserable and depressed, agitated, and irritable, and report that he can't concentrate and that his recent memory is "terrible." Such a depression can resemble major depression, but its reactive nature is revealed by it response to reality therapy, which throws the patient a metaphorical rope. In contrast, in major depression there is frequently anhedonia, lack of interest and lack of reactivity to pleasure (Klein's "endogenomorphic depression"; Klein, 1974)—"painful anesthesia." The "down" of the ADHD patient is apt to be described as disappointment, discouragement, or boredom, and he does not usually experience guilt, suicidal preoccupations, neurovegetative symptoms (decreased appetite and weight loss, decreased energy and sex drive, and diurnal variation), or sleep disruption (particularly insomnia in the middle of the night or toward dawn).[3]

The symptoms of mild chronic depressives, which may have been lifelong, have developed so insidiously that they *seem* to have been with the patient forever—a situation analogous to that of color-blind people, who are unaware that others see the world differently. Such patients may experience some mood shifts superimposed on their chronic state, but these differ from the ADHD patient's description of rapid and brief mood shifts.

The personality characteristics of the ADHD patient are almost polar opposites of those of Akiskal's patients with "subaffective dysthymic disorder" (i.e., chronic, less severe major depression). Akiskal (1983; after Schneider, 1958) describes these patients as (1) quiet and passive; (2) gloomy and incapable of fun (rather than being overtalkative, restless, having brief "highs"); (3) self-critical and self-demeaning (versus psychologically obtuse); (4) hypercritical and complaining; (5) conscientious and overly self-disciplined; (6) brooding and worrying; and (7) preoccupied with negative features of their lives. The premorbid personality of the depressive-to-be is often described as conscientious, eager to please, guilt-prone, deliberative, sensitive, and having been easy to "socialize" as a child.

With respect to age of onset and natural history, the patient with ADHD will describe affective symptoms that antedate adolescence and that may extend back as far as he can remember. They may vary in magnitude as the realistic difficulties of life increase and decrease, but they do not disappear. ADHD patients are thus unlike patients with major depression, who *usually* have had some depression-free intervals and whose ADHD-like symptoms—such as impaired concentration and memory, agitation and irritability—disappear when they are not depressed. In addition, unlike the patient with ADHD, the depressive *usually* does not remember such symptoms as part of his earliest childhood. However, this difference between the disorders is not a reliable one. In the past, biological depression (major depression) was considered an episodic illness of adulthood that rarely began earlier and very rarely before adolescence. Increasing clinical experience with children and adolescents reveals that biological depressions may begin in childhood and continue thereafter, so that the adult "episodes" often represent a continuation or an exacerbation of a lifelong disorder.

Although the childhood histories of the adult depressive and the adult with ADHD usually differ considerably, both disorders can coexist. As mentioned earlier, in evaluating a consecutive sample of child and adolescent outpatients (ages 7 to 17) Carlson and Cantwell (1980) found that about one-quarter of the children meeting the criteria for primary or secondary major depression also met the criteria for "hyperactivity."[4]

Family histories differ (Chapter 4 on etiology): the ADHD patients' relatives appear to be at increased risk for ADHD and *probably* for alcohol abuse and Antisocial Personality Disorder.[5] The status of somatization disorder is unclear. It might be expected to have an increased prevalence because Cloninger et al. (1975) found an increased frequency of Briquet's syndrome (somatization disorder) in the first-degree relatives of "sociopathic" men and women.

The differential diagnosis between ADHD and biological depression can pose a special problem when the chronic non-ADHD depression is mild, when the ADHD patient is seriously demoralized from continual setbacks (which may produce fairly deep and long-lived—if not anhedonic—depressions), or lastly, when major depression and ADHD depression coexist.

DIAGNOSING ADHD IN THE ADULT: SPECIFIC APPROACHES

■

The first step in diagnosing ADHD is to remember the cliché that to diagnose a condition you first must think of it. To paraphrase Pasteur, diagnosis favors the prepared mind. Consider what has happened to diagnoses that once were rare but now are common. The diagnosis—and overdiagnosis—of obsessive-compulsive disorder, multiple personality, Tourette's syndrome, and histories of sexual and physical abuse increased dramatically as soon as clinicians began routinely to make systematic inquiries. Thus, in diagnosing ADHD in adults one must remember that it is not a *rara avis* and probably affects between 2 and 6 percent of the adult population. Although the diagnosis in the adult is easy, it is usually missed. The reasons and their remedies are as follows.

Most psychiatrists treating adults obtain cross-sectional histories of behavior, not developmental ones. This is reinforced by the DSM, which focuses on current functioning. Although clinicians have been taught to inquire about a patient's childhood, the emphasis has been on putative psychodynamics and not on the patient's behavioral style. Frequently, for example, our patients recount that an older brother was favored and that the patient was envious of and angry toward the brother. What the patient may not report—and, unfortunately, what he cannot tell you even if you ask—is that the disproportionate share of negative parental attention stemmed from his misbehavior in school, his lower grades, and his parents' unfavorable comparison of him and his brother.

Thus, when one suspects adult ADHD, a developmental history is essential. Try to characterize the patient's childhood behavioral style *and* attempt to perform a retroactive psychiatric diagnosis: Did the patient qualify for a diagnosis of or have traits of Attention-deficit Hyperactivity Disorder, Conduct Disorder, Oppositional Personality Disorder, a "learning disability"? The DSM's diagnostic lists of symptoms are provided to assess the patient's *current* functioning. The clinician evaluating a child and the clinician evaluating an adult will be examining the patient's current symptoms, and on the basis of the patient's life, current relationships and roles will formulate a psychodynamic hypothesis. The clinician who suspects ADHD in an adult patient must in addition simultaneously attempt to diagnose what his patient was like as a child.

A number of features of the patient's functioning and history are "bell ringers" for ADHD and should alert clinicians if their attention has been directed elsewhere. The "bell ringers" can be divided into current complaints and symptoms; academic, vocational, and home-making performance; marital (or equivalent) functioning; family history; pharmacological history; and physical signs.

CURRENT COMPLAINTS AND SYMPTOMS

Complaints and symptoms are what the patient brings if he is coming under his own steam. Any residual problems seen by his "other" are signs.

Among the most common complaints in the adult with ADHD are depression, hot temper and inability to cope with the stresses of everyday life. (1) The depression is labile and may alternate with high or excited periods, is both spontaneous and reactive, is not anhedonic, has no physiological concomitants, is usually brief, and usually extends back as far as the patient can remember. (2) The hot temper is lifelong and easily provoked, and the patient (generally) "cools off" quickly. (3) The patient's performance in school, on the job, or in running a home and taking care of the children is impaired because minor, expectable stresses are apt to make the patient confused, "hassled," and "stressed out." This, in turn, further impairs his problem-solving efforts and produces a vicious circle.

It is important for the clinician to be aware of this symptom cluster because it is often the "squeaky wheel" that gets the interventional grease. These symptoms constitute the bases for referral and intervention while obscuring the underlying disorder, ADHD. Alternative possibilities must of course be considered. For example, the problems in a couple's ability to "communicate," to understand each other, may be due to incompatible personalities. A student's repeated dropping out of school may result from an unconscious need to fail. But both instances may also result from the patient's inability to sustain attention—that is, ADHD.

ACADEMIC, VOCATIONAL, AND HOMEMAKING PERFORMANCE

Academic or vocational success that is less than expected on the basis of the subject's intelligence, education, and opportunity suggests ADHD. Underachievement in ADHD usually begins very early and may continue throughout the patient's life. Individuals with ADHD have often done poorly in preschool, kindergarten, and elementary school (sometimes repeating grades), and are likely to have a record of "dropping out" of high school and college. Such academic inadequacy is the frequent consequence of ADHD behavioral attributes, the frequently associated "learning disorders," or both. A crude retrospective differential diagnosis is not difficult. Did the patient have difficulty learning to read, write, spell, do arithmetic? What were his grades? Was he always being told he could do better? Did he have disciplinary problems in elementary and high school? Was he often called to the principal's office? Were his parents called to the principal's office? If he has graduated from high school, is he receiving further education? If so, is he still having difficulty concentrating, remembering, doing his schoolwork? Is he a slow reader, someone who dislikes reading, a poor speller? Has he forgotten the multiplication tables, does he reverse digits when calculating with or without a calculator?

With lack of vocational success, in contrast to school performance, the problems are more likely to have been interpersonal rather than cognitive. How often has the individual changed jobs? What has been the basis of such changes? Has it been due to difficulty getting along with bosses and superiors? This is the adult equivalent of whether or not the patient "works and plays well with others."

Academic and vocational underachievement are, of course, also hallmarks of ASPD. However, as with the differential diagnosis of discipline problems in childhood, ADHD and ASPD underachievement have different psychological aromas. ASPD is distinguished by such behaviors as illegal acts, fighting, lying, and child neglect, and the person lacks remorse for having hurt others. The ADHD patient, in contrast, has no desire to violate societal norms but has difficulty in conforming to them.

A woman's vocational success is difficult to evaluate when her employment is only one of several roles she has assumed—for example, career employee, housekeeper and mother. Because of these multiple demands her employment may be intermittent, part-time and in occupations (e.g., clerical-secretarial) with limited opportunities for advancement. For women without employment outside the home, a good indicator of ADHD is difficulty in managing their roles and responsibilities as housewives and mothers (particularly of young children).

Although deficient childrearing skills and behavior are useful indicators of ADHD, they must be judged with special care because child rearing, as Freud observed, is one of the impossible professions.[6] It is without respite—children still require attention when their mother is ill, and they do not limit their needs and misbehaviors only to 9 A.M. to 5 P.M., Mondays through Fridays. Child care requires patience, consistency, organization, coolness of temper, lack of impulsivity, and stress tolerance. No woman born has had all of these requirements all of the time, but they are virtues in which the woman with ADHD is unusually deficient. To complicate her life, genetics ensures that she is much more likely than the average mother to have an ADHD child or children. As is evident from the review of their symptoms, ADHD children are often exceedingly hard to raise; the results of combining a noncompliant, difficult to discipline, short-tempered, affectively labile child with an ADHD mother are not hard to predict. The child who most requires patience and consistent treatment thus is least likely to receive them.

The ADHD mother with an ADHD child may also resort to physical abuse. The abusing mother may not only have "learned to abuse" from her own mother or father but may have in part been subject to abuse because she herself was a very difficult ADHD child (see Oliver and Buchanan, 1979, for three-generation documentation). This phenomenon is analogous to that frequently seen in schizophrenia. The abnormal parenting that schizophrenic offspring sometimes receive can be a manifestation of both the genetic schizophrenic abnormalities in the biological parents and the problems of raising a schizophrenic child.

(Parenthetically, such parenting is not the cause of schizophrenia—just as abnormal parenting does not seem to be a major factor in the etiology of ADHD [Wender et al., 1968, 1977].)

MARITAL (OR MARRIAGE-EQUIVALENT) FUNCTIONING

Another important social marker of ADHD is marital (or marriage-equivalent) strife and instability. For the patient whose childhood diagnosis was ADHD/CD, and who now manifests persisting antisocial characteristics,[7] relationships with the opposite sex may not only be unstable and frequently disrupted but increasingly disorganized and chaotic, with impulsive initiation and termination of relationships, and with an increased frequency of formal separations and divorces. Spouse abuse is undoubtedly also increased as the childhood diagnosis ranges from ADHD without CD to ADHD with CD.

Many ADHD patients have sought and received counseling or therapy because of their difficulties in relationships. Few are first referred to a psychiatrist for a diagnostic evaluation, and none are treated with medication. Most are correctly perceived to have problems in their relationships, but the underlying ADHD problems are missed. Communication problems tackled in couples therapy may be the result of not listening to or interrupting the spouse (attentional difficulties and impulsivity), ambiguous or inadequate apportionment of responsibilities (disorganization), or household budgeting problems (impulsivity, particularly impulse buying). In other words, prominent symptoms of ADHD are commonly seen as the emergent pathology of a relationship rather than as the expected problems of an ADHD individual in a relationship. The upshot is that the therapy is ineffective, while with effective pharmacological treatment the problems may resolve spontaneously or become amenable to talking treatments.

FAMILY HISTORY

The diagnosis of ADHD may also be helped by family history. Psychopathology runs in families, and patients' family histories may shed light on ambiguous clinical pictures.[8] Obviously, a history of "hyperactivity" in parents, siblings, or offspring supports a diagnosis of ADHD.

Patients may not be able to supply *diagnoses* for their parents and siblings, but they can describe their behavior, including such ADHD symptoms as irritability, moodiness and temper outbursts, impulsivity, and alcohol abuse. They can also recount the consequences of ADHD behavior in their parents' and siblings' lives, including academic and vocational underachievement and failure, marital failures and disarray, and alcohol and substance abuse. Other family symptoms that are suggestive of ADHD are antisocial personality in male relatives and, possibly, Somatization Disorder (hysteria, Briquet's syndrome) in female relatives. When both a patient and his or her spouse have ambiguous symptoms and their child has ADHD, diagnostic questions regarding ADHD must be directed at both parents.

The clinician cannot make much use of family history to confirm a suspected diagnosis if either the patient or his child is adopted. Although social influences have not been ruled out in some disorders, it is the hereditary genetic endowment that is the prime suspect when one sees recurrent patterns of mental illness in families of patients with disorders such as ADHD and schizophrenia. Without such a genetic connection, one can draw few conclusions from similar family behavior (see Chapter 4 on etiology and Appendix F).

PHARMACOLOGICAL HISTORY

A patient's response to licit and illicit drugs can sometimes be suggestive. Here are some examples from my experience: A graduate student recounted her disappointment upon trying cocaine because everyone became euphoric and she felt relaxed. A father fell asleep after taking his daughter's Dexedrine. A computer programmer found that his concentration *improved* after a few puffs of mild marijuana. Reports of this kind may be inaccurate, but they should at least make the interviewer curious. Early onset alcohol abuse *may* also be an indicator of a diathesis of ADHD.

PHYSICAL SIGNS

Physical signs include the minor physical anomalies (Deutsch et al., 1990; Fineman et al., work in progress) and Wender's foot sign (the rapidly flexing knee or foot, already discussed). The reduction of the foot sign in ADHD patients may also be an indicator of stimulant response.

THE NECESSITY OF AN INFORMANT

■

The ADHD patient often cannot describe his behavior, for he has lived with it his entire life. When his behavior is described by others, he often feels that it is not he who is being talked about. His experience is like that of a person who is seeing and hearing himself on a videotape for the first time—the person on the screen looks and sounds strange and foreign.

For example, the patient cannot describe himself as inattentive. His attention has not recently changed—it has always been this way, and he cannot contrast it with the experience of attentiveness that others have. He may be able to describe his own behavior: "Every time I sit down to study, I have to get up every five minutes and move around"; but he cannot compare it to others' behavior. By contrast, the depressed adult (at least without lifelong dysthymia) is keenly aware of the painful change in his mood. For the ADHD adult, "That's the way it's always been." In this respect the ADHD adult is probably like individuals with personality disorders or socially undesirable attributes, who likewise are apt to be blind to and to minimize, deny, rationalize or project responsibility for their maladaptive behavior.

Hence, the diagnosing clinician needs an informant. For the child patient, parents and teachers are essential reporters. For the adult patient, this role is best provided by a spouse or significant other. One study dramatically documenting the usefulness of an informant in increasing diagnostic sensitivity for personality disorders was done by Stangl et al. (1985), who evaluated a group of inpatients with the Structured Interview for DSM-III Personality Disorders. Without an informant the authors diagnosed 29 percent of the sample as having a personality disorder, and with an informant, 53 percent.

An obvious practical problem is that not all adult ADHD patients come equipped with an informant. In fact, their disorder increases the probability that they do *not* have a good *long*-term relationship and, therefore, a good informant. Furthermore, without informants many ADHD patients cannot measure the type and magnitude of their response to treatment.

THE QUANTITATIVE DIAGNOSIS OF ADHD IN ADULTS, OR "HOW MANY SYMPTOMS DO YOU HAVE TO HAVE TO REALLY MAKE THE DIAGNOSIS?"

■

Since 1980, we teachers have had to repeatedly remind trainees that the *Diagnostic and Statistical Manuals* were not given to the American Psychiatric Association on tablets of stone on top of Mt. Sinai. The symptoms described and the categories defined on the basis of their type and number are *not absolute*. Moreover, the number of signs and symptoms specified as necessary to "make the diagnosis" is not absolute. As I pointed out earlier, the medical analogy I've found most useful refers to blood pressure: What does it mean when we say that a pressure of 141/91 is hypertensive and that one of 139/89 is normal? Do we treat the former and not the latter? Why?

The Utah Criteria for ADHD in adulthood require the continued presence of hyperactivity and attention problems and 2 of 5 symptoms (affective lability, hot temper, disorganization, excessive sensitivity to stress, and impulsivity). Why at least two of five symptoms? Not on a theoretical basis. Without a totally independent method for ascertaining the presence or absence of adult ADHD, one cannot determine the sensitivity and specificity of diagnostic rules. The important questions can be formulated as follows. (1) Given a sample of "true" ADHD adults who are diagnosed by our (or others') criteria, what fraction of those patients who "really" have adult ADHD—true positives— remains undiagnosed? (2) Given a sample of patients who definitely do not have ADHD—true negatives—what fraction of those patients is inaccurately diagnosed by our criteria as having ADHD?

These are important questions to which we cannot provide an answer. We chose patients with at least two of the specified attributes because such patients have more clinically relevant areas of dysfunction than those with one or none (whose problems are restlessness and inattention).[9]

Our criteria should not imply that patients with one or none of these five characteristics should not be treated. The pragmatic decision to treat is based on the consequences of treatment of patients with and without ADHD and the nontreatment of patients with and without ADHD. A "cost-benefit analysis" or the "payoff matrix" will be discussed in Chapter 6 on treatment. This addresses the issue for an individual patient. The problem of the number and type of symptoms that predict therapeutic responsiveness remains to be studied. It is analogous to the question of which diagnostic criteria best predict the response of depression to somatic treatments.

NOTES

1. Some investigators have inquired about individuals who did not have problems as children but developed MBD symptoms in adult life. If they do exist, they are not common, and we have not studied them.

2. The Parents' Rating Scale (PRS) obviously has face validity, but more important, it has shown predictive validity. In a placebo-controlled study of pemoline (Wender et al., 1981), there was an interaction between PRS score and drug responsiveness. Patients in the 95th or higher percentile on the PRS experienced a statistically significant response to pemoline; patients with lower scores did not improve on the drug.

3. Nor the physiological manifestations of "atypical depression," hypersomnia, hyperphagia, and leaden lethargy—sleeping too much, eating too much, and feeling too tired to do anything.

4. This raises the interesting question of why the two are occurring conjointly at a much higher than predicted rate. If the prevalence of childhood ADHD is 5 to 10 percent, then 5 to 10 percent of the children with current major depression—not 25 percent—should have ADHD. Why? Some obvious answers are that ADHD can look like Major Affective Disorder (MAD) in children, that MAD in children can look like ADHD, that our diagnostic criteria are wrong, that there is assortative mating (of parents with MAD and ADHD), or that there is a disordered common metabolic pathway between ADHD and MAD.

5. Alcohol abuse and ASPD are more frequent among the relatives of CD and ADHD/CD children but not among the relatives of pure ADHD children. No one has investigated the frequency of these disorders in the subgroup of ADHD adults who had CD in childhood but did not go on to develop ASPD.

6. The others being teaching, governing, and practicing psychoanalysis.

7. Whether or not he qualifies for a *diagnosis* of CD "grown up"—ASPD.

8. This is one of my heterogeneous clinical rules (Wender's rules): "When confused about a child's diagnosis, diagnose by the parent's diagnosis, and vice versa."

9. Not only did we want "typical" "hyperactive" adults in our studies, but we also focused on patients whose symptoms were neither too mild nor too severe in order to maximize treatment effects. In mild cases, there is too little room for improvement; in severe cases, the patients may be less likely to respond (which jibes with the experiences of hyperactive *children*). We "stacked the cards in our favor"—which is acceptable if acknowledged. It was the strategy employed by Philip May in his classic, *The Treatment of Chronic Schizophrenia* (1968). In his study May chose patients with intermediate symp-

tomatic severity, because he wanted to compare several treatments (including psychotherapy alone, psychotherapy with drugs, drugs alone). The patients who were "not sick enough" might get well with any treatment, while those who were "too sick" would be unlikely to get better with any treatment. In practice, our patients' psychopathology on the Global Assessment Scale (Endicott et al., 1976) was usually in the range of 50 to 60 moderate to serious symptoms (or, in our patients, moderate to *any* serious impairment in social, occupational, or school functioning).

6

The Treatment of ADHD in Adults

■

The most effective treatment of the ADHD adult consists of education about his disorder, drug treatment, and psychotherapy focused on ADHD concomitants. Successful drug treatment must begin with education, which is necessary to the patient's understanding of his disorder. For this reason it will be discussed first, followed by a discussion of drug treatment. In the course of drug treatment I engage the patients collaboratively to observe the ways in which clear-cut biological problems produce secondary psychological problems. For these residual problems, which develop as (unsuccessful) attempts to compensate for or evade biological problems, specific psychological intervention may be helpful (support groups, couple treatment, etc.). I elaborate the kinds of educational psychotherapy that I use toward the end of the chapter.

EDUCATION OF THE ADULT ADHD PATIENT

■

Although medication is the main factor in my treatment of adults with ADHD, education and psychological management also play important roles, beginning with my first contact with the patient. Initially, I conduct a detailed, semi-structured interview of the patient, focusing on his "present illness." Since ADHD occurs in childhood, the history covers the signs and symptoms of ADHD as they have manifested themselves in early and late childhood, adolescence, and adulthood (as discussed in Chapter 5 on diagnosis). At the same time, I obtain a history of the patient's relationships—with parents, siblings, playmates, peers, teachers, bosses, sexual partners, "others," spouses, and offspring—and how they have been affected. For each major symptom of ADHD (e.g., inattentiveness, impulsivity, etc.) I try to obtain as many *concrete current* instances as possible. These will be among the target symptoms I will evaluate during treatment.

As part of the interview I obtain a family history, searching both for diagnoses and for the family resemblances, the psychological "flavor." The family history sometimes demonstrates to the patient that his ADHD problems (and ADHD-associated problems) "run" in his family and thus indicate that his ADHD may be genetic and have a biological basis. It also allows me to apply this principle: "Diagnose the patient by his relatives." If his history sounds very much like ADHD but everyone else in the family has touches of unipolar depression, I may rethink my diagnosis.

Education of the patient and, if present, his significant "other" constitutes the minimum goal of a consultation and is a mandatory basis of treatment. Until fairly recently, educating psychiatric patients about their disorders was sometimes considered déclassé. "Bibliotherapy" was, the psychodynamicists informed us, a maneuver by which patients could avoid the real basis of their problems. It was the defense of intellectualizing and was considered at best third-class treatment and at worst countertherapeutic. Psychiatrists now realize that many patients can benefit from learning about their condition. Such information is considered *de rigueur* by patients who belong to psychiatric support groups—for example, patients with mood disorders, panic disorder, and obsessive-compulsive disorder.

INITIAL CONSULTATIONS

I begin patients' education by telling them about the signs and symptoms of ADHD, emphasizing that different symptoms are more or less prominent in different people and that the pattern of symptoms may vary from person to person. On the basis of the symptoms we have discussed, I illustrate the form they have taken in the patient's life and suggest that we continue to examine them and their effects. In doing so, I often make comments of this kind: "Many but not all people with the temper problems you described do such and such . . . or cause their spouse to feel, to respond thus and so . . . ," or "I have seen a number of people who suddenly became aware of. . . . How does that make you feel?"

I am here not attempting to lead the patient. I am trying to expedite the collection of information. One of the beneficial side effects of so doing—anticipating the patient's symptoms or their consequences—is confirmation of the patient's expectation that you are an expert (Harry Stack Sullivan defined the psychiatric interview as an expert-client two-group [1954, p. 4]). Another is that your awareness of symptoms he has not told you about suggests that his problems really are identifiable and expectable, and are like symptoms of any other disease. Demonstrating knowledge of a patient's illness can often be reassuring to the patient even though the knowledge is of something undesirable. For example, inquiring of a patient who has very likely just experienced a "heart attack" whether the pain felt "crushing," whether the pain has moved down his left arm, or whether he broke into a sweat and leaned over can reassure the patient that the doctor understands what is happening.

After discussing his symptoms with him, I try to communicate the following points to the patient: (1) We regard ADHD as a hereditary disease, probably mediated by alterations in the functioning of the brain. (2) In a very large number of instances the symptoms can be suppressed by medication. (3) Psychological interventions are, to the best of our knowledge, ineffective in controlling the basic symptoms. (4) Some of the symptoms (such as affective lability) are obviously painful to the patient himself, while others (such as his "short fuse") obviously impair the relationship with his spouse; still others (such as disorganization and inconsistency) may generate friction with his children or produce problems at work. (5) His awareness of the ADHD symptoms he manifests will enable us to gauge the effectiveness of drug treatment and allow him to understand both the direct and the indirect effects they have had on his life.

I try to separate the patient's ADHD core symptoms from other problems he is currently experiencing that may have been generated by the symptoms. I also try to separate these from two other sources of human unhappiness: learned maladaptation and reality. It is important to recognize that the ADHD symptoms may generate secondary symptoms that persist even when the ADHD symptoms are gone (as in the "functional autonomy" described by Gordon Allport [1937]). In some patients these secondary problems resolve fairly quickly; in others, slowly. The situation is analogous, I tell them, to that of a person who breaks his leg and has a cast put on, which stays on for several weeks. A few months later the bone may be as good as—or better than—new, but while the bone has been taking care of itself, his muscles may have been atrophying. When the cast is removed, his leg may be weak. Strength may come back simply by using it, but if this is not enough, physical therapy may help him to regain function more rapidly. Similarly, counseling or "therapy" (broadly construed) may help the ADHD patient to unlearn "habits," behavioral patterns and attitudes that had developed as a result of and in response to his ADHD. Accordingly, if medication, counseling, and possibly psychotherapy are effective, he may be relieved of additional painful and self-engendered unhappiness with his family.

I ask all patients about problems they may have had and may continue to have in reading, spelling, and arithmetic computation. If they had or have such problems, I discuss "learning problems" and dyslexia. Many adult ADHD patients experienced considerable difficulty in school, are poor readers and spellers, have had trouble with arithmetic, and have considered themselves to be stupid. I explain that they aren't dumb but have a poorly understood condition that is not a sign of being retarded (many recall having had that label applied to them). This can be a huge relief. I remember one very bright, depressed 15-year-old who had an immediate elevation in her mood when she was diagnosed as dyslexic. Her mood lifted further when she called all her friends to report, "I'm not dumb, I'm dyslexic."

All of this material is explained at a level appropriate for the patient's background and education, and in all instances, I try to tie it to concrete examples chosen from his history. I inform him of what I propose to do, how long the various components of the treatment should last, and how he and I (and often his significant "other") will determine how he is progressing. It should be obvious that the preceding catalogue of possible human woes does not apply to all ADHD patients, and that it should be varied in terms of individual differences. It is also important to introduce the material at a rate that the patient can accommodate and digest.

EDUCATION ABOUT DRUG THERAPY

Having reviewed the nature of the illness, I turn to a discussion of the drug treatment itself. Many patients who have been referred to me expect drug treatment. A few do not want to take drugs and want to see if they can manage their problems through some form of psychotherapy. To those I emphasize that in my experience it does not decrease the central ADHD problems, but that if it does, they are "home free." If it doesn't work, they are free to call me—I am not leaving town.

In discussing drug treatment with a patient, my approach varies in terms of the type of patient and how he or she reached my office. Before describing the content of my discussion of drugs with the patient, I will describe here several types of patients.

The Patient Referred by His ADHD Child's Physician

Many patients who appear under their own steam do so on the basis of a referral from their child's physician, who probably has asked if either parent used to have similar symptoms when he or she was a child. In many instances this question is answered by a spouse who responds, "What do you mean, used to have?" In some instances the parent in question has already consulted with his parents or other caretaker in childhood about *his* behavior as a child.

This patient is obviously the easiest to deal with. He recognizes that he has problems, believes that they are ADHD problems, and readily accepts the hypothesis that ADHD is a hereditary disorder, mediated by differences in biological processes (unknown) in the brain and frequently responsive to medical treatment. The only important point to make to the patient is a cautionary one. The patient may have reported ADHD-like problems (concentration difficulty, irritability, etc.) and he may have been correct in referring himself, but he may be incorrect in his self-diagnosis. He may have a major depression accompanied by concentration difficulties, irritability, etc. All that is required of the diagnostician is that he bears this possibility in mind.

The Unwilling or Doubtful Patient

Unwilling or doubtful patients resemble to some degree ADHD children brought by their parents. Such a child often perceives his visit to a psychiatrist as a punishment for various misbehaviors and failings, academic and otherwise, many of which he does not acknowledge or, if he does, feels have been exaggerated. The child psychiatrist has to work with the family and the child to convey to the child that there are problems, that he is the child's friend, and that he will be working with the child to make him happier—that the psychiatrist is not an agent of his parents empowered to punish him, quite possibly with drugs.

Similarly, patients referred by an importunate spouse (sometimes with the support of a minister, sibling, or other family member) often deny the existence of problems. Often the spouse has made the diagnosis of "hyperactivity" and wants treatment because, for example, "He is harsh and inconsistent with the children. I can't take any more. If he doesn't get help I'm going to leave." If these quasi-coerced potential patients do acknowledge problems, I tell them that the first order of business for us will be to sort out what the symptoms are. I mention that there are psychiatric look-alikes and that the diagnosis of ADHD is not a foregone conclusion. If the symptoms indicate ADHD, we will also decide whether they are serious enough to warrant treatment.

The Patient Referred by a Nonphysician Therapist

Sometimes a patient is referred for "medical management" by a nonphysician therapist. The implication of such a referral is that the central problems are being handled by the current psychotherapist and that pharmacotherapy may temporarily control the patient's symptoms and enable him to derive even greater benefits from psychotherapy. As I have mentioned, ADHD can engender secondary psychological problems, but often the ADHD patient has been referred *for core ADHD symptoms* that the psychotherapist is mistakenly treating. In this instance, the psychiatrist must convey to the patient that many of his major symptoms indicate the presence of ADHD and are likely to respond best to medication. I educate him in the same manner that I do other patients, pointing out that symptoms that are not "cardinal ADHD symptoms" may indirectly be the consequence of those symptoms, and that some of them may gradually disappear as the basic symptoms are controlled by medication. I leave the door open for my psychotherapeutic colleague by using the "broken leg" analogy—that is, that residual problems that developed consequent to the underlying medical problems may profit by psychotherapy.

Treatment with Medication: Pros and Cons, Costs and Benefits

For patients who agree to try medication, I provide a brief course in applied psychopharmacology. Since there is a lot to communicate and a lot to be learned by the patient, I have transcribed my talk so the patients can review this material at their leisure. The information for adults grew out of my work with hyperactive children. The longer I was in the business of educating parents, the longer my presentation became. Eventually, the elaborated material became a concise book (Wender, 1987). The important points about medication are:

1. Treatment is symptomatic, not curative: Treatment suppresses or controls the symptoms but does not eliminate their underlying cause(s). I point out to patients that this is usually the case in the medicinal treatment of disease. We do not cure epilepsy but give anticonvulsants; we do not cure high blood pressure but give antihypertensives; and so forth.

2. We have a number of effective medications. It is impossible to determine beforehand which will be most effective for any particular patient, and finding the best medication may require trying several. Failure to find the "right" drug right away does not reflect ineptitude in the physician.

3. The stimulants are still the most effective drugs in the treatment of ADHD in children and adults. Though stimulants may be abusable by non-ADHD people, drug abuse is not a problem in the doses we prescribe. Nevertheless, many patients feel that the prescription of stimulants (or other medication) will cause them to develop an addiction. In discussing drug dependence, I distinguish between abusive psychoactive drug dependence and obligatory medical dependence, such as that of the diabetic on insulin or of the person with pernicious anemia on vitamin B12.

4. I also address the subtle concern of many patients about "chemical control." This is the concern, hard to articulate, that drug treatment will somehow impair their freedom of will. This is reminiscent of the concern expressed by ostensible "protectors" of children that Ritalin was being prescribed as a chemical straitjacket to contain the naturally ebullient spirits of young children reacting to a repressive educational system. I make two points: First, many patients with ADHD report that medication has given them more freedom, because they are no longer the victims of uncontrollable moods or temper, impulsive decision-making, and so forth. Second, the decision to take medication is not irrevocable and binding for life; if they wish, they can discontinue medication at any time and see how they do without it.

The pros and cons of medical treatment can be summarized in the following *payoff matrix*.

The payoff matrix weighs *the risk of treating with medication and the risk of not treating with medication* those patients whose ADHD diagnosis (by our arbitrary Utah Criteria) may be uncertain. The important question for the patient, and one which should be addressed at the outset, is what the advantages and disadvantages are of the four possibilities:

1. The patient has ADHD and is treated with medication.
2. The patient does not have ADHD and is treated with medication.
3. The patient does have ADHD and is not treated with medication.
4. The patient does not have ADHD and is not treated with medication.

I explore each of these four possibilities.

1. The patient has ADHD and is treated with medication. Here a patient has a 60 percent (or more) chance of obtaining an immediate and substantial reduction in or disappearance of his primary symptoms. He can also anticipate that, in time, his secondary symptoms will decrease, so that altogether he can look forward to noticeable improvements in his life. The changes in primary symptoms can lead to such direct effects as reduction or elimination of restlessness, moodiness, and anger. As the secondary symptoms abate, the patient may see such indirect effects as an increased ability to cope with stress and to solve problems, and improved relationships with others at school, on the job, as a partner, as a parent, and so forth.

Such benefits must be weighed against the *possible* physiological toxicity from long-term administration of drugs. The amphetamines have been used for more than 50 years and are very rarely allergenic, but they do increase heart rate and they often increase blood pressure. As mentioned earlier, if stimulants are the most effective agents for a particular patient and if they increase blood pressure to an undesirable degree, the physician *may* want to continue to use them and add antihypertensive medication. There may be a parallel problem with tricyclic antidepressants, which can have similar cardiac effects. They increase heart rate, and although they usually produce *hypotension*, in some patients they produce hypertension. If the patient wants continuing control of his symptoms, we must often administer these drugs for years. On the other hand, patients have told me that when treated with stimulant medication they have been able to change patterns that were physiologically detrimental, substituting healthier ones, for example, changes in diet and exercise (initiating jogging), drinking less or stopping smoking, and driving less recklessly. Such reports, of course, are only anecdotal.

2. The patient does not have ADHD and receives stimulant medica-

tion. If he does not like stimulants, there is little problem, because he will probably soon stop taking them. But what if he does like stimulants? How likely is he to become an iatrogenic (the creation of additional problems resulting from the activity of physicians) stimulant abuser? How can one know? If he initially has a "good" response, finds that he works more effectively (has a slight elevation of mood), and gradually becomes tolerant to the therapeutic drug effects, one may have to worry. Situation "2" is the one of concern to the physician. Tolerance to the medication does not always indicate nonADHD because some ADHD children and adults initially experience *mild* tolerance; when the medication is increased, they become stable and do not require further increases. An experienced physician should be able— *almost* always—to determine if the patient's response is a typical ADHD patient's response. Sometimes he will not be able to do so, since there are non-ADHD adults with a variety of psychiatric problems who continue to benefit from continued treatment with amphetamines (Chiarello and Cole, 1987). The physician may have to be content with benefiting the patient even if he cannot be sure of the diagnosis.

3. The patient has ADHD and is not treated with medication. As one frustrated psychotherapist said, ADHD patients who are untreated "are able to screw up their lives in ways I never thought of." Not treating a potential responder with medication is doing the ADHD patient a disservice.

4. The patient does not have ADHD and does not receive treatment with stimulant medication. Fine.

The physician can quickly determine whether or not the patient responds to stimulants, and the physiological risks for a brief trial are minimal. But the physician's personal payoff matrix also plays a role in treatment. The failure—or reluctance—to offer patients a trial of the amphetamines or methylphenidate often does not have a *scientific* basis but is related to the fact that these are Schedule II drugs; physicians are afraid to prescribe them not because of concern about toxicity or producing an iatrogenic addiction but because of the regulatory agencies. However, just as it is possible to employ methadone in a special administrative setting, it should be possible to work out a method of dispensing stimulants to ADHD adults that will relieve physicians of this extraneous concern. Comparably effective drugs would never be used so sparingly in internal medicine.

DRUG TREATMENT

■

The drug treatment of ADHD, with stimulants and with other medications, is of both practical and theoretical importance. The practical importance of stimulant medication is that, as with children, it frequently produces a near complete remission of symptoms. In psychiatry and in other branches of medicine, drug treatment usually restores a patient's functioning to the *status quo ante*. However, drug-responsive adult ADHD patients (like children with ADHD) often function better than they ever have in their lives. Long-term treatment of patients responsive to stimulants often produces major changes in scholastic, vocational, and personal functioning. When the stimulant drugs are effective, the ADHD individual may experience a temporary period of psychological maturation. Stimulant medication appears to be working at a very early point in the etiological chain. Still another advantage of medication is related to the fact that ADHD patients may have other psychiatric disorders. ADHD sometimes conceals such disorders, and the successful treatment of ADHD symptoms may reveal them. Attention can then also be directed at their psychological and biological treatment.

In these instances drug treatment almost appears to be replacement therapy—as if administration of, for example, amphetamine were correcting "congenital hypoamphetaminemia" secondary to hypoplasia of an imaginary gland. When drug treatment is effective, it is analogous to giving vitamin C to a patient with scurvy. This contrasts with treatments that remedy secondary effects (treating pneumococcal pneumonia with penicillin) or tertiary effects of a disease (e.g., treating complications of hypertension, such as myocardial infarction and congestive failure, with antihypertensives, diuretics, and digitalis).

The response to stimulant drugs is of theoretical interest because of the presumed mechanism of action of these drugs. The drugs increase dopaminergic (and possibly noradrenergic) activity, which leads to the hypothesis that decreased dopaminergic or noradrenergic functioning plays a role in the etiology of ADHD, as discussed in Chapter 4 on etiology.

Before discussing the practical clinical aspects of drug treatment, I will first review the studies of drug treatment in ADHD adults. I will also include the few related studies on adolescents, which provide supportive data.

STUDIES OF DRUG TREATMENT
IN ADHD ADULTS

The use of stimulants in the treatment of ADHD-like problems in adults was first reported by Hill in 1947, ten years after Bradley's (1937) report on the behavior of children receiving benzedrine. Hill decided to use amphetamine with eight "adult psychopaths" because "it seemed possible that the predominantly aggressive psychopath . . . developed from the same constitutional background as the behaviour problem child extensively studied by the Canadian and American workers" (p. 50), and because he and his colleagues had "immediate success" in the treatment of such children. The adult patients Hill reported most likely to respond were characterized as aggressive, bad-tempered, responding hostilely whenever they encountered frustration, impulsively irritable, fickle, irresponsible, inclined to moral lapses, *but also* (and this distinguishes them from the usual concept of a "psychopath") as "capable of warm interpersonal relationships." Additional symptoms included "motiveless petty pilfering" and alcoholism. Secondary consequences of their behavior were loss of jobs and ruined friendships and marriages. Hill's report is somewhat unclear, but it appears that his eight patients had a diminution in their symptoms with treatment and that the favorable drug response was maintained for "over four years." Three of the eight had problems with alcoholism, petty theft, and arson. All "remitted completely after amphetamine therapy was started."

Although Zimmerman and Burgemeister reported in 1958 that methylphenidyl acetate (Ritalin) might be effective in the treatment of adult "behavior disorders," the usefulness of amphetamines in treating some adult "behavior disorders" seems to have been totally forgotten until the 1970s, when case reports began to appear. In all instances the patients discussed had not been diagnosed in childhood. The patients described are heterogeneous, and their clinical pictures vary—which is not surprising because of the primitive stage of nosology at that time. Arnold, Strobl, and Weisenbert (1972) described a 22-year-old "hyperkinetic" man whose restlessness and anxiety were decreased by D-amphetamine but whose depression was worsened. The authors pointed out the usefulness of studying "hyperactive adults," who could provide better reports of subjective changes than children could. Huessy (1974) reported anecdotally on his successful use of stimulants and tricyclic antidepressants in a group of adult patients with histories of childhood hyperactivity and with prominent adult symptoms of impulsivity and emotional overreactivity (but some of these patients had been diagnosed as schizophrenic). Mann and Greenspan (1976) described two cases of "adult brain dysfunction," one of whom was described as "hyper" in childhood and both of whom responded to small doses of imipramine.

The uncontrolled studies are obviously only suggestive. Controlled experimental studies are necessary to demonstrate scientifically the effects of medication on the symptoms of persisting ADHD.

In discussing the findings of the systematic studies of drug treatment of ADHD in adults, I describe the drug studies summarized in Table 6.1 (which is at the end of the chapter) and begin with the work done by my research group at the University of Utah.

Our group has conducted three placebo-controlled trials of stimulant medication in adults with ADHD, and is now involved in a fourth. Overall, about 50 to 60 percent of the adult patients in the first three studies experienced moderate-to-marked improvement in their symptoms in response to one or another drug. I should emphasize that we have employed methylphenidate rather then D-amphetamine or methamphetamine in our crossover trials. As discussed below, methylphenidate is not superior to the amphetamines, but it currently is the prototype drug for the treatment of ADHD.

It is important to emphasize at the outset that our patients have been drawn from a population with a number of unique features. Virtually all our patients were of Anglo Saxon ancestry, were native born with English as their first language, and were high school graduates. More than half of our patients were active members of The Church of Jesus Christ of Latter Day Saints (Mormon) and obeyed their religious proscription to abstain from alcohol, tobacco, and drugs.

Our first study (Wood et al., 1976) consisted of a trial of a number of medications, including methylphenidate and pemoline, in a sample of 15 adults with "minimal brain dysfunction" (MBD). In this group, most had received unsuccessful trials of drug therapy (tricyclic antidepressants). Five of the responsive patients had previously received individual or couple therapy without appreciable benefit. All who participated in the study appeared to have had prominent MBD symptoms in childhood and manifested what appeared to be adult metamorphoses of the childhood symptoms. Two-thirds of them were retrospectively characterized by their parents in a way that placed them in the 95th percentile of childhood "hyperactivity"—the approximate cutoff point used in drug studies of MBD children. Eleven of 15 patients were given a random assignment, double-blind, placebo-controlled trial of methylphenidate, and the other 4 were given open trials of methylphenidate or pemoline.

Eight of the 11 double-blind patients experienced moderate or marked improvement and an obvious decrease in symptoms, and 2 others manifested a good response later. The patients who responded to treatment with methylphenidate manifested a drug response similar to that seen in ADHD children. The effects on target symptoms were the same: there were decreases in restlessness and attentional problems, depression and lability of mood, irritability, hot temper and impulsivity, and the patients became more effective in organizing their lives and solving practical life problems. They did not experience euphoria with the doses of methylphenidate employed (up to a maximum of 60 milligrams per day), and they did not develop tolerance to methylphenidate's effects—in contrast to the tolerance seen in adult abusers. Those who responded to stimulants maintained their improvement at their last follow-up, which represented an average of 13 months of treatment. Their *lives* had been significantly benefited, which was especially heartening because patients with these personality traits and diagnoses are generally considered refractory to psychological therapies.

The important question that remained was whether we had *demonstrated* a selective therapeutic response to methylphenidate or whether we had found that administering a euphoriant to a heterogeneous group of unhappy people had made them feel better. A critic might have argued that our results were similar to those we might have obtained if we had treated patients who suffered from realistic life difficulties with alcohol or heroin. In a sense the question is a pseudo-question because our patients manifested continued benefit in a large number of areas and, unlike abusers, continued to maintain the same response to the same doses of methylphenidate.

In another study we examined the effects of pemoline, a Schedule IV drug[1] with minimal "street value." The purpose of the pemoline study (Wender et al., 1981) was to address three methodological weaknesses in the first study: (1) The absence of specific diagnostic criteria for "minimal brain dysfunction" in adults; (2) the uncertainty of the childhood diagnosis of "minimal brain dysfunction"; and (3) the use of methylphenidate, a euphoriant drug that can be and has been abused.

To address these problems we planned to: (1) establish more specific diagnostic criteria; (2) obtain norms for the measure of childhood hyperactivity, the Parents' Rating Scale (PRS); and (3) employ a stimulant drug, pemoline, which has been shown to be effective in hyperactive children and which has not been considered a euphoriant in normals (Dren et al., 1971; Schuster et al., 1969; Wilson and Hitomi, 1969).

The inclusion criteria in the pemoline study were that the patient had manifested a history of longstanding inattentiveness *or* restlessness or both,[2] impulsivity, irritability, and emotional lability. The presence of *both* prominent hyperactivity and inattentiveness was not mandatory nor was it mandatory to have both symptoms in childhood *and* adulthood. The current Utah Criteria require the continuing presence of *both* symptoms. We attempted to obtain the PRS on all of our subjects, but the PRS was evaluated in a nonpatient population only after the study had begun.

We conducted a six-week, random-assignment parallel trial of pemoline and placebo in 48 patients. An initial examination of the data showed no difference in outcome between pemoline and placebo. When the PRS data were analyzed, we found that only 54 percent of the subjects had a score that placed them in the 95th percentile of "hyperactivity." A *post hoc* analysis of this subgroup (the "true hyperactives") revealed that slightly less than half of these patients experienced moderate-to-marked improvement on the Physician's Global Assessment of Change on pemoline while only one patient experienced such a response in the placebo condition.

Since the pemoline study showed treatment effects only on the basis of a *post hoc* analysis, we decided to conduct a study introducing several modifications (Wender et al., 1985). First, we made the Utah Criteria more restrictive, requiring the combined presence of *both* restlessness and inattentiveness in and since childhood. Second, we made the *ante hoc* prediction that a "high" rating on the PRS scale (a percentile score > 95) would be a predictor of greater drug responsiveness. Third, based on our experience in the pemoline study, we made the presence of an "other" as informant a necessary inclusion criterion. Fourth, we decided to employ methylphenidate rather than pemoline, because our clinical experience had been that methylphenidate was tolerated better (had a lower incidence of side effects), that the drug response was immediate rather than delayed, as often occurred with pemoline, and that a greater percentage of patients responded to methylphenidate than to pemoline.

Thirty-seven patients were entered into a random-assignment, double-blind, placebo-controlled crossover trial of methylphenidate and placebo, with each trial lasting two weeks. On the Physician's Global Rating Scale, 57 percent of the patients experienced moderate-to-marked improvement on methylphenidate while only 11 percent of those on placebo did so. On the Physician's Target Symptom Scale (hyperactivity, short attention span, disorganization, depression, and anger), the patients improved significantly. The degree of clinical improvement was probably best captured by the Global Assessment Scale. In the 21 patients showing a moderate-to-marked response to methylphenidate, the mean pretreatment Global Assessment Scale score was 59 ("moderate symptoms . . . generally functioning with some difficulty, e.g., few friends . . . depressed mood and pathological self-doubt . . . moderately severe antisocial behavior"); their average posttreatment Global Assessment Scale score was 76 ("minimal symptoms or no more than slight impairment in functioning"). Significant differences between methylphenidate and placebo conditions were also detected on the Profile of Mood States (POMS): The patients reported significantly less tension-anxiety, depression-dejection, anger-hostility, confusion, and fatigue during treatment with methylphenidate than in the placebo condition.

These three drug studies were of brief trials of medication, but because ADHD is a chronic disorder, we had no systematic data about its long-term effectiveness. On the basis of informally following many of these patients and other, nonstudy patients over many years, we have observed two important phenomena. First, almost all stimulant responders did not appear to become tolerant to those medications; second, if the drug relieved or diminished their ADHD symptoms, they made gradual but substantial improvements in psychological, academic, and vocational functioning and in their relationships with parents, spouses, "others," and children. The changes in their long-term psychological functioning were related to those that they experienced daily: restlessness diminished, concentration improved, labile mood stabilized, and temper and irascibility decreased. They learned to postpone gratification; they handled stress more effectively; and when tasks demanded it, they became focused and persistent. They organized their offices and households more efficiently and became less impulsive; they received A's and B's at college rather than flunking or dropping out; they stayed at their jobs and got promoted rather than quitting or being fired; and household managers were often able to function effectively both at home and in part-time or *full*-time work outside the home. Personal relationships gradually improved; spouses established better equilibria; and ADHD parents learned to handle their frequently ADHD children. These observations were provocative but of course not scientifically compelling. We were observing the numerator, but not the denominator; our follow-ups were nonsystematic, and we may have been following the successes while the failures dropped out.

Our long-term observations needed to be tested, since there may have been several reasons why the patients succeeded. First, they may not have had ADHD at all. We may have misdiagnosed them, and the other condition may have spontaneously remitted without any relationship to the stimulant medication. Second, we might have treated them for what *we* thought was a chronic problem but what was in fact a temporary perturbation; if so, we attributed their recovery, as doctors often do, to our ministrations—*post hoc ergo propter hoc*—but the medication may have functioned as nothing more than an active placebo. Third, our "successes" may have initially responded to drug treatment, but by the time they became tolerant to their medication, they may have learned new adaptive habits that combined with nonspecific, unplanned effects of the reality-oriented and supportive contacts of our medication management. Finally, stimulant treatment may indeed have produced the benefits we observed—the medication may have continued to relieve their symptoms and to improve their behavior, allowing delayed normal psychological growth to occur, which in turn elicited "normal" and "better" responses from the real world—a "virtuous cycle."

To try to sort out these possible causes, we undertook a long-term study (Wender et al., in preparation) on a sample of 120 ADHD adults who met our current diagnostic criteria for ADHD, and who experienced a moderate-to-marked improvement on a placebo-controlled trial of methylphenidate. We followed these patients for a minimum of one year in order to answer two questions. The first was whether a favorable response to stimulants persists—that is, whether or not adults with ADHD become refractory to drug treatment with methylphenidate. Almost all the patients continued to do well but a possibility existed that the disease had remitted during treatment and no longer required medication. To test this possibility we divided our group of patients (double blind) who responded well to methylphenidate into one subset in which the medication was maintained at the same level or another subset in which the medication was gradually tapered. When symptoms recurred in the group receiving tapered medication, at their pretreatment severity, we interpreted that to mean that the drug therapy was still effective. Our analysis to date has shown that those subjects in whom the methylphenidate was tapered reexperienced—with equal severity—the same symptoms that they had had before they had been treated with methylphenidate.

The second question was to what extent drug-responding patients experience improvement in interpersonal and occupational functioning. Such improvements were assessed by independent raters who evaluated the patients every six months with a structured interview schedule, the Social Adjustment Scale. We found that the patients receiving methylphenidate experienced a moderate-to-marked improvement in interpersonal and occupational functioning.

Two other groups of investigators have conducted placebo-controlled studies of the treatment of adult ADHD with methylphenidate (Mattes et al., 1984; Gualtieri et al., 1985). Mattes et al. did what is by far the larger of the two studies. They initiated their research with several goals: (1) to determine whether adults with putative MBD responded more favorably to methylphenidate than placebo; (2) to determine "whether [methylphenidate response] reflects nonspecific effect of the drug, or a specific drug-diagnosis interaction"; (3) to determine if there was a difference between drug response in subjects with both adult and childhood symptoms of ADD (the experimental group) and drug response in those with adult ADD symptoms but without the childhood ones (the control group).

Mattes et al. entered the 66 subjects (33 men, 33 women) in a double-blind, crossover trial of methylphenidate and placebo. Each trial lasted three weeks. Although the authors found a trend ($p < .07$) for the subjects with a history of ADD in childhood to respond more favorably to treatment with methylphenidate, overall there were no significant drug-placebo differences, except for a psychiatrist-rated decrease in impulsivity with the drug. Unlike the Wender et al. study (1985) of methylphenidate, there were no differences in Profile-of-Mood-States ratings between the methylphenidate and placebo results. The authors' major conclusion was that they were unable to confirm "the existence of a group of adult psychiatric patients with residual ADD who respond to stimulants" (p. 1062).

Because this is the largest attempt at replication by an independent group of researchers, it is important to discuss several reasons that may account for their failure to observe stimulant-treatment effects. There are differences in the sample, their diagnostic criteria, and the method of assessment that may cast light on the difference between their overall results and those of the Utah group. First, their subjects differed from ours in an important aspect: their scores on the Parents' Rating

Scale (PRS), which is a measure of childhood "hyperactivity." They judged only 41 percent of their subjects to have been definitely or very likely to have had ADHD in childhood. In their study, the mean PRS scores for presumptive ADD adults with and without a childhood history of ADD-H were 10.7 and 6.7, respectively; 7 of 29 (24 percent) of those clinically diagnosed with childhood ADD had a PRS score >12. These figures are critically important because in the pemoline study we found that only subjects with scores of 12 or higher (the 95th percentile or higher) showed a therapeutic response to pemoline.

The Utah Criteria exclude individuals suffering from current major depression, Borderline Personality Disorder (BPD) and Borderline Personality Disorder traits, and current alcohol and drug abuse. Mattes et al.'s exclusion criteria did not. Mattes et al. provide total diagnoses only (each patient could have more than one). The sample includes patients with substance abuse, 35 percent; Borderline Personality Disorder, 24 percent; and major depression, 29 percent. Of the 7 patients with PRS scores in the 95th percentile, 3 would be excluded by the Utah Criteria—that is, of their 66 subjects only 4 met our current diagnostic criteria.

There are two other possible sources of error. First was the use of less sensitive techniques of evaluation. We found that patients' ratings of ADHD symptoms were often insensitive as compared with those of "others" living with the patient (see Wender et al., 1981). Such informants apparently were not employed in this study. Lastly, they gave methylphenidate in two daily divided doses. Our experience is that most subjects require four to six divided doses and that b.i.d. (2 doses per day) dosing controls symptoms for half or less of the day.

Gualtieri et al. (1985) reported on the effects of methylphenidate in eight men who were participating in a group of studies investigating biological and psychological correlates of ADHD. No formal childhood or adult diagnostic criteria are cited. The subjects received a twice-daily fixed dose of methylphenidate for five days and of placebo for five days. All eight were reported to respond favorably to methylphenidate during the brief trial but not in a three to six-month follow-up. It is impossible to draw any conclusions from this small sample since the authors do not report patient diagnoses, adjustment of the drug regimen, frequency of follow-up meetings, and so forth.

Although, as our studies show, the stimulants are effective in the treatment of adult ADHD, they are not ideal. First, since they are Schedule II drugs, physicians are apprehensive about prescribing them, fearing investigation by state and federal licensure agencies if they prescribe them to a substantial number of patients. Second, they are not long-acting. Patients are without pharmacological control before their morning dose has taken effect, and to avoid insomnia they must take their last dose several hours before bedtime, which means that as the drug effects wear off, they may reexperience their symptoms. We, therefore, decided to investigate certain monoamine oxidase inhibitors (MAOIs) because they have a long duration of action and because they are not scheduled. We selected pargyline (Wender et al., 1983) and L-deprenyl (Wood et al., 1983) because in low doses both (particularly deprenyl) are believed to be relatively pure MAO-B inhibitors (Murphy, 1978; Pickar et al., 1982), which we hypothesized might be specifically effective in the treatment of ADHD (see Chapter 4 on etiology). In addition, deprenyl in low doses appears to have little or no "cheese effect" (the MAOI side effect in which a sudden rise in blood pressure accompanies the eating of certain foods) and so might prove useful in impulsive patients who might not adhere to a rigid dietary regimen.

We administered pargyline to 22 patients, 6 of whom dropped out because of side effects. Pargyline produced moderate-to-marked improvement in 68 percent of the remaining 16 patients. Patients were maintained and their symptoms controlled by pargyline for periods of up to seven years, during which they developed a gradual tolerance that could be overcome by increasing doses.

We administered L-deprenyl (now selegiline) to 11 patients for a period of up to twelve weeks. Two dropped out because of side effects. L-deprenyl produced moderate-to-marked improvement in 6 of 11 cases (55 percent) but produced annoying side effects in all instances and no patients wished to stay on it. This was very probably a result of excessive dosing (an average of 30 milligrams and up to 50 milligrams a day; we would recommend trials of 5 to 15 milligrams a day). Use of L-deprenyl has also been reported by Jankovic (1993), who used it in the treatment of ADHD associated with Tourette's syndrome in 29 children (ages 6 to 18). Ninety percent were reported to experience moderate or greater improvement on doses of 5 to 15 milligrams a day (and tics were aggravated in only 2). Further trials of L-deprenyl are warranted because it appears to be effective, its effects are relatively long-lasting, and possibly (this must be fully documented) dietary restrictions can be less stringent for patients on the lower doses.

Zametkin et al. (1985) reported on the treatment of 14 ADD boys in a double-blind, placebo-controlled, crossover trial of D-amphetamine and either of these MAOIs: clorgyline, a MAO-A inhibitor, or tranylcypromine, an inhibitor of MAO-A and MAO-B. They reported that the stimulants and MAOIs were equally effective. Since the number of subjects was small, there is the recurrent problem of a Type II error—failing to detect an actual difference. Another problem is that the study covered a short period. We had reported that the two MAO-B inhibitors pargyline and L-deprenyl were effective in ADHD adults but that the response to pargyline decreased over time; in contrast, it is our experience that few patients become tolerant to stimulants.

Another ostensibly long-acting nonstimulant that we elected to try was bupropion (Wender and Reimherr, 1990), an antidepressant. It is a unique antidepressant (an aminoketone) since its mechanism of action has been hypothesized to be dopaminergic (Cooper et al., 1980). Although it is currently marketed as an antidepressant, earlier trials had shown it to be effective in some ADHD children. We conducted an open clinical trial of 19 ADHD adults who had previously shown a moderate-to-marked response to stimulants $(N = 16)$ and monoamine oxidase inhibitors $(N = 3)$ and who had been maintained on these drugs for an average of 3.7 years (range 9 months to 11 years). Five patients could not tolerate the lowest dose of bupropion (150 milligrams a day). Of the remaining 14, 8 showed marked benefit and 6 moderate benefit; 10 of these (71 percent) chose to continue on bupropion.

Bupropion appeared to have a fairly rapid onset of action—within days or a few weeks (as compared with the prolonged latency—4 to 6 weeks—of traditional antidepressants and the serotonergic specific reuptake inhibitors in the treatment of major depression). In some patients all seven of the target symptoms were controlled, while in others only mood and temper were improved. Overall bupropion seemed to be most effective in controlling or eliminating temper and mood problems. It appeared to be less effective in the treatment of concentration difficulties, hyperactivity, hyperreactivity, disorganization, and impulsivity, although the latter symptoms were controlled in some patients. In my own clinical experience some patients seem to benefit most from combined therapy of a stimulant and this drug.

In the treatment of ADHD with the precursor amino acids (L-dopa, DL-phenylalanine, and L-tyrosine) (Wood et al., 1982, 1985; Reimherr et al., 1987) neither DL-phenylalanine nor L-dopa produced sustained therapeutic effects. In an open trial of L-tyrosine on 12 patients, 2 experienced marked and 6 moderate improvement within one to four weeks, but all quickly developed tolerance by eight weeks. Because toxicity has been described in chronic administration, the use of larger doses is not warranted. We have no data on whether these amino acids would be synergistic or would amplify the effects of the other drugs mentioned.

The last report on drug treatment of ADHD in adults that I would like to review is that of Hans Huessy and his colleagues (Huessy et al., 1979), who have reported their uncontrolled clinical experience in the drug treatment of a large number of patients with "minimal brain dysfunction" over many years.

Huessy's report summarized the findings of drug trials on the first 64 (32 male, 32 female) of over 200 patients with "minimal brain dysfunction." The patients treated were much sicker than those we have studied. Eighty percent of them had one or more admissions to psychiatric hospitals, and "many" were drawn from a private residential therapeutic community. The sample was diagnostically heterogeneous, and the concept of MBD very broad. Less than half had "histories suggestive of MBD," so that half the sample would certainly not be currently diagnosed as having met DSM-III or DSM-III-R criteria for adult ADHD (for which childhood ADHD is a mandatory criterion). Comorbidity included schizophrenia, 53 percent; "depressive disorders," 25 percent; "CNS organicity," 14 percent. The men were characterized by antisocial behavior and aggressive acts, the women by suicidal gestures and mood swings. The most common signs and symptoms included impulsivity, temper outbursts, emotional overreactivity, distractibility, mood swings, hyperactivity, and drug and alcohol abuse. Huessy had his own criteria for "minimal brain dysfunction," which do not include a childhood history of ADHD. He defines MBD as consisting of a "basic triad" of emotional overreaction, emotional lability, and impulsivity, and states that evidence of any of the three, if interfering with performance (and no matter what their other diagnoses), "warrants a trial of medication" (Huessy et al., 1979, p. 21). The drugs his group employed were the stimulants and, more frequently, the tricyclic antidepressants (TCAs). They prescribed amitriptyline and imipramine in low doses (as little as 5 to 10 milligrams a day of imipramine), and they suggest that both be tried because they feel some patients may respond to one and not the other, and that the treatment response is immediate (as with children). They do not comment on the drugs' long-term effectiveness, although it is my experience that tolerance to the TCAs usually develops in initially drug-responsive ADHD children.

In this report, all trials of medication were open. Responses were evaluated clinically. Approximately 50 percent had a "positive response" to imipramine, amitriptyline, D-amphetamine or methylphenidate. The magnitude of the responses was apparently substantial.

The authors state: "We look for just as dramatic a response in adults as we have seen in children" (p. 28).

Although the sample was diagnostically heterogeneous, the authors' results warrant systematic evaluation since they claim that half of a sample with severe and persistent ADHD-like psychopathology—patients who did not respond to other treatment—responded to treatment with the tricyclic antidepressants or stimulants, or both.

DRUG TREATMENT OF ADHD IN ADOLESCENCE

During the years since we published our 1976 paper on the treatment of "minimal brain dysfunction" in adults, child psychiatrists have increasingly recognized that ADHD persists into adolescence and that ADHD adolescents exhibit the same drug responses as ADHD children. These studies constitute an empirical bridge and increase the plausibility of the results of our studies. The following are the more important studies.

Biederman et al. (1989) conducted a placebo-controlled trial of desipramine (DMI) in 31 children and adolescents (ages 6 to 17), 69 percent of whom had not responded to stimulants, and reported that 68 percent of the patients receiving DMI and 10 percent of those receiving placebo were much or very much improved. Kaplan et al. (1990) conducted a placebo-controlled trial of methylphenidate in 9 adolescent boys (average age 14) with both Conduct Disorder and Attention Deficit Disorder with Hyperactivity and reported a significant reduction in aggressiveness and a trend for reduced hyperactivity scores (on the Conner Teachers Rating Scale). In the largest study, Klorman et al. (1990) reported on the efficacy of methylphenidate in 48 adolescents. The design was a random-assignment, double-blind crossover of methylphenidate and placebo. Thirty-six were comorbid for Conduct Disorder or Oppositional Disorder. Fifty percent of parents reported total, good, or general improvement, 12.5 percent reported a lesser degree of improvement, and 37.5 percent reported their children as unchanged or showing a dramatically bad response. That 50 percent responded favorably to methylphenidate is consistent with our findings. That about one-fifth did worse may be due to the dosing schedule. For two weeks out of the three-week trial the last dose was at noon, with parents possibly observing the "rebound" exacerbation of ADHD symptoms that occurs in the late afternoon and evening with such dosing. The results may also be related to different drug responsivity in oppositional and conduct-disordered children. Nonetheless, the authors' results indicate that an appreciable number of a difficult-to-treat subgroup sustained noticeable improvement. Furthermore, informed observers reported that the improvement continued and, in some, increased over a period of months.

DRUG TREATMENT OF ADULT ADHD: PRACTICAL CONSIDERATIONS

This summary of the practical aspects of treating ADHD is based on more than 300 patients treated openly and in studies by Fred Reimherr, David Wood, and myself.

The stimulant drugs are generally the most effective and should be the first tried. Despite their brief duration of action, their abuse potential by others and *possibly* by some patients, and the inconveniences and concerns of prescribing Schedule II drugs for long periods of time, two amphetamines (D-amphetamine and methamphetamine) and methylphenidate are currently the most effective agents in the treatment of most adults with ADHD. The amphetamines and methylphenidate appear to be equally effective. (For detailed accounts of patients' experience on methylphenidate, see Chapter 7.) Since some patients do better on one and some on others, the only way to determine if the patient has experienced the maximal positive benefit is by offering a trial of all three medications. If the response to either methylphenidate or one amphetamine is good but not optimal, the patient should be tried on the other two agents. It is not known whether there are important differences between D-amphetamine and methamphetamine. A few patients have reported that methamphetamine was somewhat sedating and that in equivalent doses D-amphetamine was not, so trials of both seem indicated—that is, one might offer a trial of methamphetamine if the patient is too stimulated on D-amphetamine and of D-amphetamine if methamphetamine is too sedative. The merit of this procedure has *not* been confirmed. Many patients who are overstimulated by the amphetamines can tolerate methylphenidate, and many who are too sedated by methylphenidate will experience normal arousal with D-amphetamine. Pemoline is effective in a smaller number of patients than are the other stimulants.

After discussing the stimulants in greater detail, I describe the possible uses of other drugs in the treatment of ADHD in adults. Before turning to psychological management, I also discuss such aspects of drug treatment as informants, quality control, costs, abusability, and the evaluation of medication effects.

Stimulants

1. General principles

Stimulants should be started at a low dose and increased until the benefits reach a plateau (the level of maximum therapeutic effect) or the side effects become unpleasant. Even if the patient has shown a positive response, the dose should not be kept constant. He may respond more with a further increase in dose. Short-acting stimulants must be spaced throughout the day so that their effect is relatively constant. The dose and timing must be worked out individually for each patient. A rigid dosage schedule should be set for the patient based on when both he and his other observe the waxing and waning of drug effects. For example, an ADHD father should be reminded that if in the evening he begins to shout at routine misbehavior of his children, it may be because his medications have worn off. In all cases, *electronic timekeeping, with an appropriate multi-alarm watch or pill container, is mandatory.*

2. Amphetamines

The most useful amphetamines are D-amphetamine (Dexedrine, available as a generic) and methamphetamine (Desoxyn, no generic available). The duration of action of D-amphetamine is approximately 3 to 4 hours; methamphetamine is available only in a long-acting formulation, "Desoxyn Gradumets," which last 6 to 12 hours. Known as "meth crystals," methamphetamine achieved notoriety during the 1960s in the Haight-Ashbury area of San Francisco as the preferred amphetamine for "highs." I begin D-amphetamine at 2.5 milligrams 3 times a day and increase the dose by 2.5 milligrams every 3 to 4 days. The median daily dose is usually between 15 and 45 milligrams divided into 3 to 4 doses 3 to 4 hours apart, for example, 7.5 milligrams every 3 hours 4 times a day or 10 milligrams every 4 hours 3 times a day. Although some patients require 4 daily doses, D-amphetamine is usually given 3 times a day.

Dexedrine is marketed in a (purported) long-acting formulation (Dexedrine Spansules) of 5, 10, and 15 milligram sizes. The long-acting form sometimes produces an initial spike that may be experienced as unpleasant agitation or sedation, suggesting that too large a bolus is released at once. It is easier to start with D-amphetamine tablets, which are typically begun at 5 milligrams, 3 or 4 times a day. In switching to the long-acting formulations, one begins with approximately the total daily dose and increases the dose by 5 milligrams every 3 to 4 days. However, again, the exact dose and dosage regimen must be determined empirically. Of the two, the Desoxyn Gradumets appear to have a longer duration of action, but this has not been demonstrated. If single dosing is decided upon, both the Dexedrine Spansules and Desoxyn Gradumets should be tried and evaluated in terms of gradualness of onset (i.e., fluctuation of symptoms during the period of drug action) and duration of action. The usual total daily doses of either the regular or long-acting formulation are between 15 and 45 milligrams. The usual dosing of the long-acting preparations is in the morning only, but if drug effects wear off in the early afternoon, a second dose in the early afternoon may be necessary.

3. Methylphenidate

Methylphenidate produces effects similar to those of D-amphetamine and methamphetamine. Because it appears to be approximately half as potent as the amphetamines, the dose is usually twice as large. Methylphenidate is available in 5 milligrams and in scored 10- and 20-milligram tablet sizes; the proprietary 20-milligram long-acting form ("slow release") is Ritalin-SR. The package insert for Ritalin-SR claims that duration of action is 8 hours. Most clinicians have found it to be shorter, about 4 hours, although the duration should be determined by trial and error.

The usual dose range is between 15 and 90 milligram a day. Our procedure is to begin with 5 milligrams taken every 3 hours, 4 times a day, and to increase each dose by 5 milligrams every 2 to 3 days. The duration of action of methylphenidate is appreciably shorter than that of D-amphetamine, and doses must be given much more frequently (every 2 to 3 hours). Typical schedules are 10 milligrams every 2 hours, 7 times a day; 15 milligrams every 2 1/2 hours, 6 times a day; 20 milligrams every 3 hours, 4 times a day. To avoid a "roller-coaster" effect during the day—as the drug effects wax and wane—methylphenidate must be taken on a very precise schedule. This requires the patient's use of either a wristwatch with an alarm or a medication box with a "countdown feature." Useful devices are watches that can either be set for several alarms a day or have a button that will reset the watch at the time that it turns off the sound of the alarm. A timed pill dispenser is carried by some electronics stores. Even with carefully planned schedules, accurately timed frequent dosing is difficult for our patients. The ironic problem we face with ADHD patients is that although they are chronically disorganized, we expect them to regulate their dosage obsessionally. The benefits of once-a-day dosing are obvious. The instructions I employ with patients receiving methylphenidate are provided in *The Hyperactive Child, Adolescent, and Adult* (1987).

4. Side effects of the amphetamines and methylphenidate

Excessive doses of D-amphetamine or methamphetamine usually produce agitation rather than euphoria. Too large a dose of methylphenidate *may* produce excessive sedation and fogginess. This subjective effect reported by adults may correspond to the response to excessive doses seen in children who are described as "dazed" or as "zombies."

The side effects of D-amphetamine in the dose ranges we employ and of methylphenidate are these characteristics of sympathometic drugs: increased systolic and diastolic blood pressure, short-lived depression of appetite, dry mouth, and insomnia (if taken too late in the afternoon). The major side effect of concern is hypertension. If the patient experiences a moderate-to-marked response, one should consider the use of alpha-adrenergic blockers (see section later in this chapter). The other side effects can usually be minimized or eliminated, without appreciable decrease of the therapeutic effects, by a careful adjustment of dosage.

In patients for whom late afternoon doses are necessary and in whom they produce insomnia, the physician can consider the use of small amounts of sedative neuroleptics—for example, 10 to 25 milligrams of thioridazine. Obviously, one is concerned about cumulative neurological toxicity, although the risks are low in this dose range. The risks of neuroleptics should be discussed with the patient. Benzodiazepines are obviously an unsatisfactory treatment for insomnia on a long-term basis because of tolerance and dependence. (See also the discussion of clonidine below.)

Methylphenidate-SR, the long-acting form, has been associated with hypersensitivity reactions (presumably produced by the excipient). We have no experience with its use in ADHD adults. Since both methylphenidate tablets and the amphetamines are rarely associated with idiosyncratic or allergic reactions, and since the more expensive long-acting form is available in only one dose size, SR seems of little value.

Some patients receiving stimulants may gradually become withdrawn, suspicious, and anxious. With the powers of hindsight we now think that they may be diagnosed as having had symptoms in the "schizophrenic spectrum" although they may not meet diagnostic criteria for schizotypal or paranoid personality disorders. An association between apparent ADHD and schizophrenic disorders has been reported by Mednick and Schulsinger (1968), who observed an increased frequency of ADHD/CD-like symptoms in the adolescent sons of schizophrenic mothers. This response to stimulants may be that of a pharmacological challenge, a provocative test, which *reveals* "latent" schizophrenia—that is, the stimulants may be an operational test for "latent" schizophrenia. The phenomenon is important: Some schizotypal patients become clearly worse—in a schizophrenic way—when treated with the amphetamines, methylphenidate, or pemoline (Schulz et al., 1988).

5. Pemoline

Pemoline is the most recently introduced of the stimulant drugs. It differs in several respects from the amphetamines and methylphenidate. Pemoline is effective in a smaller fraction of ADHD patients than the other drugs, although a few patients respond best to it. Another advantage is that once-a-day treatment may be effective. While the amphetamines and methylphenidate are classified as Schedule II drugs, pemoline is a Schedule IV drug. It is apparently not used "recreationally."

Pemoline is available as scored 18.75, 37.5, and 75 milligram tablets. In treating patients, we begin at a low dose (e.g., one-half of the 18.75 milligram tablet) and increase the dose as tolerated every few days. The average dose of pemoline for good responders in our controlled study was 65 milligrams, with a range of 18.75 to 150 milligrams a day.

Side effects—to which tolerance may or may not develop—include anorexia, abdominal discomfort, headaches, and insomnia. Whether or not the drug has a delayed onset of action is uncertain since it must be begun at a low dose and gradually increased. The response is delayed, but the time required to increase the dose to a therapeutic level and the latency of response once therapeutic level is obtained are confounded. After pemoline has been administered for a few weeks, twice-daily dosing may occasionally be necessary. An important difference be-tween pemoline and the other stimulant drugs is that periodic labora-tory screening is necessary for pemoline (at uncertain intervals), since hepatotoxicity (with elevated liver enzymes, hepatitis, and jaundice) and aplastic anemia have both been reported. The manufacturer's pack-age insert states that "liver function tests should be performed prior to and periodically during therapy."

6. Abuse potential of stimulants

Patients responsive to stimulant drugs rarely require increased doses after they reach their benefit plateau. Tolerance is the exception rather than the rule. Most patients experience no decrease in efficacy even after years of use.

Euphoria does not occur with orally administered stimulant drugs in the dose ranges we have employed. Euphoria may occur if the drugs are taken in large doses, intravenously or "snorted" (see Goyer et al., 1979; Jaffe, 1991). I will say more about dealing with such patients later in this section. Because stimulants have the potential for serious abuse (with the probable exception of pemoline), it is important for clinicians to know about other effective drugs.

The maximum doses of D-amphetamine (45 milligrams a day) and methylphenidate (90 milligrams a day) are not absolute. However, most patients who will respond do respond at or below these doses. If tolerance begins to develop so that the patient's symptoms respond only to increasing doses of stimulants, one must consider the possi-bility that he does not have ADHD,[3] and that he is experiencing a "normal" euphoric response to stimulants. For such a patient stimu-lants are not the treatment of choice.

Antidepressant and Mood-Stabilizing Drugs

1. Monoamine oxidase inhibitors

Monoamine oxidase inhibitors are possible candidates for long-acting, nonabusable drugs that can be used in the treatment of ADHD. Since our studies of pargyline and selegiline (formerly L-deprenyl) in open trials, pargyline has been taken off the market. Because of the absence of the familiar MAOI "cheese effect" in the lower dose range, selegiline might be a particularly effective MAOI in the treatment of ADHD adults. As mentioned earlier, in our trials we probably pushed the dose too much (the minimal dose was 30 milligrams a day). Trials of lower doses (<20 milligrams a day or perhaps 5 to 15 milligrams a day) would be worthwhile. Although the duration of action of MAOIs is generally thought of as "long," many patients require both a morning dose and one in the early afternoon.

We have successfully treated patients with phenelzine (Nardil) and tranylcypromine (Parnate), and they may be effective in producing 24-hour symptom control. Such control is useful in patients who need behavioral controls before the morning dose of stimulant takes effect or when the dose wears off in the evening—such as the 14-year-old who burned down two chicken houses, one at 5 A.M. and one at midnight. However, there have been several problems in their use. In addition to dietary limitations, the patient on an MAOI is subject to such unpleasant side effects as hypotension, dependent edema, weight gain, insomnia, and decreased libido. Furthermore, tolerance often develops to any therapeutic effects and usually cannot be overcome by increasing doses. To reduce the risks of a sudden increase in blood pressure, I have my MAOI-treated patients carry the calcium channel blocker nifedipine (Procardia) and instruct them to take 10 to 20 milligrams if a headache develops.

2. Bupropion

Although we have found bupropion to be an effective drug, we have tested it only in patients who were responsive to other agents (Wender and Reimherr, 1990). Its efficacy in children was evaluated by Simeon et al. (1986), who conducted an open six-week trial of bupropion in 17 children (ages 7 to 13). They reported that the drug produced moderate-to-marked improvement in 71 percent of the subjects. It appears more effective than the stimulants in controlling affective lability and depression, but less effective than the stimulant drugs in improving concentration and in decreasing motor hyperactivity, overreactivity, disorganization, and impulsivity. When it is effective for concentration, the drug appears to have a relatively short duration of action and must be taken every 4 to 6 hours (that is, three times a day). Effective doses range between 50 and 150 milligrams 3 times a day. The drug is proconvulsant, and daily doses of more than 450 milligrams are not recommended. Bupropion is available in 75 and 100 milligram tablets, but some patients cannot tolerate an initial dose of 75 milligrams twice or three times a day. My policy is to divide the tablets with a pill cutter and begin patients at 37.5 milligrams twice a day, gradually increasing the frequency to three times a day, dosing as required and tolerated. The advantages of bupropion, like those of the MAOIs, are that it provides 24-hour a day "coverage" and is not abusable. Bupropion has a major advantage over the MAOIs in that it does not require dietary restrictions.

It is my clinical impression that bupropion may be more effective than other antidepressants (including the "selective serotonin reuptake inhibitors" described below) in ADHD patients who suffer from a concurrent chronic major depression. In some of these patients it is not effective in controlling concentration problems, motor hyperactivity, disorganization, and possibly overreactivity to stress and impulsivity. In such patients the use of a stimulant combined with bupropion can be effective in controlling both groups of symptoms.

Some patients respond to bupropion in very low doses. An example is a 49-year-old man who reduced his dose to the optimal level of one-quarter of a 75 milligram tablet (18.75 milligrams) twice daily. Since the lowest formulation available is 75 milligrams, accurate administration of low doses constitutes a practical problem.

3. Other dopaminergic drugs

Other dopamine agonists might be effective in the treatment of ADHD. The only systematic study reported thus far is of nomifensine (Shekim et al., 1989), which is no longer available. Of 18 adult patients with ADHD, 15 responded in an open trial, but the side effects were unacceptable. Other possible dopamine agonists are bromocryptine in the treatment of ADHD in chemically dependent patients (Cavanaugh et al., 1989; $N = 2$) and amantadine. They are of interest since they do not produce euphoria and they are direct agonists, that is, they stimulate the postsynaptic receptor directly. The amphetamines and methylphenidate are indirect agonists increasing the release of dopamine from the presynaptic cell. As a cautionary note, there are at least five dopamine receptors, so that all such drugs loosely grouped together may have appreciably different effects.

4. Tricyclic antidepressants

Tricyclic antidepressants (TCAs) have not been systematically evaluated in ADHD adults. Because of the dysphoria that many ADHD patients exhibit many have been treated with TCAs or lithium and have failed to respond. Our sample is thus biased toward TCA failures—we do not see the successes. Nevertheless, it is interesting that most of these patients report the same effects: perhaps an initial response within hours or days, followed by tolerance that does not respond to increasing doses; ADHD patients also seem to be more sensitive to TCA side effects than depressives, particularly dry mouth, constipation, weight gain, and decreased libido and impaired sexual functioning.

The TCAs have been demonstrated to be effective in ADHD children but not as effective as stimulants. The pattern of response they produce is different from that in adult depressives. In ADHD children, their onset of action often occurs in hours, while in adults it takes a few days. At about the length of time the TCAs "kick in" in adult depressives, the children often become tolerant. Gittelman-Klein has observed that "instead of a resurgence of hyperactive signs occurring over time with imipramine treatment, new difficulties emerged such as temper outbursts, aggressiveness, and antagonistic behavior" (1980, p. 659). She continues, "Curiously, this particular pattern has also been reported in adults with imipramine-treated emotionally unstable character disorder who *often have a history of hyperkinesis*" (my italics).

Huessy reports the use of both imipramine and amitriptyline and suggests that if either is ineffective the other should be tried. He states that some patients respond to as little as 10 milligrams a day and that patients rarely require more than 100 milligrams a day. The duration of drug effect is brief, and patients require twice-daily dosing. Unfortunately, Huessy has not reported how long the therapeutic effect lasts.

5. Selective serotonin reuptake inhibitors (SSRIs)

Fluoxetine. Our experience has been limited, but fluoxetine appears to be generally ineffective. I have seen a few ADHD adults whose affective problems did improve initially but who became tolerant after a few months. The fact that tolerance in controlling ADHD symptoms seems to develop for the TCAs, MAOIs and probably fluoxetine (we do not know about bupropion) and not for the stimulants would be informative if we knew the mechanisms of action of the antidepressants. I have treated three ADHD adults with SSRIs when they developed a concurrent major depression. The antidepressant could be discontinued when the depression had remitted, but the stimulant had to be continued.

Because major depression and ADHD in adults seem to occur with a greater than chance frequency, it should be noted that the treatment of such patients with fluoxetine and stimulants is worth trying.

Sertraline and paroxetine. We have no experience with sertraline or paroxetine. Sertraline appears to be similar to fluoxetine but with a much shorter half-life. Compared with fluoxetine and paroxetine, it does not interfere with drug metabolism. Because interference in drug metabolism may affect the levels of other drugs, making their titration difficult, sertraline may be preferable for use with a stimulant for patients with a major depression and ADHD.

6. Lithium

We tried lithium because Rifkin and Quitkin (1972) had described the effectiveness of lithium in "emotionally unstable character disorders," who they speculated might be *formes frustes* (an atypical or minimal manifestation of a disease) of bipolar affective disorder. Since such unstable conditions were ostensibly characterized by hour-to-hour affective lability—an ADHD characteristic—we tried several ADHD patients on lithium and found that it produced no clinical benefit. We have seen many ADHD patients who had been incorrectly diagnosed as having cyclothymic disorder and had received trials of lithium without benefit. Lithium had previously been found to be ineffective in stimu-
lant-nonresponsive "hyperactive" children (Greenhill et al., 1973), and this has been our experience with adults.

7. Adrenergic drugs

Clonidine. Clonidine, an alpha-2-agonist, decreases noradrenergic outflow from the locus caeruleus. It has been used in the treatment of ADHD children by Hunt (1985, 1987, 1990), and there are some reports that it may be helpful when combined with stimulants in the treatment of aggressive ADHD children. The dosage schedule that Hunt employs in using clonidine *with children* is as follows. Because of the side effects of sedation and hypotension, it is begun at a low dose (0.05 milligrams at bedtime) and increased as tolerated every third day. One medication is also available in skin patches that release doses of 0.1, 0.2, or 0.3 milligrams a day for a period of a week. Hunt reports that it requires approximately two weeks to obtain the desired effects and that the maximal effect of clonidine may not be reached for two to three months. We have no experience with its use in adults. It could be useful in low doses (e.g., 0.05 to 0.1 milligram) at bedtime for patients who must take stimulants in the evening to control symptoms, with resultant insomnia. Its side effects in normotensive patients can include hypotension (with the danger of falling) and withdrawal rebound hypertension, which has been observed when it has been used in antihypertensive doses and discontinued abruptly rather than tapered; rebound hypertension has also been reported even with gradual discontinuation. Since insomnia can be a significant problem with the stimulants, clonidine may be a useful medication. It should obviously be tried with caution.

In Chapter 4 on etiology I discuss the evidence that supports the role of decreased dopaminergic functioning in the etiology of ADHD. However, as the following single case suggests, adrenergic factors may also play a role. The patient was a 48-year-old academic who was diagnosed as having Attention Deficit Disorder, Residual Type. He participated in a placebo-controlled trial of D-amphetamine, manifested an appropriate and stable therapeutic response to 10 to 15 milligrams a day, and did not require an increase in the basic dose over a period of five years. Prior to stimulant treatment, the patient had developed mild hypertension for which his internist prescribed antihypertensive drugs. Because of various unacceptable side effects attributable to these agents, several different drugs were used. The fact that some of the following drugs prescribed for hypertension in this patient changed the effects of D-amphetamine is of interest, although it is hard to judge the evidence provided by only one patient.

1. Propranolol (80 milligrams per day), a beta$_1$- and beta$_2$- adrenergic-receptor blocker, antagonized the beneficial response to amphetamine, requiring an increase in dose to 20 to 25 milligrams a day during the period of administration of propranolol.
2. Metoprolol (100 milligrams per day), a beta$_1$-adrenergic-receptor blocker, similarly affected the D-amphetamine response.
3. Clonidine (0.1 milligram per day), an alpha-adrenergic-receptor and partial agonist, nearly doubled the duration of the action of D-amphetamine, but tolerance rapidly developed to this prolongation.
4. Prazocin (1 milligram per day), a postsynaptic alpha$_1$-adrenergic-receptor blocker, changed the central effect of D-amphetamine from stimulation to depression.

5. Alpha-methyldopa (1 gram per day) or hydrochlorothiazide (100 milligrams per day) exerted no detectable interaction with D-amphetamine.

It is also significant that the patient rapidly developed tolerance to D-amphetamine's pressor effect; therefore, the stimulant drug did not appear to interfere with the therapeutic efficacy of the antihypertensive drugs. The alteration of amphetamine's therapeutic response by the antihypertensive drugs, however, may shed some light on the mechanism of action of D-amphetamine in the treatment of Attention-deficit Hyperactivity Disorder. The results of the metoprolol interaction suggest that the therapeutic effect is, at least in part, mediated by beta$_1$-adrenergic receptors. In addition, the results of the prazocin interaction imply that the central stimulant properties of amphetamine are dependent on alpha$_1$-adrenergic receptors. Ratey et al. (1991) have reported three cases of ADHD in adults that were treated with methylphenidate and nadolol, a beta$_1$- and beta$_2$-antagonist. They found that the beta blocker decreased feelings of inner tenseness, anxiety, and temper that were not suppressed or were aggravated by methylphenidate. These four cases suggest that altering noradrenergic functioning with beta blockers may be helpful in the symptomatic treatment of adult ADHD.

Naldol is among the less lipid soluble and more hydrophilic (preferably absorbed by water rather than lipids and thus having relatively higher concentrations in the blood versus the brain than lyophilic beta blockers) beta blockers, and it has been suggested that these drugs have fewer central nervous system effects. However, there are limited data from controlled trials to support this contention (Hoffman et al., 1990, p. 35).

8. Neuroleptics

Neuroleptics were formerly used extensively in the treatment of ADHD in children. They are no longer employed. They have a modest usefulness in counteracting the insomnia produced in some patients by stimulants, and, as mentioned, small doses (e.g., 10 milligrams of thioridazine, Mellaril®) an hour or two before bedtime may be useful. Their chronic use would be expected to diminish the effect of stimulants, since the neuroleptics have a very long half-life. The long-term hazards of their use should be recognized and discussed with the patient. Some of my patients who found neuroleptics useful but who reported an increased appetite were given trials of molindone because of claims that its use has not been associated with "excessive" weight gain. It is unclear whether its effects on weight differed from those of other neuroleptics.

Informants

Good treatment requires a good informant. The informant must be living with and know the patient. The "other"—significant or not—is as necessary for monitoring drug treatment as she or he is at the time of an initial evaluation. As I have repeatedly said, ADHD adults often have as little insight into changes brought by treatment as they had about their pretreatment behavior. They often fail to observe the connection between medication and changes in their behavior, feeling, attitudes, work and social relationships. They are the adult equivalent of the effectively treated ADHD eight-year-old whose grades go from C's to A's, who stops spending every other day in the principal's office, who begins to be invited to birthday parties, and who, when queried, reports that not much has changed, and if it has, that he doesn't know why. Two vignettes will illustrate the importance of an informant.

During our study of pemoline, a nurse I did not know stopped me in the hospital corridor. She told me that her husband had been involved in one of our studies and that he had changed remarkably, as had their marriage. Their marriage had been progressively deteriorating for several years, and their problems had not responded to individual, couple or group therapies. They had been contemplating separation, but first her husband had reluctantly agreed to participate in the study, expecting little from it. Among the surprising and welcome changes the nurse reported was that he now listened to her without interrupting, virtually never lost his temper, and had started disciplining their children rationally; in summary, "It's been the difference between night and day." Afterward I returned to the office and reviewed the case chart. According to notes made by a colleague, the patient had been "slightly improved." The nurse had been unable to come to the interviews during the drug trial because she had to return East to care for her sick mother. Without the wife's comments, the patient's own reports about symptomatic change indicated to the clinician much less progress.

When interviewing another methylphenidate-treated patient and his wife, I queried him about our target symptoms (moodiness, temper, disorganization, etc.). The patient declared himself slightly improved on each of the items and mildly improved overall. With this statement his wife's jaw dropped, she put her hand on her husband's knee, looked him in the eye, and then turned to me and said, "Slightly improved! It's like being married to a different man!"

Without an informant, treatment is extremely difficult. The informant should be someone who lives with the patient—a spouse, significant other, adult child, or parent would all suffice. Patients not only fail to assess their symptoms accurately but are frequently unable to report accurately on drug effects. Without such information it is almost impossible to adjust medications.

Quality Control and Costs

Unbeknownst to the lay consumer, the quality control of drugs is not perfect, and on occasion, patients may fail to respond to a refilled prescription (the physician must always worry—pharmacists, like automobile dealers, often receive recall notices). For example, once we noticed that a number of patients appeared to regress despite continuing treatment with a particular stimulant. When we switched these patients to an elixir of the same drug or to other stimulant drugs, they responded promptly. Changes in the response to a drug may also occur when changing from the brand name formulation to a generic formulation. This is best evaluated by again employing the brand name drug. Generics may be substituted, but they may require adjusting the dose up or down or at a different dosing frequency.

Cost

The costs of the various stimulants vary considerably. At a large local pharmacy, monthly costs for the drugs in 1994 were as follows:

D-amphetamine: 10 milligrams 3 times a day = cost unavailable
Dexedrine: 10 milligrams 3 times a day = $47.00
Methylphenidate: 10 milligrams 6 times a day = $61.00
Ritalin: 10 milligrams 6 times a day = $74.00
Desoxyn: 30 milligrams (two 15 milligram tablets in a long-acting formulation) each day = $159.00
Cylert: 75 milligrams a day = $57.00

The Problem of Abusability

A major legal and administrative problem in the treatment of adult ADHD is that the amphetamines and methylphenidate, which are in general the most effective drugs available, can produce euphoria in many people. They are "popular" recreationally and have been heavily abused. Physicians are understandably hesitant to prescribe them for long-term and sometimes indefinite treatment. The problem is further aggravated by the fact that the potential recipients, patients with ADHD, are at greater than average risk for syndromes such as conduct disorder and antisocial personality disorder. Persons with these proclivities are more likely to be abusing or to have abused drugs and alcohol, and a rational physician, understandably, is even more unwilling to prescribe amphetamines or methylphenidate to such patients. Physicians who maintain a sizable number of adults on Schedule II drugs are more likely to be investigated by state licensure boards. The justifiable concerns of licensure boards are that the physician either is running a "speed clinic" or is naively being exploited by drug seekers who are falsifying their histories.

It is uncertain whether all ADHD patients will respond with a "high" to large doses of intravenously administered stimulants (that is, will experience the same effect as a non-ADHD individual). In one instance, a patient was helped by small doses but became addicted to large intravenous doses. More recently, Jaffe (1991) reported the case of an adolescent who stockpiled methylphenidate for several days and then "snorted" 100 milligrams to produce "a high." Even if the patients themselves do not abuse stimulant drugs, they have a high "street value" and can easily be sold. Accordingly, we use amphetamines and methylphenidate only in individuals we believe are responsible, and generally only in those with partners. In "high-risk" patients, we use pemoline and sometimes MAOIs and bupropion, and do not employ the amphetamines or methylphenidate, even if patients fail to respond to the former agents.

Depending on the local concern about the prescription of Schedule II drugs (usually considerable), the prescribing physician is well advised to support his position legally and medically. From a practical standpoint, it is a good idea to get an independent confirmation of the diagnosis of ADHD from another physician and also, probably, to have the latter discuss the rationale for using stimulants in an adult. If one plans to treat more than an occasional patient, it may be helpful to contact the local branch of the Drug Enforcement Administration and ask what special safeguards should be employed and whether the agency wants the physician to institute any special procedures.

Evaluation of Medication Effects

The evaluation of medication effects is best accomplished by using the Targeted Attention Deficit Disorder Rating Scale (TADDS; see Appendix E). With the use of a semi-structured interview and the probes provided, one should inquire systematically and rate the seven target symptoms: hyperactivity, inattentiveness, mood lability, temper, disorganization, stress sensitivity, and impulsivity. It is wise to request and record concrete instances of difficulty in these areas (e.g., Where does inattentiveness show up in the patient's daily life?) prior to and throughout treatment. These can serve as individualized anchor points for this patient.

In administering medication, the physician can expect to see the following changes in the target symptoms in drug-responsive patients.

Hyperactivity

Both fidgeting (finger tapping and leg kicking) and restlessness decrease. One ADHD woman, who described herself as "nationally ranked in useless energy," stated that when she had broken her leg and had to remain in bed, "I tossed and turned all the time and nearly went crazy." Later, when she had been placed on stimulant medication, she was able for the first time in her life not only to sit quietly in front of the television set for an hour but also to read a book! Similarly, the lawyer mentioned in Chapter 2 would work at his desk for a while, then rush down and up 18 flights of stairs in order to be able to resume desk work. With medication he was able to work efficiently for hours at a time when it was necessary to do so, and he felt very pleased that he could use his energy profitably.

Inattentiveness

Patients report greatly improved concentration, a change that may have significant life effects. It is not only the ability to concentrate better, but to have conscious control over attention. The patient can make himself concentrate when he wants to. Stimulant responders report decreased daydreaming, wool-gathering, and distractibility. One patient had started a college education on six separate occasions but was unable to complete even one quarter. He was totally unable to concentrate for more than 5 or 10 minutes at a time and frequently read and reread the same pages without registering or remembering information. On stimulant medication, with increased attention, he has completed one year of college with A's and B's. A woman whose housework suffered because she was distracted by the noise of the cat coming through the door, the ice maker dropping cubes, and the leaves rustling on the roof found that she became unaware of these sounds when she responded to stimulant medication.

Mood lability

Patients report decreased "lows" and "highs," increased interest and increased motivation. Demoralization is decreased. They feel able to deal with problems that they were formerly unable to tackle. The extent to which initiative and interest are increased may be dependent on specific dose schedules which are highly individualized and arrived at by trial and error.

Temper

The threshold for outbursts is raised, the patient's "fuse" is lengthened, and sensitivity to provocation diminishes. Angry outbursts become much less common, and their magnitude is decreased. Patients who hit, screamed, and broke things now express their unhappiness in words. Patients whose anger is greatly diminished by medication may report when the medication is begun that they are not having temper outbursts and then, as the dose is increased, that they are no longer irritable. Sometimes patients recognize such changes even though they have experienced lifelong irritability.

For example, a high school teacher had chronically been verbally abusive to his students and eventually was asked to resign before he was fired. His temper with his own children was so severe that his wife frequently had to prevent him from injuring their younger children or to keep the older children from fighting back and injuring him. Several months after his resignation he obtained a menial civil service job and enrolled in the university night school to take mathematics courses. With medication his concentration improved markedly and his temper was completely held in check. He made very rapid progress in his civil service job, got A's in intermediate and advanced algebra, and enrolled in a calculus class. He was very surprised and pleased by his mathematical accomplishments, which he found "easy."

Disorganization

Disorganization is diminished. Messy desks and kitchens become neater; patients work at projects systematically rather than rushing from one partially completed task to another. An extreme version of this is sometimes seen in ADHD children receiving excessive doses of stimulants (and in stimulant abusers), where organization and drive become purposeless repetitive activity. "Speed freaks" have been reported to take the same mechanical alarm clock apart and put it together repeatedly. A very hyperactive and distractible nine-year-old, who could be neither induced nor terrified into studying for more than 15 minutes at a time, proved unusually responsive to medication. A few weeks after having been started on a small (but later recognized as excessive) dose of D-amphetamine she misheard her teacher and thought that the class assignment was to write the Roman numerals from 1 to 1,000 rather than those from 1 to 100. She began doing her homework after supper, and at bedtime her flabbergasted parents discovered her in her room still patiently plodding away.

Stress sensitivity

This is a poorly defined dimension but one to which patients continually refer. With medication they describe themselves as thicker-skinned, less readily "hassled," better able to tolerate stress. Improvement in the target symptoms is often accompanied by improvement in more complex areas of functioning. Treatment-responsive patients may experience substantial life changes, gradually developing better vocational functioning and improved relationships.

Impulsivity

Impulsivity decreases. People begin to "plan ahead" and to listen to others rather than interrupting, a phenomenon sometimes described as "improved communication skills." A husband and wife described the changes in impulsivity and conversational skills produced by medication in this way. She stated that previously she used to wait until the other person had spoken without listening very much, sometimes interrupting to respond. She now found herself listening more and reflecting on what she heard before replying. Her husband reported: "It's just as if she were starting to process things—she listens to them, absorbs them, and then responds."

Interpersonal behavior in relationships is better not only because of stable mood, decreased temper, and improvement in the faculty of actually listening to other people, but also probably because of more subtle changes in behavior that may be more easily observable in ADHD children. ADHD children are often overtalkative, bossy, controlling, domineering, and intrusive, and these qualities sometimes diminish or disappear in stimulant responders. Such attributes are not calculated to win friends and influence people in childhood, and they are no more successful in adult life. Diminution in these personality characteristics helps adults to work and play better with others.

What does *not* improve is also of interest. Learning disorders, particularly "dyslexia" ("reading disorder") and problems with calculation ("mathematics disorder"), are not improved. Whether memory improves for such material needs to be evaluated. Handwriting improves in ADHD children, but we have not examined this in adults.

Some addictive behaviors *may* be altered. Several patients reported that they spontaneously cut down their drinking substantially while on pemoline and methylphenidate (i.e., from one or two six-packs per night to three or four cans a week) and that they relapsed when they discontinued stimulants (see also Heiman, 1983; Turnquist et al., 1983). Two subjects spontaneously reported that they had done without their "maintenance dose" of cigarettes. These observations need to be explored systematically.

TREATMENT OF ADHD SPECTRUM DISORDERS AND OF ADHD IN COMBINATION WITH OTHER DIAGNOSES

The Utah Criteria were constructed to be diagnostically *specific* rather than diagnostically sensitive—to identify clear-cut instances of ADHD and to increase interrater reliability. We were concerned lest vague criteria prompt promiscuous dispensation of stimulant medication to inappropriate patients. However, it is obvious that the symptoms of ADHD occur along a spectrum of severity, as in schizophrenia (Kety et al., 1975) and other psychiatric disorders. To further complicate the diagnostic picture, it is important for the clinician to be sensitive to the possibility that ADHD patients may also be suffering from some other disorder, and that patients with a different diagnosis may also have ADHD symptoms.

An important question arising from these complexities is the extent to which lesser forms of the disorder—*formes frustes* of ADHD or "ADHD spectrum disorder"—or ADHD symptoms in combination with other disorders respond to the drugs most effective in treating the full-fledged syndrome. A related question is to what extent single residual symptoms of ADHD—such as inattention—respond to such drug treatment. The following case histories indicate possible answers to these questions.

Concentration Difficulties and Hyperactivity without Additional ADHD Symptomatology

The patient was a 35-year-old high school English teacher who was requesting treatment because she had read that concentration difficulties were now a recognized and treatable problem. She described her ability to function professionally as due solely to her wits and compensatory mechanisms. She found it difficult to concentrate on the printed page for more than ten minutes at a time. "I squeaked through teacher's college using my brains—I was much smarter than my colleagues but got worse grades—I remembered what I heard, and I can write well—I kept a journal from age 12 to age 25. Anyhow, you won't believe this, but I taught English on the basis of movies and college study guides."

Her mood was equitable, she was even-tempered, her house was immaculate and well organized. She was always busy, doing two or three things at one time. Her family saw her as having prodigious physical energy. Her family doctor responded to her reports of anxiety (reactive and appropriate) by treating her with benzodiazepines, which aggravated her concentration problem. Later a psychiatrist treated her reactive anxiety with low doses of tricyclic antidepressants, which were ineffective, and then with MAOIs, which produced improvement in her concentration but which had to be discontinued because of side effects. I placed her on methylphenidate, which was sufficiently helpful to enable her to earn a Master's degree in English.

ADD without Hyperactivity

The patient was a 42-year-old lawyer working in his father's firm. The fifth of five children and the only boy, he was indulged by his mother while his father expected great things of him. As a child he was an inattentive, lost-in-the-clouds, lovable bumbler. He received no treatment but by considerable effort did fairly well in elementary and high school. By very hard work he achieved middling grades both in his state university and at law school. His grades were affected by his concentration difficulties, by his tendency to hand in assignments late, and at times by severe examination anxiety.

Following graduation he went to work with his father. His major asset as a lawyer was his genuine interest in and concern for his clients. His major deficits were his persistent procrastination, disorganization, and tendency to "fold under pressure": "I am easily discombobulated, Doctor, easily fazed, I overreact to all kinds of stress." The patient clearly perceived both his father's disappointment and his own disappointment with himself. With stimulant treatment his concentration improved and, more strikingly, he became more resilient in the presence of stress. Medication did not change him into an energetic, brilliant defense attorney, but it did allow him to perform adequately in civil law.

ADHD and Emergent Major Depression

The Utah Criteria exclude major depression, but as indicated, I have had several patients who appeared to develop such a depression in the course of extended treatment with stimulant drugs. One woman with prominent ADHD symptoms, who had been physically abused until her teenage years, had a sleep pattern of multiple anxious awakenings throughout the night. She was not anhedonic, guilty, or suicidal. On methylphenidate both her ADHD symptoms and her abnormal sleep pattern were resolved. A year and a half later, while still doing well on stimulants, she began to develop symptoms of a biological depression with anhedonia, guilt, suicidal thoughts, and neurovegetative symptoms. Bupropion controlled her depressive symptoms, but methylphenidate had to be continued in order to maintain the improvement in her concentration and motor restlessness.

In a similar case the combination of tricyclic antidepressant and methylphenidate controlled both depressive and ADHD symptoms but seemed to produce a moderate tachycardia (heart rate = 112). A switch to bupropion did not relieve the depressive symptoms, but they were subsequently controlled by sertraline, administered along with the methylphenidate.

Depression and ADHD

A 35-year-old woman came to me after having been in and out of multiple psychotherapies during the previous 12 years. Her problem had been recurrent, seemingly reactive, "neurotic" depression. Initially, it had been interpreted as a response to a bad marriage and two difficult children. However, her depressive hyperresponsivity continued when she divorced and remarried, this time happily. In discussing her childhood, she focused on her father's alcoholism and its effects on the family (she was not sexually, physically, or emotionally abused) and mentioned her childhood temperament only in response to direct questioning. She described herself as a tomboy, not much of a student, and "tough"—stubborn and bossy. Because her depression was reactive, short-lived, and had occasional "microhighs," I decided to treat her problem as ADHD. She was placed on pargyline and did well until the drug was withdrawn from the market. She was then placed on stimulants, to which she responded well and to which she did not develop tolerance. Currently, she is being maintained on bupropion and is without depressive symptomatology.

Borderline Personality Disorder and ADHD

One is reluctant to offer a therapeutic trial of stimulants to most patients with Borderline Personality Disorder (BPD) because of concerns about abuse and overdose. However, some symptoms in some borderlines do respond to stimulants. One major problem with the stimulant drugs is their on-again, off-again treatment control (symptoms occur before medication is taken in the morning and after it wears off in the evening). One must constantly weigh the hazards of drug treatment against the severity and hazards of the illness. Which drugs might be useful in treating such patients is unclear. D-amphetamine, methamphetamine, or methylphenidate are usually unwise for patients who have frequently misused similar drugs in the past and are often continuing substance abusers. The MAOIs are unacceptable because the dietary restrictions are apt to be violated by the impulsive, and pemoline is ruled out in alcoholics because of its known hepatotoxicity. Bupropion should be considered in these groups because *to date* there have been no reports of abuse. The reversible inhibitors of MAO, such as meclobemide, might also be tried because they require minimal dietary restrictions.

One can have occasional success in recommending an "anti-ADHD medication" for these difficult patients. Here is an example. One borderline woman of 30 had been very "hyperactive" as a child and had become a serious self-mutilator as an adult. She had been wounded in an altercation with a policeman, had cut herself badly enough to interfere with her movements, and had produced septicemia and severe endocarditis in herself through subcutaneous insertion of contaminated matter. On a combination of bupropion and methamphetamine both her thoughts about and impulses to commit self-harm were appreciably diminished. This was the more striking because she had failed to respond to adequate trials of tricyclic antidepressants, antipsychotics and lithium.

PSYCHOLOGICAL MANAGEMENT

■

INTRAPERSONAL AND INTERPERSONAL CONSEQUENCES OF DIAGNOSIS AND TREATMENT

There are important and predictable psychological "side effects" from the diagnosis of ADHD, both for the patient himself and for the patient's relationships with others. To the patient, the diagnosis and any changes produced in his functioning by medication can be disturbing. This is the consequence of his realization that he had previously been looking at the world through "astigmatic" glasses.

For patients who are brought to treatment at the request of others, one of the consequences of diagnosis and prompt drug-produced remission of symptoms is the patient's feeling that he was "wrong" and that others were "right." Specifically, the others were "right" when they ascribed certain undesirable ADHD attributes to him—for example, that he was stubborn, bossy, and hot tempered. In addition, there is an implication that there always had been something abnormal about the patient's functioning. This is an obvious blow to the patient's self-esteem. If he likes the way he functions on medication, he may look back unhappily on his "preconversion" behavior and, sometimes, on wasted years. In many instances, he had, like most of us, accepted or resigned himself to the way he was; he may even have regarded himself as being the way he wanted to be. The realization that the changes in his behavior are obvious to others emphasizes the differences that treatment has made. If one is feeling righteously indignant about what one has perceived as unjustified criticism, it is embarrassing to find that one's spouse has made accurate observations. If he likes the way he is now—regardless of whether or not he was self-referred—he must acknowledge that medication has turned him from Mr. Hyde into Dr. Jekyll. In trying to counteract such feelings, I point out that with the help of medication he is *more* in control of himself and has an increased ability to change himself.

If the patient responds to medication, after some time he will usually request a drug holiday to determine if he still needs it. The best way to do this is with prearranged double-blind tapering. Stimulants are short-acting so that an abrupt discontinuation is immediately recognized by the patient. However, a gradual double-blind decrease is almost impossible in ordinary practice. Stopping the medication, which must always be with the consent of the patient, can be traumatic, but it is always informative. One man—who had improved his marital, parental, and vocational functioning dramatically over three years—ran out of medication and nearly drove off his daughter-in-law to be. His wife recalled that she had lived 17 years with these inappropriate outbursts and told him she would seriously consider divorce if a similar episode ever recurred. Another man, who was involved in a study with double-blind tapering of the dose, nearly lost his job when his medication was diminished and he returned to his previous level of dysfunction. In both instances the experiences had a marked impact and made the patients much more aware of how they had functioned before treatment.

SELF-MONITORING

When medication is effective in reducing the patient's target symptoms, I strongly encourage the patient to learn to monitor it himself—another illustration of the important point that treatment gives him a greater degree of self-control. In the course of such monitoring, he may learn which of the symptoms of ADHD cause him the most difficulties in everyday life.

The ADHD patient's lack of self-awareness is often attributed to his psychopathology (he is egocentric, narcissistic, etc.). Perhaps to some degree that is true. However, it is very important to remember that most of us do not have the ability to self-observe even the simplest nonconflictual aspects of our behavior. When tape recorders were introduced and became widely accessible, most people's reaction to hearing their own voice was one of unpleasant surprise; they asked if they *really* talked like that. A similar blow to self-esteem has been one of the consequences of widely available videotaping. For most people it was bad enough to look that way in candid photographs and to sound that way, but to have those odd facial expressions *and* to move that way was an even tougher nut to swallow. But these blows are minor compared to those affecting the ADHD patient. If other people have been telling you that you are misguided, wrong, and frequently unpleasant, defensive denial is highly likely to amplify the normal human lack of self-awareness. Most of us can get by without developing an awareness of how we appear to others, but the ADHD patient cannot. Robert Burns may have been a little off the mark when he wrote that "would some power the giftie gie us to see ourselves as others see us"— our lack of awareness may actually be a giftie.

PSYCHOTHERAPEUTIC GOALS AND APPROACHES

Many of our patients had been in psychotherapy or "counseling," often with several therapists, in the past. By and large it did not seem to help—although it should be remembered that those whom it did help did not contact us. Many had received trials of whatever medication was popular at the time they sought help and, in general, experienced little benefit—although, again, those whom it helped we didn't see; we see only the failures. Stimulants had rarely been tried because most psychiatrists, aware of the Drug Enforcement Administration looking over their shoulder and concerned about generating drug abuse and possible dependence in their patients, were reluctant to prescribe them.

In discussing the treatment of ADHD in adults, I have focused on what is novel about its possible biological correlates and its response to treatment with specific medications. Many medication-responsive patients are able to handle related psychological problems on their own. It is as if medical treatment allows psychological homeostasis to take effect so that such patients learn *by themselves* new techniques of avoiding problems and problem solving, and gradually correct their own deficiencies. However, I do not want to minimize the roles of learned maladaptions and the unfortunate reality of the disease as contributors to the ADHD adult's difficulties. For a number of reasons that I describe below, the ADHD patient is more likely to have had a difficult childhood and a realistically unhappy childhood and adulthood. On the other hand, we cannot extrapolate from our sample to the population at large—obviously, we have been seeing patients with marked problems—and it is possible that individuals with ADHD genes but nontraumatic upbringing do not suffer the kinds of consequences detailed below.

Since ADHD is largely genetic, the patient is likely to have had a parent or parents who themselves had ADHD and were at increased risk for traits characteristic of Antisocial Personality Disorder. Such parents tend to be disorganized (inconsistent), hot tempered, impulsive, and punitive, and to project blame. They are also more likely to be alcoholic, which in turn increases the possibility of uncontrolled, abusive behavior. In addition, ADHD parents are more likely to be vocational and academic underachievers and, all other things being equal, to earn less than their ability would merit. The ADHD patient is likely to have endured a family life similar to that described by many of the adult children of alcoholics. But the problem does not stop there. Because of their ADHD, they were more likely—compared to their non-ADHD sibs—to be the recipients of parental abuse. The personality characteristics of the ADHD child make him a "difficult" child, and the combination of such problems and the low frustration tolerance of the parents increases the probability that the adult patient was the target of abuse as a child. In our long-term trial of methylphenidate, about 45 percent of our long-term patients were physically abused.

In addition to gross physical abuse, ADHD patients are even more likely to have been the target of parental and school criticism because they have been underachievers. They have been accused of not paying attention and of not working hard enough, and their parents and teachers frequently let them know that their school performance was disappointing. We are beginning to document that such early childhood traumas may produce lifelong distortions in personality. We do not have any information about the effects of nondramatic chronic psychological trauma. An obvious question is, "What are the long-term consequences to the ADHD child of the low self-esteem that he experiences in childhood and adolescence as a result of evaluation by others?"

In the realm of self-inflicted reality problems, our patients are likely to have experienced academic and vocational underachievement. They are likewise apt to have had problems with interpersonal and preferential reality—such as an unsatisfying marriage or job. The marriage (or other close relationship) may have started out on the basis of an impulsive decision. Whatever its origins, the patient's behavior will frequently have antagonized, driven off, or depressed the partner, and he will be responding to self-generated difficulties with his other. He is likewise at high risk for impairing the relationship with his children. His children are more likely to be victimized, in part because of his temper and impulsivity, in part because he may be reacting to inherited ADHD in his children, and in part because parental abuse of him in his childhood may have affected his learned behavior in gross and subtle ways. At the very least, his children will have learned to distance themselves in the service of self-protection—for example, hiding in the basement when their father's car pulls into the driveway. With such a history of unrewarding accomplishments and relationships, the ADHD patient is often realistically depressed. Even when medication produces beneficial change—as when the patient's improved temper means the children no longer hide—the behavioral legacy of the past takes a long time to dissipate.

Patients with ADHD thus can benefit from psychological intervention that focuses on the consequences of the core symptoms of the illness. As I mentioned before, when untreated, such patients have a tendency to fall into self-dug holes; while a metaphoric rope ladder may help them to extricate themselves, they are very apt to dig new holes and fall into them.

Resolution of the persisting problems involves explaining what has happened to the patient and offering him what might be called "general insight." If the patient does not bring up material in these areas, I do. I begin in a general way, stating that most ADHD adults had a difficult time with their parents, sibs, and teachers while they were growing up. I tell them what I have been told by other ADHD adults and wonder out loud whether these are applicable to him or her. An example I frequently begin with—particularly if the patient has described a very strict or severe upbringing—is the consequences that can follow when a "hyperactive child" has a "hyperactive parent." If the patient has described himself as having been noncompliant, forgetful, and disobedient, I describe the usual effect such behavior has on the hyperactive parent. Discipline was likely to have been administered inconsistently, sometimes with inappropriate severity. If the patient's behavior to his own children is similar to that of his father to him, I emphasize that the hyperactive disciplining parent may love his offspring but still behave in such a manner that the message does not "get through." It is often useful to help the patient to understand that if his parent was ambivalent toward him, he may be ambivalent toward his own ADHD child. The spousal and parental roles he learned in his ADHD family may affect his behavior toward *his* spouse and *his* children in predictable ways.

His relationships with non-ADHD siblings are also likely to be affected. They probably did better academically and were more popular among their peers. His parents no doubt compared his unfavorable performance with that of his siblings, sometimes in anger, sometimes with feelings almost of desperation. I point out that it is understandably difficult to experience warm feelings toward siblings who are chronically held up as your betters.

I thus explain to patients that the origin of much of their low self-esteem is understandable on the basis of experience. I add that as their functioning and performance improve they can expect their self-esteem to rise. Some of our patients are so chronically unsuccessful in their endeavors that one would expect them to be pessimists and to recognize that they frequently need help that others do not. However, perhaps defensively or as a show of bravado, many ADHD patients say that things will get better and disavow any need for assistance (except, perhaps, for certain tasks delegated to the spouse, such as compiling their income tax).

With regard to those ADHD adults who are at increased risk for alcohol and substance abuse, we have anecdotal evidence (as mentioned earlier) that some patients experience a decreased urge to drink when responding to pharmacotherapy. It is possible—though this has not been tested—that medication might increase the efficacy of 12-step programs such as Alcoholics Anonymous and Narcotics Anonymous, and of related psychological support groups. Realistic interventions other than psychotherapy are also often helpful—for example, debt consolidation, vocational retraining, obtaining medical help for a child, even declaration of bankruptcy. The therapist is a functional alter ego, but the patient needs help in learning to use problem-solving techniques. The therapist has helped the patient solve his major symptomatic problems, but many old and new problems remain. Finally, counseling may help the patient to continue with the medication and thus avoid the recidivism that frequently follows without it.

COUPLE TREATMENT

Many of the patients we see have been in unsuccessful couple therapy (again, we do not see the treatment successes), but pharmacotherapy seems to make couple therapy much more effective. In many instances a major problem of the previous couple therapy had been impaired communication. When that was a result of the patient's failure to listen or interruption of his spouse when she was talking, the increased attention and decreased impulsivity in drug responders can produce a quantum leap in improved communication. The rapid change in one partner can produce a significant change in the relationship.

At times the improvement of a patient is followed, at least temporarily, by an increase in marital friction. The nonpatient finds that she has been right all along in her belief that her spouse was difficult. As I commented earlier, the responding patient has to contend with "a new identity" and acknowledge that he made serious contributions to marital, vocational, and academic dysfunction. Not uncommonly, the

Table 6.1 Drug Treatment of ADHD in Adults: Systematic Studies of Several Types of Medication

Study	Study Focus	Sample N (m = males; f = females)	Average Age	Design	Results (Good = moderate-to-marked improvement)
Stimulants					
Wood et al. (1976)	Methylphenidate	15 (6 m, 9 f)	28 ± 5	11 in double-blind crossover with placebo, 4 in open trial	8 good early response, 2 good response later (67%)
Wender et al. (1981)	Pemoline	48 (22 m, 26 f)	28 ± 5	Double-blind parallel with placebo	For 26 subjects with PRS scores[1] ≥12: good response in 8 of 17 (47%) given pemoline, and in 1 of 9 given placebo. For 22 with PRS scores ≤12: no significant difference between pemoline and placebo.
Wender et al. (1985)	Methylphenidate	37 (20 m, 17 f)	31 ± 7	Double-blind crossover with placebo	Good response in 21 of patients when given drug (57%) and in 4 patients when given placebo. For patients with PRS score ≥12, significant difference in treatment response to drug and to placebo. For patients with PRS scores ≤12, differences not significant.
Mattes et al. (1984)	Methylphenidate	66 (33 m, 33 f)	—	Double-blind crossover with placebo	Trend for subjects with ADD in childhood (PRS ≥10.7) to respond more favorably to drug. No overall drug-placebo significant differences

Gualtieri et al. (1985)	Methylphenidate	8 m	—	Double-blind crossover with placebo	All 8 responded favorably in brief trial, but not in follow-up.
Monoamine Oxidase Inhibitors					
Wender et al. (1983)	Pargyline	16 (13 m, 3 f)	32 ± 6	Open trial[2]	Good response in 11 patients (69%)
Wood et al. (1983)	L-deprenyl	11 (8 m, 3 f)	32.9	Open trial	Good response in 6 (54%), but annoying side effects
Other Medications					
Wender & Reimherr (1990)	Bupropion (antidepressant)	19 (14 m, 5 f)	39 ± 6	Open trial in excellent responders to stimulants or MAOIs	5 unable to tolerate minimum dose. Good response in remaining 14 (74% of original sample).
Wood et al. (1982)	Levodopa (precursor amino acid)	8 (5 m, 3 f)	—	Open trial	Intital positive response, but no sustained response
Wood et al. (1985)	DL-phenylalanine (precursor amino acid)	13 (5 m, 8 f)	27.6	Double-blind crossover with placebo	Some initial improvement, but loss of all benefits within 3 months
Reimherr et al. (1987)	L-tyrosine (precursor amino acid)	12 (6 m, 6 f)	30 ± 7.5	Open trial	Initial good response in 8 (67%), but loss of all benefits within 8 weeks.

[1] PRS = Parents' Rating Scale.

[2] Most of our open trials were done after elimination of some patients in placebo washouts.

treated patient is concerned with the question of, "Who is the real me?" These concerns also extend outside his marriage and involve his relationships with his children, fellow employees, boss, and so forth, and these changes, in turn, can put more pressure on the marriage. The fixed, although frequently maladaptive, pattern of relationships is disrupted. As has been observed in other psychiatric areas, a relief of symptoms in one partner can produce a worsening of the relationship (Satel and Southwick, 1987). However, if the patient and spouse enter couple therapy at this point, the patient's improved functioning often allows couple therapy to work. The cognitive, behavioral, and emotional changes that the patient has experienced can make him a more rational and thoughtful person, with whom psychological techniques can work more effectively.

Effective drug treatment can also worsen relationships in ways that are hard to change. One treatment-responsive patient reported that she could now think about her husband in a rational, well-organized way and, because of her new and better perception, could perceive his limitations accurately. She now understood what she had only felt before: that her husband did have manifold defects and that "our relationship was, is, and will probably continue to be lousy . . . it was hard for me to see when I was focusing on *my* problems."

UNANSWERED PSYCHOLOGICAL QUESTIONS

Although the efficacy of medication has been documented, the usefulness of psychosocial treatment, counseling, support groups, and couple treatment remains to be explored. My impression is that psychological therapies are of limited benefit unless drug treatment is effective. The interaction of medication and psychological treatments should be of much interest to both the researcher and the therapist. The question to be decided is which psychological treatments are helpful with which types of ADHD patients who respond to medication. The answers to that question would be enormously illuminating to the therapist who must make recommendations for approaches to persistent difficulties following drug treatment.

NOTES

1. The federal government has, under the Drug Enforcement Administration, established laws governing the prescription of certain "controlled" drugs.

These are drugs which produce a dependency, "a cluster of cognitive, behavioral and physiological symptoms . . . which the individual continues use of . . . despite significant substance related problems" (DSM IV, p. 176; associated with tolerance, requiring larger and larger doses of a medication to produce a given effect, and physiological and psychological symptoms when the medication is discontinued). The "Schedule" ranges from I to V. Schedule II drugs are those regarded as at greatest risk for dependency and abuse among those clinically available; these include morphine, meperidine (Demerol), the amphetamines and methylphenidate. Prescriptions must be presented to a pharmacist for dispensing within ten days of the date the prescription was written. The maximum number of pills that can be dispensed is one month's supply: a new prescription must be written each month; renewals are not permitted. Schedule IV drugs are considered to pose a comparatively small risk for dependency of abuse and include codeine with aspirin, diazepam (Valium) and pemoline. Prescriptions may be renewed up to a six-month maximum. Because of the paperwork and the concern about how they may be perceived by the regulatory bodies in their states, many physicians are reluctant to prescribe Schedule II drugs.

2. Inattentiveness without hyperactivity we felt to be too nonspecific. ADD without hyperactivity is believed by some to be a different group from ADD-H and to respond less well to stimulant medication; and inattentiveness itself is seen in Generalized Anxiety Disorder and in Major Depression.

3. Safer and Allen (1989) found that 6 percent of school age children followed for an average of six years developed tolerance to methylphenidate. When tolerance to methylphenidate occurs, patients apparently do not develop cross tolerance to D-amphetamine and should receive a trial of that drug. The same probably obtains for patients who become tolerant to D-amphetamine.

7

The Experiences of Adult ADHD Patients on Stimulants

■

The following accounts by four patients (Daniel P, Caroline G, Sonia D, and George F) and two spouses (writing about Bruce C and George F) communicate a sense of the relief some adult ADHD patients and their families experience when treatment with methylphenidate (Ritalin) begins. The history by Sonia D conveys an idea of changes experienced on both amphetamine and methylphenidate. All of the accounts also vividly describe what it is like to be afflicted with ADHD.[1]

DANIEL P

■

CLINICAL BACKGROUND

Daniel P is a 31-year-old married father of two who referred himself to the clinic with complaints that "More and more I am aware that I am different from other people—I can't get things done—I have no stick-to-it-tiveness." He stated that he rarely lasted in any job for more than 6 months. He was not fired—he got bored and would go away. His easy susceptibility to boredom penalized him at college, which he had begun on several occasions, never lasting more than a few months.

He stated that he has had chronic difficulties in his associating with other people. He had never had a close friend or a confidant. In company he always found himself doing things inappropriately and was embarrassed by his own behavior. When invited by other people he felt they didn't like him. He also felt that he could not participate in the conversational trivia of parties and social gatherings.

Boredom has been a chronic problem. He will watch a movie and read at the same time. While watching television he continually flips the channels. He has had chronic difficulty with anger. As a child he stole powder from his father's shotgun shells and used it to make cannons. He chased his sisters with knives until the age of 15 or 16: "I thrived on making them cry." The other things he would do to upset them was to put his fingers in their food and twist their arms. He learned to turn anger inward as a child and apparently sublimated his hostility with imaginative, gory science-fiction-like inventions. As an adult, when angry, he has put his fist through the wall. His marriage has lasted because his wife is very calm and obliging.

Despite his social isolation and what sound like early (primitive) fantasies, he does not manifest any other symptoms of schizotypal disorder.

His course in the study has been as follows: in the placebo-controlled trial he showed a moderate-to-marked response to methylphenidate and has continued in the study for the past two years on a dose of 50 mg per day (10 mg every 3 hours, 5 times per day). On medication his temper has been controlled, he is not bored, has shown little affective lability and has become extremely well organized. As a consequence his relationship with his wife has improved substantially and he has been able to obtain and function well in a position of a religious teacher. His score on the Global Assessment of Functioning has risen from 50 to 77, and his score on the Social Adjustment Scale has improved from moderate maladjustment (4) to excellent (1).

STATEMENT BY DANIEL P

"Apples and Oranges and Bananas"

It is difficult to know where to begin. My goal is to explain what it is like to have Attention Deficit Hyperactivity Disorder Residual Type. But I believe it is impossible for "normal" people to understand the frustration, anger, confusion, and eventual hopelessness that comes with failure at every turn. I will do my best, but please understand, I am attempting to tell apples and oranges what it feels like to be a banana.

I am an adult male of 31 years. About three years ago I met Dr.

Paul H. Wender for the first time. The meeting was painful. Whether he intended it or not, I don't know, but his questions became increasingly irritating. Not for content, but because of the seemingly unimportant gibberish. I have come to realize that those questions were important, but the experience illustrates the frustration that comes with the inability to focus or understand. This was a very common experience throughout my life.

Inevitably, this frustration leads to fits of acting out and even violence. While these results seem related the causes are different. The acting out comes from a need to do something. The something could be anything that crossed the mind. On one occasion in high school my science teacher had assigned us several pages of text book busy-work. Everyone was working so hard and the class was so silent, but the work was so senseless that I stood on my desk, screamed at the top of my lungs and ran across the tops of the desks, then returned to my desk and continued the assignment. The teacher was either too shocked, too amused (along with the class) or too stupid to do anything about it. I, on the other hand, was mortified at my actions. When I said there was a "need to do something" that need is genuine. So overpowering that it forced me to do things I normally would not. There is no rhyme or reason, it simply had to be done.

The other result of frustration—violence—was actually the release of anger that I felt at all times. Always just below the surface, I had a seething volcano of anger and violence ready to explode. I played football in Little League and again in high school and I enjoyed hitting and hurting others. There was such a tremendous sense of relief to hit and to hurt. When someone would limp off or have to be carried off the field the feeling was near ecstasy. Even now as I write this I can remember those feelings. I don't understand them, but I remember them.

The anger also caused me to constantly look for a release. I wanted someone to provoke me so I could hurt them. This anger could not be eaten up by physical exercise or other releases. It typically was just there, and I was forced to deal with it. My parents, being very strict, forced me to learn control. Which I did, but the anger was always there, waiting.

Another effect that I can now recognize was an inability to read and study. On countless occasions I would attempt to study for school and fail miserably. After only a few minutes I would become so irritated that I would throw the book across the room and watch television instead. The biggest problem was my inability to stay focused. I could read pages in a text while my mind was elsewhere, settling an old argument I had had with a friend two years ago, or beaming aboard the Star Ship Enterprise. I could read the words, I just couldn't attach any meaning.

Much of this led to the last effect that I am aware of, and that is guilt. I have felt guilt for everything I have ever done and many things I didn't do. Please do not suppose me guilty of any great wrongdoing, but things like hitting one of my sisters, lying to my mom, saying the wrong thing at a party or simply being the life of the party. Afterwards, even after admitting my lies or apologizing, I was still racked with guilt. Similarly, in situations when I should have done something and didn't, the guilt was also very real. Like remembering when I meant to tell a foul-mouthed man on the bus to shut his yap, but didn't, can be a particular source of pain. My mind would return me to the instance time and time again. I would imagine that I acted properly each time, but it never helped. Some of these moments are decades old. There was an incident where I embarrassed myself on stage when I was in elementary school in front of the entire student body that had bothered me until I met Dr. Wender.

Hopefully, I have given some kind of an understanding of my experience. Although most illustrations were from my younger years, rest assured they continued well into adulthood. In fact, things had gotten so bad that I was becoming a recluse and refused to mingle with other people. It was then I realized I needed help and was eventually introduced to Dr. Wender. As I said, his first interview was almost more than I could stand, but after being placed on Ritalin 10 mg, 5 times daily, I have sincerely enjoyed our meetings and even looked forward to them. My wife told Dr. Wender that the change had been dramatic. I was a little slower to recognize the change. Frustration was only a memory, the "need" as well as the seething anger were gone, and for the first time I opened a college text book and read it from cover to cover with good understanding. Not just reading it, mind you, but outlining and taking notes. The experience frightened me because I was actually understanding nearly all of it. That gave me the courage to return to college full-time and finish my degree, which I have done. I can think clearly, I can discuss without getting frustrated, I can argue without losing control, and most wonderful of all, I can read! I have discovered the wonderful world of literature. But that's not all; for the first time *since my first job when I was 14, I have kept a job longer than six months and actually have a professional career.*

There is one more thing, for lack of a better word, that Ritalin has changed. There were times that my mind would seem to engage without my knowledge or consent. And I would be stranded on a run-away locomotive that would crash through any barrier I would erect in attempts to gain control. This would happen most often as I lay in bed waiting for sleep. The mental locomotive might take a trip that lasted all night. Sometimes it might engage in the middle of the night and wake me from a dead sleep. Ritalin stopped this. On more than one occasion I have asked Dr. Wender to convince me that Ritalin is a stimulant because on those nights of the thought express, I take Ritalin and it's like the calm after an ocean storm. The waves are slowly subdued until the surface is like shimmering glass and sleep comes so naturally that I enter REM easily. Sometimes I will wake up exactly two and a half hours after taking the first dose and need to take a second. Again the storm passes and sleep returns. On rare occasions I might awake having not taken any Ritalin before bed, but a dose then has the same calming effects.

There is no way to explain what Dr. Wender and his treatment of me with Ritalin means to me. Ritalin is a true miracle drug. It saved my education, my marriage, and quite possibly my life. Ritalin has given me what I thought was impossible, control of my life. And although I'm still a banana, at least I'm a little more spherical and can roll with the punches.

CAROLINE G

■

CLINICAL BACKGROUND

Caroline G was a 32-year-old mother of two boys who contacted our clinic after reading an article given to her by one of her son's teachers. She had enrolled in a community college computer program, but homework was a terrible problem since she could not stick with it. Caroline experienced chronic distractibility, impulsivity, an explosive temper, and an inability to sustain long-term relationships. During the entire initial evaluation she was swinging on her chair.

Caroline met the criteria for a diagnosis of Attention-deficit Hyperactivity Disorder and was entered into the five-week double-blind portion of the study. She showed a moderate-to-marked improvement on methylphenidate and was then entered into the open phase of the study. After one year in the study she reported that she had quit smoking and drinking on her own. She continued for three years on a dose of 50 mg of methylphenidate per day (10 mg every 2¹/₂ hours, 5 times per day). Her score on the Global Assessment of Functioning has risen from 55 to 68, and her score on the Social Adjustment Scale has improved from moderate maladjustment (4) to good (2).

STATEMENT BY CAROLINE G

I've been asked to write this letter to describe how Ritalin has helped and changed my life. Before I can describe the changes, I feel it necessary to give a little background on myself so that you can better understand how I have benefitted from the use of Ritalin over the last two years.

I grew up in a very dysfunctional home as a child. Although my family, specifically my parents, tried to keep up the appearance of normality, it was anything but a normal childhood.

My father was an alcoholic. Although I can never remember him staggering drunk, he was always drinking. As a loving parent, he was totally lacking. He never really involved himself in raising us, except when he had to, as in physically disciplining us.

My mother, on the other hand, did everything that was expected of a middle-class housewife—the PTA, Girl Scout Leader, Cub Scout Leader, etc . . . although her heart wasn't really in it. She admitted to me several years ago that she hated it, she only did it because it was expected of her to keep up appearances. She portrayed the perfect loving mother to the world, while at home she showed us very little affection or love. I'm not even sure if my mother really loved any of her children, or even wanted us, and I think that even as a child I sensed this.

While I was growing up, my mother described me as her free spirit. I was always happy and on the go. Always getting into trouble, I did things on impulse without regard to the consequences of my actions. Most of the time I believed I wouldn't get caught, and if caught I would lie about it. I thought if I kept up the lie, they would eventually have to believe me. I was like a whirling dervish, always on the go, I couldn't sit still for any length of time, and if I had to stay in one place, I always had a body part moving, such as shaking my leg or fiddling with my hair.

As a child, I was very emotional, to the point of being overly dramatic. I would laugh too loud, cry constantly over little things, stupid things, my voice could carry over any conversation, and I was extremely aggressive with a very violent temper. My emotions ruled my life, making it difficult to fit in very well with my peers. I constantly would say inappropriate things to try to fit in, but I was basically a loner.

I didn't really do well in school for the first three years, although I was above average intelligence and could read before I entered Kindergarten. I nearly failed in second grade. I can remember being frustrated with how slow the other children were. I would finish the lesson the teacher and class were doing and go on to the next lesson. Then when called on by the teacher to read or do a problem, I wouldn't be able to because I didn't know where we were. This caused the teacher to become very frustrated with me because my test scores were always very high but I couldn't keep my attention on what the class was doing. In the fourth grade I was lucky enough to get a teacher who recognized my problem and my potential and put me into an individual study program. At this time I started to get straight A's. By the time I was in sixth grade, I was doing eighth-grade-level-work. I managed to keep my grades up and graduate, although if I had been an average student, I probably would never have made it out of High School.

These problems followed me into my teen and adult years. Although I did extremely well in school, I still had trouble socializing with my peers. I was an overactive, talkative teenager, I was impulsive and I blurted out inappropriate things at the wrong time. Basically, I irritated other people. When I was 14 years old, I started to drink alcohol and when I was 15, I sought out the local drugs on the street. I started smoking marijuana first, then progressed by the time I was 17 to painkillers (Percodan, Demerol), LSD and cocaine. It wasn't until I started using drugs and alcohol that I was able to actually socialize with other teenagers. Not just those who partied, but also the kids who didn't. The use of marijuana slowed me down enough to stop and think before I acted. I became more comfortable in situations that used to be very stressful and difficult for me.

As an adult, I had problems with any kind of relationship. I could be friends with men, but on a dating-relationship level, I could never stay in one more than 3 or 4 months. I was still impulsive, spending money earmarked for bills. I had a serious drug and alcohol problem, and my self-esteem was in the basement.

After I had children, I found that I had another serious problem. I had no patience and no control over my temper. I became fearful of hurting my own children. I took parenting courses, and had several classes in child and adolescent psychology in college, but even with all these courses, it didn't help when disciplining my children. There were times when I actually felt like beating my kids senseless. I couldn't understand how I could feel this way when I loved my children. It got to the point where any little thing would make me break into tears. Sometimes, I would cry for no reason. I knew I wasn't depressed because I was always happy. But my mood swings were driving me crazy. One minute I would be mad, the next a raging maniac, then I would start crying and then I would be fine as if nothing had happened all in the span of five or six hours. I would get depressed, but it would never last more than a day or two. Sometimes I felt as if I was going crazy.

Since I have been involved in the Ritalin study at the University of Utah Medical Center, my whole life has changed for the better. I finally feel normal. My mood swings are not as severe as they used to be. They could almost be considered normal. I don't explode or blow up over little things anymore. I have more patience with my children and have been able to institute a more consistent form of discipline without the physical violence that permeated my discipline before.

I have better control over my impulsivity. My financial situation has improved considerably and I no longer find myself spending money recklessly. I have even stopped my drinking and use of drugs without having to go through any kind of counseling or rehabilitation. I find that I just don't have the desire to do them anymore.

But the most important change of all is in my self-esteem. For the first time in my life, I can actually say that I like myself and I can accept who I am, with all my faults and my assets.

The Ritalin has changed my life for the better and I will challenge anyone who says that it is not an effective medication for adults to use. I don't want to go back to what my life was like before and I hope that I will be allowed to continue the use of Ritalin for my ADHD.

BRUCE C

■

CLINICAL BACKGROUND

Bruce C was a 54-year-old teacher and sports coach who left his job after more than a dozen years at the same school because of an accumulation of complaints both at school and in the community. He describes himself as having been very restless and inattentive during elementary school, where he had a difficult time learning. He described himself as a troublemaker. When he was four years old he told his parents that his brother had drowned, "just to get a rise out of them." As a six or seven-year-old he got annoyed and broke all the windows in his father's car. He had very low feelings of self-esteem. Not only was he a recognized problem in the school but his father was the town drunk. His Parents' Rating Scale was 22 (over the 99th percentile). There was a family history of alcoholism. Both his parents, his brother and one sister were alcoholics and the patient said he would have become one too had he not vowed (successfully) not to drink. At the time of admission the patient had just left his teaching job and was in the process of looking unsuccessfully for another job. Under this pressure his ADHD symptoms had become more severe. He was having chronic difficulty with his wife and was estranged from his two older children. During the placebo trials he had a marked beneficial effect from methylphenidate. The dose has been standardized at 90 mg per day (15 mg every $2^{1}/_{2}$ hours, 6 times per day). He has been continued on the drug for five years without development of tolerance. His score on the Global Assessment of Functioning has risen from 53 to 78 (at 48 months follow-up), and his score on the Social Adjustment Scale has improved from moderate maladjustment (4) to good (2).

COMMENT BY SPOUSE OF BRUCE C

When I met and started dating Bruce in the 1960s, he was in the U.S. Army. I dated him and got to know him pretty well over the next year. I also knew his parents, and his four brothers and sisters. As I got to know his family better I noticed that most of his family members were very "quick tempered" and seemed to act quite impulsively. While dating Bruce, I lived with his sister, while we were both in the process of getting a divorce. One of the most common examples of his sister's behavior is that she never allowed enough time to get ready for work and almost always ended up throwing either the iron or her clothes across the room and bursting into tears and usually blaming whatever, or whomever, she could. The family thought of themselves as "outspoken." I thought they acted without much thought or common sense. In most circumstances Bruce and I got along quite well. We were not in very many stressful situations, even though I did observe that Bruce had a "quick temper" usually directed at the "idiots" on the road that didn't know how to drive. He was also very sensitive and thought people were talking about him, but often they would be, to comment on his "quick tempered" behavior.

All of the C family liked to consume alcohol and this habit seemed to enhance all of these negative behaviors. Both of his parents drank regularly, his father daily, his mother usually all weekend. All of his family drank more than occasionally and Bruce's only brother and one sister have been in several programs for alcoholics. Bruce quit shortly after our marriage, or I'm positive we never would have made a life together. Whenever under the influence it was common to have verbal and physical confrontations dancing at a local club. Bruce felt like the bartender was not putting the amount of alcohol he should have been putting, so he took a drink of it and threw it across the room into the jukebox. When the waitress came over he told her he wanted a drink with some alcohol now.

The thing the C's were most successful at was excusing each other's and their own behavior, always claiming that if "they hadn't screwed up" or if "he would have shut up" or if "she would have just did what she should have" then they wouldn't have become angry or lost control. This behavior bothered me a lot. However, Bruce and I decided not to consume much alcohol, which helped greatly, and until after we married in 1967, I didn't observe this behavior very often. Since Bruce was and is a very intelligent and caring person, it seemed I could overlook the other behavior, and like every woman in the world, I thought he would improve with time—Bruce didn't improve with time. I observed very belligerent, impulsive behavior whenever a near crisis situation would come up—for example, arriving in a large West Coast city and having Bruce under the wheel and trying to survive his outrageous out-of-control behavior when he couldn't find the address, which was always. He would, as I called it, pull his big "R&R" (ranting and raving) until I could visualize somehow getting him out of the car and then either running over him or driving off and leaving him and never seeing him again.

There are literally hundreds of similar examples over the years. Instead of carrying out either of the examples I just used, I chose to distance myself from Bruce. By the early seventies we had four small children. I spent a lot of my next years keeping every stressful situation from Bruce that I could, covering for the kids so they didn't make Daddy angry, and even though Bruce was quite successful at blaming me for his behaviors, I tried never to let him do it to the *kids and handled everything that I could alone. I learned to resent and feel unhappy and lonely most of the time. I tried to invite family or friends to our home when Bruce had to work, because when people were visiting were the times he would always manage to have a reason to be out of control and usually yell at me and usually throw something or just be generally rude. Every time we had events we had to go to I would try just to leave Bruce home. My salvation, so to speak, was that along with his working full-time and part-time, when he was home he wanted to be left alone and spent all of his time at home watching TV.*

Bruce spent over a dozen years teaching. At this job and his part-time job, even though he was always very qualified, he continued over the years to have personality conflicts with unruly kids and their parents and though very educated and knowing what he wanted to communicate to people, it never worked out. Bruce was the "most unlucky," "misunderstood" person in the world, and he always ended up losing his temper and letting the other person know the problem belonged to them, and that they were idiots. Bruce went through hell, because of these problems, and finally over the years Bruce even started realizing as I did that these were "his problems." Finally in the late 1980s, he was given the choice to resign or be fired from teaching, and he resigned. He felt very "picked on" and had a very hard year out of work and found it impossible to get another job that was very impressive, or paid very much. We were barely staying married and were both very unhappy, but now with eight children we didn't have too many choices. I am positive if Bruce hadn't gotten into the ADD study, I would have divorced him.

About his situation in life. One day while he was listening to the radio he heard someone talking about a federal study in ADD. They talked about the symptoms and effects this could have on some-one's life—Bruce quickly called me to listen and asked me who this might sound like. It described Bruce exactly. *We got on the phone and made an appointment and went in.*

The first 2 weeks Bruce was on Ritalin I could tell a great change in him. Instead of him barely being able to concentrate on one conversation or one telephone call, he could watch TV and listen in on my phone conversation, which I never had to worry about all of the years I knew him. I found him being able to communicate with the kids and follow through with reasonable discipline. One son commented that he liked Dad better before he "knew what was going on" because now he would follow through when he grounded them or whatever he was doing with them. Soon he could even talk to our oldest son with no tempers flaring, and being aware of how he would have reacted earlier in life. For the first time I dared to count on Bruce to help me with our large family. I slowly started to confide in him about a few things, and found I could even vent a little anger about my life.

There is no, none, no way that ours would still be an existing family if it weren't for this medication and counseling therapy that has gone along with it. I feel that Bruce's improvement is both medication and behavior modification. However, if a crisis of any dimension comes up when he hasn't had his meds, we have a very painful recall of past times. Bruce is different in almost every way. He has always wanted to be someone we could count on and talk to and have those he cares about and works with value and respect his opinions; this happens often now.

Bruce works for the government doing a job that is very detailed and takes more concentration than he ever could have had anytime prior to this study. He stayed totally away from computers, because they drove him crazy. Now at his job Bruce helped change his department over to computers, and is a very well-respected, valued employee. He contributes ideas and several of his ideas have been incorporated as policy. His communication skills have improved drastically at home and at work. Several years ago Bruce went back to a state university and received an advanced degree and updated his teaching certificate, and while working full-time and going to school full-time graduated with a 4.0 in his major and a 3.7 overall. Bruce seems to have gained a lot of confidence and isn't afraid people won't respect or listen to him. His life has improved in every way possible.

SONIA D

■

CLINICAL BACKGROUND

Sonia D was the first patient I diagnosed as having "minimal brain dysfunction"[2] persisting into adult life. When I first met her and she presented her history, I felt that she was an unhappy woman who had had an exceedingly difficult childhood and who had discovered that she felt better when she drank in moderation or took sympathomimetic drugs. As we talked about her symptoms and life history it gradually became clear to me that she was a "minimally brain dysfunctioned" child grown up. She gave a detailed account of the metamorphoses of her symptoms as she grew older and their response to stimulants, which she responded to in an atypical way—she became calmer, less angry, more trusting. She convinced me that she was what I then thought a *rara avis*, an "MBD" adult who responded to stimulants as did MBD children. Her history follows. I have now followed her for the past 17 years. Her dose of medication has remained constant at 30 mg per day (10 mg of D-amphetamine every 4 hours, 3 times per day). Her score on the Global Assessment of Functioning has risen from 52 to 80, and her score on the Social Adjustment Scale has improved from moderate-to-marked maladjustment (4.5) to good (2).

STATEMENT BY SONIA D

I am a 61-year-old American woman of Russian extraction. I have no physical impairments, and I am reasonably healthy despite being slightly overweight. I have a Ph.D. in Medieval History, I am a member of Phi Beta Kappa, I speak two foreign languages fluently and have a working knowledge of several others. I am a free-lance writer and editor. I have been married for 40 years to a medical science professor, and I have had no children.

Because childhood ADHD is so frequently equated with school difficulties, it would seem unlikely that the above-described "achiever" had ever been afflicted with ADHD. I, however, having spent a lifetime in the skin of that individual, have no doubt that I was an ADHD child. Besides the overt "hyperactivity"—including terrible difficulty falling asleep and, once asleep, waking up—I had many of the other signs: impulsiveness, stress intolerance, hot temper, garrulity, bossiness, stubbornness, unpopularity—and I was easily distracted. Moreover, I am not drastically changed from that child—except to the extent that I am medicated. Attila the Hun on tricycle wheels did not undergo a startling transmogrification at the age of 13 or 14. I did not suddenly become a tractable, well-behaved, rational and controlled adolescent; I merely withdrew. I became a sullen, fearful, unpopular teenager with periodic episodes of explosive temper. In young adulthood I was unconventional in my behavior, "pushy" in my dealings with others and still subject to explosive temper. Since my early forties I have been medicated with amphet-

amine, which has given me the control that makes life reasonably peaceful and productive—but the child is still there and, even as a successfully medicated adult, I have no difficulty identifying with her.

But why, then, did I not fall into the usual life pattern of one failure after another? I suppose my first advantage was being bright. Reading—most learning in fact—came easily to me, and I think I learned how to compensate for my lack of attention span in one way or another; for instance, somewhere, sometime, early in life, I apparently discovered two techniques for facilitating any kind of rote learning: (1) I could concentrate better if my pencil was engaged (taking notes, scribbling in margins, underlining key words) and (2) most abstractions could be learned if they could be reduced to a concrete image (a graph, a chart, an outline, a diagram, a fanciful cluster of shapes, a technicolor picture on the blank screen on my brain). Numbers, lists, abstractions, then, never became easy, but at least they became manageable. And, because school was my joy from the first day, I became easily obsessive about any form of learning.

Another factor could well have been my much maligned "stubbornness": Each time I was told, "You never finish anything," I responded to the challenge, and the "I'll show you" attitude kicked in, so that I remember being tenacious about many tasks that required a good deal of attention span. But then I ask, is it truly "attention span" or is it a compulsive, obsessive desire to compensate for a native distractibility that wears you out and drives you crazy and makes your day-to-day existence a painful experience from waking (catastrophe) to sleeping (collapse)? Much of the anguish is trivial, of course: I cannot bear to have someone read over my shoulder or watch me do anything that requires some concentration. I cannot tolerate anyone in the kitchen when I'm preparing a meal. I cannot carry on a conversation or drive if the radio is on. All day long I hear everything and mechanically identify each sound: the mail truck, the cat coming through the swinging pet door, the click in the furnace, the robins in the pyracantha, a sudden shift in the wind. My brain is never on automatic pilot. My husband and I long ago decided that on long trips it made sense for me to do all the driving, since I drove the whole way in any event—whether I was behind the wheel or not. I am incessantly noting and recording facts—important and trifling indiscriminately: the state of the gas gauge, the shaggy brown and white dog on the corner of High Street and the Cornmarket, the position of the town in the relationship to the river, the cop in the white Jaguar squad car in Aberdeen. I'm handy to have around on a second trip to anywhere, because I never forget a place, I know how to get from one side of town to the other, and I'd be a perfect traveling companion if I weren't so habitually uptight, if I didn't gasp look out! to the driver, if I didn't bark out orders and directions and become shrill when they weren't carried out to my satisfaction, if I didn't have to stop at the gas station "rest room" so often, if I didn't keep mentioning the funny little rattle in the engine that wasn't there yesterday. . . .

And I cannot bear a wind that lasts longer than three or four hours: It drives me wild and wears me down and sets my teeth on edge and makes me impossible—more impossible—to live with. It impinges, intrudes, makes demands on my consciousness, and concentration is then quite out of the question. To put it another way, I feel as if my brain has no filtering system for the massive sensory barrage that relentlessly assails it.

All the other characteristics of ADHD children—impulsiveness, disorderliness, temper, hyperreactivity, unpopularity—I recall well and, in retrospect, I believe they all stem from an overpowering impulse to act. The mot clef is urgency. Everything is urgent. There is no letup. Life is an endless, relentless series of white-knuckle events. All of the miscellaneous dysfunctions (low frustration tolerance, poor planning and judgment, recklessness, disregard for injury, antisocial behavior) are reducible to an urgency that brooks no delay, no postponement, no obstruction to the fulfillment of a necessary goal, which is usually an urge to act. I believe it is a hyperactivation that is not susceptible to reason, to suppression, to socialization, to inhibition—it is a force that is compelling, distressing and uncontrollable; and it manifests itself in an urgency that cannot be ignored—a kind of "tunnel vision" of life.

Because of a number of chance circumstances, I have had doctors' prescriptions for amphetamine at various times during my life: When I was an undergraduate I consulted the student-health physician for extreme fatigue (we called it my "sleeping sickness" or "hibernation" because it was most prevalent in the fall and winter); she prescribed small doses of amphetamine, which I found fairly miraculous. Parenthetically, all during my undergraduate years I consumed enormous quantities of coffee when I studied. I don't now remember how long I took amphetamine during that period, but I do remember that I was very favorably impressed with the results. When I was in my mid-to-late twenties my husband and I thought we'd like to begin a family; I, however, suffered from endometriosis, a condition that is frequently associated with barrenness. At that time endometriosis was susceptible to a great many tentative—trial and error—courses of treatment, and, having undergone a course of basal-temperature recordings, Cytomel® (triiodothyronine), estrogen, progesterone, myriad combinations thereof, and, as somebody's last resort, D-amphetamine, I was no nearer motherhood than I had ever been—or ever would be. I was, however, about to embark upon a decade of remarkable creativity, productivity and relative contentment: I explained to my gynecologist that the amphetamine made me feel very good, and he obligingly assured me that there was no harm in my continuing to take the drug. I can no longer remember the trade-name of the compound or the dosage, but, as I recall, I had a prescription for 100 tablets, which I had refilled every three months for ten years. I was scrupulous about never exceeding my allotment of drug—perhaps because I sensed that it would be taken away from me if I abused it, perhaps because I never felt a need for more. During that period of purposeful activity, I researched and wrote my first novel, I undertook several major landscaping and decorating projects in the home we had purchased, and I quit smoking—three packages a day. I continued to pursue my intellectual and literary interests, and in 1965 I decided to return to school, this time to earn a degree in History, which I had found to be more broadly appealing than Romance Languages, my undergraduate major. I finished my M.A. in 1968, and in 1970 I successfully passed the qualifying exams for a Ph.D.

In that year the cause of a slow but troublesomely persistent weight gain was traced to moderately severe Gull's disease (hypothyroidism). I was—and am still—treated with L-thyroxine, but the amphetamine was judiciously discontinued. It was not a happy decision: While my hypothyroid symptoms—dry skin, edema, hoarse voice, etc.—disappeared, I continued to gain weight, I was depressed and I was unable to work on my dissertation. After a few months I consulted an internist who specialized in "weight control." He prescribed a reducing diet and issued a prescription for—wonder of wonders—Didrex! I eagerly took the drug, followed the diet, lost 20 pounds and was, once again, happy and purposeful. Unfortunately, when I failed to lose more weight, my physician scolded me and withdrew the Didrex, and I ceased to consult him. Again I was depressed, again my weight soared, again I was unable to work on my dissertation. In addition, my alcohol consumption rose sharply *and there were severe recurring conflicts with my husband. In January of 1972 I decided to finish my dissertation by June—or die trying. Without telling my metabolics doctor or my husband—who had always objected to my taking Dexedrine—I again appealed to the "weight specialist" I had seen before. Motivated by desperation and reliant on native craftiness, I managed to lose just enough weight to keep the drug coming, and I carefully husbanded whatever excess drug I could squeeze out of my monthly prescription. My credibility with the weight man ran out in May just as I finished the dissertation.*

From 1972 (when I received my Ph.D.) until the summer of 1977, I desperately stuffed myself with No-Doz, my weight continued to rise, my inability to make any significant progress on a second novel (begun in 1973) began to be anguishing, my uncontrolled alcohol consumption became debilitating and frankly terrifying, my relationship with my husband deteriorated steadily, I developed a siege mentality, and somewhere within that disordered period I found myself consulting a psychiatrist for depression and frustration at my inability to cope with almost every facet of life—big or small.

Under my psychiatrist's supervision, I began taking methylphenidate (later D-amphetamine) in June 1977. In September I finished my novel. (From January 1973 to June 1977, I wrote 250 pages; from June to September 1977, I wrote 400 pages!) I remember feeling that my life had been saved. From that time to this (July 1994) I have taken amphetamine, and if the most reliable proof of the disorder is whether the medication works, than it is clear to me that I do have ADHD because the medication definitely works!

The most noticeable effect of both methylphenidate and D-amphetamine is a cessation of my normal agitation—physical and mental. The methylphenidate has a truly "calming" effect: a serenity that has nothing to do with sedating or euphoria, but seems rather to be a conscious feeling of control *over irrelevant and intrusive motions and thoughts. Amphetamine, on the other hand, appears to give a purposeful direction, a meaningful channeling to the intensity of one's drive; in other words, it, too, gives* control, *but it appears to be a more dynamic, more decisive control. When I take methylphenidate I become aware of the fact that, unmedicated, I habitually clench my teeth and rhythmically move my foot and frequently clutch the arms of my chair; I am aware of these habits by the simple fact of their* absence. *Amphetamine also removes this desultory muscular tension or motion, but it is less noticeable be-*

cause there may still be activity, but now it has some purpose. In these—admittedly difficult-to-describe—examples I hope to convey the notion that the "good," purposeful activity may be mental as well as physical, because one of the next immediate reactions that I get to either drug is an exquisitely satisfying awareness of the ability to concentrate, to focus, to blot out the massive, indiscriminate sensory input that continuously besieges my brain.

Another striking effect of both drugs is to remove the frightful intensity and urgency of my day-to-day life. This effect is noticeable not only to myself but also to those who know me well and is one of the changes which my husband particularly perceived at an early stage: I become uncharacteristically patient—both with people and things. My "short fuse" is considerably lengthened. I cease to monopolize all conversation. Incidents which once would have driven me to rage and hysteria can now be viewed with a certain objective—help!—humor.

In a general way, my interpersonal relationships are also greatly improved. For example, with medication I am free to be warmer, more affectionate; I say free to be, because, once my irritability is removed, I no longer have to resent the putative source of irritation, to wit, whoever is in closest proximity to me. My abandonment of domineeringness is equally dramatic after medication; it is even possible for me to regard my uncharacteristic patience and tolerance with some degree of amazement, for it is still easy for me to imagine vividly how I would normally behave toward the people around me—outrageously dictatorial and impossibly irascible. Now, it seems fairly unimportant to insist on my way, on my point of view, on my desires. The life-or-death intensity with which I normally operate is absent, and the potential areas of confrontation appears to be either trivial or childish.

On the negative side, my sleeping problems have not been alleviated: If anything, the sleeping problem is exacerbated by the amphetamine and, as a result, some evenings are most unsatisfactory. If I take my last dose of medication at 3:00 p.m., I may be able to sleep by midnight, but between 8:00 and 12:00 I am sometimes beset by an agitation (rebound hyperexcitability?) that causes me to pace, to become irritable and hostile, to eat compulsively and to consume too much alcohol. Unfortunately, this agitated state is difficult to describe and it is equally difficult to separate out the component parts: How much is ADHD? How much is drug withdrawal? How much is alcohol (which has never had a depressant *effect on me until the near "passing out" stage)? During the past 17 years I have tried to observe myself and to analyze my actions and responses, and I have come to believe that there is a curious paradox in my behavior: I welcome the control that amphetamine gives me because it permits me to work, because it permits me to maintain decent relationships with others, because it gives me some surcease from the terrible intensity of my daily existence; on the other hand, this controlled state is not my natural one, for I think that, at heart, I am a kind of incorrigible savage. In other words, my normal ADHD behavior is overlaid by control, but the normal state is, in a strange way, more comfortable, perhaps because it is familiar. In some ways it is a relief to return to the state of hyperactivity, irritability, etc. It must be said that I do, after all—even without medication—exert some control over my disorder, however faulty that control may be. Thus, it seems to me that the use of alcohol gives me the license to throw off my inhibitions (my learned control) and to revert to my normal (excitable, aggressive) state; that constitutes relief and, of course, enough alcohol permits me to sleep at last. So, then, the end of my day is most always comfortable.[3]*

In addition, the positive effects of the drug therapy (concentration, equanimity, domestic tranquility) are so miraculous that it is easy to be stampeded into over-optimism. Alas, there are some negative aspects of your life that do not go away: It's terribly difficult to believe in an "illness" rather than your essential "badness." The tendency to overt self-denigration never really disappears, nor does the guilt: When you are 61 your opulently developed sense of guilt is no longer negotiable—especially when you revert to "ADHD behavior." There is a helpless consciousness of transgression before, during and after the event that usually results in a pathetic eagerness to atone, to make amends. When one adds these difficulties to the evening problems, it is obvious that the miracle is not whole. Fractional as it is, however, it is enough to render one—me—inalterably grateful. At my age I think I'm dispassionately resigned to living with many of my reactive patterns: guilt, lack of self-esteem, nighttime agitation. These less-than-desirable attributes I can overlook, if I can have control and purposeful activity for the greatest part of my day. A day of serenity and creative accomplishment is a shining reward that makes all "difficulties" pale into insignificance.

GEORGE F

■

CLINICAL BACKGROUND

George F is 49 years old and had been in the methylphenidate study for three years. George is adopted, and his family history is unknown. His symptoms at intake were varied and severe. He loved to read but was unable to do much, owing to attention and concentration difficulties. Professionally he has lost numerous jobs because of failure to complete important projects on time, and restlessness and fidgetiness that caused him to (literally) jump around. Extreme disorganization at work and at home were major chronic problems; in fact, he and his wife have separate bedrooms because she can't stand his messiness. His wife describes him as chronically irritable, hyperreactive to sounds that don't bother most people and periodically explosive at home and at work. "The kids never know when or at what he's going to explode."

Emotionally he was mildly depressed, expressed feelings of guilt and inadequacy about letting his family down, but seemed *not to worry* about problems his wife felt he should be worrying about. She was particularly upset about his pattern of making impulsive, inappropriate remarks in social settings that his few close friends put up with and that he didn't understand were inappropriate until much later, if at all.

These severe difficulties continued to plague George even after seven years of psychotherapy. He has been receiving 40 milligrams of methylphenidate per day (10 milligrams every 3 hours, 4 times per day), and after three years in our study showed these changes: his score on the Global Assessment of Functioning has risen from 56 to 80, and his score on the Social Adjustment Scale has improved from moderate maladjustment (4) to good (2).

STATEMENT BY GEORGE F

The controversy surrounding Attention Deficit Disorder is certainly understandable. Those who haven't experienced it personally or through their children are only aware of the various issues through the simplified media coverage. I know. Even though I have the disorder, it took me a long time to realize that my various struggles could be much more than mere lack of self-discipline. From my under-

standing of the disorder through the press, I initially felt I didn't suffer from ADD since I didn't manifest the most obvious symptom: hyperactivity. After all, the other symptoms seem common to everyone to some degree for some of the time. It is hard for most people to comprehend that for a few of us these symptoms are constant and debilitating. It is not a simple disease like the measles or the common cold. We who suffer are so used to the struggle that we are unaware that we are not functioning at a level that others take for granted.

Like most critics, I thought that ADD was just another fashionable trend in medicine. I felt that taking a magic pill that could change the way your mind works was naive. It was the easy answer for those who were merely avoiding the hard work of learning the skills of concentration, developing good work habits, and simply taking responsibility for one's immaturity. I distrusted drugs in general. Unlike most of my friends in the sixties I didn't take marijuana or LSD. I didn't want to give up what little control I had over my behavior.

For most of my life I held onto the belief that I could change my poor work habits if I could just find the right method of self-discipline. When I began to realize that all the efforts I had made to try to become more efficient, more focused, and more attentive were not working, I reached a level of profound despair. Nothing worked. To make things worse, my wife shared that despair. My marriage and family life were on the verge of failure and I had lost all hope.

Like many adult sufferers of ADD, it took outside pressure from my spouse to force me to submit to diagnostic tests. Even after I was accepted into the University of Utah's ADD study group, I had lingering doubts about its worth. I was relieved to have a medical explanation for what I had considered serious personality flaws. However, a lifetime of dashed hopes had left me skeptical of much benefit from a mere pill. I took part in a double-blind test for four months. Neither the doctor nor I knew if I was taking placebos or Ritalin.

The first two months were discouraging, since I figured that at least one of the monthly supply of pills must have been Ritalin. There was no discernible difference in my behavior in either month. I received the third bottle of pills in November of 1992. Without much confidence, I took the first pill of this group that evening before I relaxed in my bedroom to read a difficult book that had stymied me for over a month. I didn't feel anything at all from the pill. Somehow I expected a palpable rise in my awareness, a change in my mood or a bit of a high since Ritalin is, after all, a stimulant. So I forgot about the pill, dismissing it again as worthless. Soon my wife called me to dinner, a little earlier than usual, I thought. I looked at my watch and realized that nearly an hour had passed. As I marked my place in the book I noticed with shock that I had read 30 pages without once losing my train of thought. This may not seem significant to most avid readers but to me it was astonishing. Although I read a great deal, it has always been a struggle for me. Only truly good fiction holds my attention for more than a paragraph. But I had read this particularly turgid nonfiction at a much faster rate than I had ever read any of my favorite books.

I became a believer in the miracle drug Ritalin. Why don't people accept such a possibility when we all know that other drugs are equally amazing? We take aspirin for granted as one of the most effective medicines for pain, but no one has been able to discover how it works. This cheap, simple drug is now being recognized as helpful in controlling heart disease and preventing strokes.

During that next month other subtle changes occurred that were much more apparent to my wife and children. Before I describe the many ways this drug has affected my life, I have to give you an idea what my struggles were like for the previous four decades.

The first clear memory I have of my lack of attention was in fifth grade. I know it was obvious earlier because my mother told me that even my second grade teacher commented on my "daydreaming." But in fifth grade I remember a specific day when we were reading silently in class about Mexico. As I was reading, I remember feeling anxious that I wouldn't finish the assignment before the class day ended. I kept looking at the clock to see how much time was left and trying to push myself to read faster. I looked at my neighbors' books and noticed they were much farther ahead than I. There was a wonderful photograph of a lush mountainside with a man taking a loaded donkey down a narrow trail. I began to think about being there on that trail, feeling the hot Mexican sun, and hearing the birds in the trees.

Soon I was thinking about the canyon near my home that cuts into the city from the foothills of the Wasatch Mountains. I remembered seeing the Denver-Rio Grande train going past the swimming hole one day of the previous summer. I looked out the window to see if the weather was good enough to go down there that day right after school. My teacher noticed me gazing out the window and asked me if I had finished already. She became angry when I said no and took me out into the hall. She gave me a stern lecture about my lack of "stick-to-itiveness" and embarrassed me deeply. I remember vowing to never let that happen ever again. But, despite all my efforts, it occurred over and over again, even through college. Every time I caught my mind wandering from the text, I would try to force myself to focus. It never worked. In minutes my mind would be on another track. It was apparent that the harder I tried, the more anxious I became, which inevitably caused me to think about not getting finished and imagining the consequences instead of focusing. It never occurred to me that there was anything I could do besides vowing to learn how to change my bad habits. But none of the study techniques I tried seemed to help. I generally approached my work in a state of panic, spending late hours trying to catch up, and developing a chronic case of diarrhea.

All through school I never finished a single textbook. I specifically recall being desperate about chemistry. Despite my intense determination to do well I was only able to read two of the 17 chapters assigned for that year. I still managed to get a C in the class. In most of my classes, I survived purely by my wits. Fortunately, my memory for facts has been phenomenal and compensated for my inability to focus on my reading. Taking notes was a disaster since it got in the way of my listening. Since I got good grades, my parents never worried about my work and never pushed me to do better. They were just happy that I wasn't a poor student like my three brothers. They didn't suspect that I was having difficulties.

They didn't have to push me because I already did so myself, mercilessly. I would consistently stay up to one or two in the morning to work on assignments which should have taken half the time. I would come to school exhausted, often with my work unfinished. Teachers regularly gave me good grades on my incomplete papers because it was obvious that I understood the assignments. Report cards would usually comment on my incompletes, that I was capable of doing much better.

Because I loved literature, my favorite class was English. I eventually majored in English in college. I often came early to my favorite high school English teacher's class to talk about what we were reading in class and about other fiction as well. Despite my constant lack of full preparation I would still find time to read other things. She told me near the end of the year that I had a wonderful mind for *literature but it was too bad that I didn't work hard enough. I remember thinking that I couldn't possibly work any harder.*

One symptom I never had to any great degree was hyperactivity. Perhaps if I had, my ADD would have been recognized earlier in life. Of course, in the 1950s and early 60s hyperactivity was not yet considered anything more than poor behavior. The most I would do was bounce my leg rapidly in my chair or tap my pencil. This would irritate my parents, and later my wife, but I was only admonished to quit doing it. I could sit at my desk without jumping up and running around like other ADD kids.

However, I was very impulsive. When my mind wandered away from the immediate tasks at hand I would think of other things I needed to do and drop what I was doing and pursue the distracting interest. Too many things had the capability to distract me from the more crucial tasks. In a perverse way this was often beneficial to my education. For instance, whenever I read an unfamiliar word, I would immediately look it up in the dictionary. Words have always fascinated me. However, once in the dictionary, I would look up synonyms, antonyms, and the etymologies of the word I was researching. Often the simple goal of looking up a single word would take half an hour or more. Although my vocabulary and spelling skills grew to be impressive, I wouldn't be able to finish reading anything within a reasonable time. Distractions would also benefit my later interest in architecture. The tendency to go off on a different angle would aid my designs because my divergent thinking often led to unique ideas and other possibilities that could not be predicted in a strictly linear approach. Unfortunately, precious time would be lost and I would have to work long hours to synthesize these ideas into a coherent whole. Usually this would leave me exhausted and many of the details needed to complete the design would be poorly thought out.

Usually the content of my reading would stimulate related but diverging thoughts. This helped me to gain better insights about literature through analogy. Mention of an unfamiliar event, topic, or person would drive me to my encyclopedia in another time-consuming digression.

This was also particularly noticeable in my speech. If I were talking with someone about some idea I would often veer off the track in mid-sentence with a related point. This would generally lead to yet another diverging explanation until I would lose all sense of my original direction. While listening to others, I would be thinking of my next thought, which I feared would vanish before I had time to respond. I would blurt it out before the speaker had a chance to finish his point.

Since my mother also had this annoying tendency, our conversations were particularly chaotic. She would complain that I didn't have a clutch on my tongue, that my speech would jerk into motion before I engaged my mind. Of course, her habit of finishing my sentences for me while I was searching for the right words drove me crazy.

Needless to say, my social skills did not develop in a normal manner. Many people would gradually drift away from me while I tried to talk to them. I tended to keep quiet whenever I met new people. Parties were never much fun. I was particularly uncomfortable when I met anyone who spoke with grace and ease. By the time I graduated from high school I was so resentful of the popular students that I was becoming bitter, sarcastic and deeply depressed. I not only had not gained any confidence in myself but I began to lose hope that I would ever be able to perform the tasks necessary for success in any field that I wanted to pursue. When teachers or employers would give me instructions, my mind would often be racing along unproductive directions. I would try to take extensive notes during and after instructions but they were inevitably chaotic and difficult to read.

My attempts to organize my work led me to try many different techniques that would have been effective for the average person. But they rarely worked for me. I would be thinking of too many things at the same time and be frustrated about learning how to make priorities. Despite the many files I organized, I would usually lose some crucial bit of information and waste my energy trying to recover it. I became fanatical about having all the information I needed to finish a project. If I didn't know an answer to some matter, its importance would grow into an obsession. I grew more and more unable to make simple decisions.

Despite all my problems I managed to receive a degree in English Literature and later a Masters in Architecture. After I got my professional license, I began to believe that maybe I had grown out of my bad habits. However, they continued to persist and even got worse.

Becoming an adult did not end my ADD. Of course, I didn't realize that my problem had a neurological basis. I continued to feel depressed about the pervasive nature of my problems. Nothing seemed to work for me. In 20 years of professional practice, I did not advance to the level of income, performance, and ability that I knew I was capable of achieving if I could only work productively. I resented my colleagues who did much better than I, those whose design abilities were less than mine. Of course, I rationalized, they knew how to use the system better than I. I became very adept at finding excuses for losing jobs, blaming others for my failures.

I turned this on to my wife as well. My negativity almost destroyed my marriage. I blamed her for being too difficult, too demanding. I realize now how badly I abused her trust and love. Even though I knew she had the right to expect me to be home when I said I would be, my inability to predict how long a project would take drove her to despair. It was so hard to keep my work timely and give her and our children the attention they deserved. My frustration with work left me irritable with my family. Often, I would explode in unpredictable anger. Thankfully, they kept their faith in me long enough for me to discover the possibility that I had ADD.

It would be an exaggeration to claim that my life has changed overnight into a wonderful dream since I have been on Ritalin, but the long nightmare is at last over. Although I still have a lot to relearn about organization, time management, social skills, and obsession with detail, I no longer feel despair or anxiety. I can now make reasonable estimates about the time necessary to complete projects and finish them without resorting to long anxiety-ridden nights. My relationships with my employers and fellow workers have improved significantly. I'm more cooperative and attentive to their needs. Architecture has now become the delightful profession I had long ago wished it would be. I no longer drag myself to work late and exhausted because I stayed up late trying to catch up.

Ritalin literally saved my marriage and my relationships with my children and close friends. I pay attention to them without getting defensive, critical, or insensitive. The last three years with my wife have been a marvelous restoration of our initial love for each other. We share much more time with each other and her trust in me continues to grow. I no longer keep her waiting up for me past the time I have told her I would be home. I don't make us late for movies or parties because I always know where I leave my keys now. She tells me her feelings now without fear that I will criticize them as irrational, which they never were.

Distractions still occur, of course, but I do not impulsively respond to them. I have limited my nonarchitectural interests to those that are important to me. I have enjoyed researching a particular social problem (not ADD) that I have deeply cared about for eleven years. My writing about it has received recognition from the international press and a growing audience of those intimately involved in it. One of the rewards of this effort has been several opportunities to travel and speak to the public. Last year I went all the way to Melbourne, Australia, to speak to the Victorian Parliament, several other groups, and to the press.

This is amazing to me since I had never been comfortable speaking about ideas for fear that I would make a complete fool of myself. I can confidently speak to many people at once and maintain a coherent direction without confusing them with digressions. This is immensely satisfying after a lifetime of being unable to express myself.

As I said at the start, I can understand the lack of acceptance of ADD as a neurological disorder and the effectiveness of its treatment through a mere drug. Unless someone has gone through the agony of my experiences, it is difficult to accept. I can only hope that critics can suspend judgment about this until more evidence is gathered. I am confident that it will be appreciated in the near future and that the medical profession will finally recognize the validity of the diagnosis and its treatment. Scientific revolutions have often been dismissed as false, even blasphemous. Galileo, Darwin, Pasteur, and many others had suffered the outrageous criticism that ADD researchers are now receiving from reactionary groups like the Church of Scientology. For the sake of the thousands of sufferers of Attention Deficit Disorder, both children and adults, I hope that sympathy and understanding will soon prevail over the hysterical forces of ignorance. They deserve the right to experience a life relatively free from confusion and despair.

COMMENT BY SPOUSE OF GEORGE F

It's always been hard to put my finger on exactly what was so difficult about living with George. By all standards, he was the ideal mate: he worked hard, was faithful, wasn't abusive, was highly intelligent and extremely good-looking.

My complaints were those of every married woman: he was uncommunicative; he kept me waiting for hours; he didn't care about my feelings; our ways of managing money and disciplining children were diametrically opposed; etc.

The problems were run of the mill but abnormal in the sense that they were extreme and unrelenting: e.g., he would estimate that he had three or four hours of work before coming home but it turned out to be 18 hours, an "all-nighter."

My emotional history made me very vulnerable to someone not showing up. I would be in a state of panic for hours. Even though I told George how much I suffered when he kept me waiting, he never changed his behavior.

I could never count on him to be on time, to help me with decisions or with the children. He just could not attend to his inner world and to the rest of the problems of living.

One night we came home at midnight and our 13-year-old son was playing catch at the corner. I yelled at him to come home. He didn't. I asked George to deal with the problem and he got furious with me for yelling, thereby disturbing the neighbors.

An angry tone of voice always irritated him. Once he got mad because the sound of my daughter chewing croutons irritated him. It took hours of discussion for me to convince him to be reasonable. I thought that I was the one who was lacking in relating and communicating skills. This eroded my self-esteem.

His behavior was unpredictable, impulsive and almost completely unresponsive to outside influence. Raising my voice, confrontation, asserting my needs, explaining, getting angry, moving out twice, not only failed to get my needs met but resulted in his asserting that I was the "bad guy."

A typical scenario occurred the summer our 12-year-old daughter was in a recital at a music camp in St. George. After the five-hour drive George arrived rather disheveled and his appearance caused our daughter some embarrassment.

The next day we were attending the recital and after examining the program, George assumed that he would have time to go get a hair cut before Jennifer's turn. After 16 years of marriage I knew that it was useless to advise him not to do this. So he went and of course missed her performance. After everything was over, he insisted that she go to the piano and play the piece for him so that he could get a picture. She was upset and uncooperative and George was irritated.

As my psychiatrist put it, being around George was like "having to walk on egg shells."

The stresses of any change in his routine (like a vacation) exacer-
bated his condition: Once he lost a contact lens while taking it out
at dusk at a windswept roadside stop; another time, he left his
wallet on top of the car and lost it, thus ruining our skiing holiday.
In France, he got so angry when a driver tailgated and passed us,
that he had to follow the driver and do the same thing.

He was not a mean person and as long as I left him alone and
didn't need anything from him, he was fine and quite mellow. He
couldn't tolerate the mildest of stresses of family life. The unremit-
ting nature of his impulsive and irrational behavior and the inabil-
ity to grow and develop into a fully sharing partner are the factors
that made our problems different from the usual marital difficulties.

After 23 years of marriage plus three years of courtship, and after
George had been in psychoanalysis for seven years, I was ready to
die: I had gotten nowhere in my various careers and I couldn't love
the man to whom I had committed so much of my life.

And then one final crisis and the miracle of the ADD diagnosis
and the Ritalin cure occurred.

I had left my job when George had managed to hang on to a job for
two years. Our daughter had been accepted at Yale and then, once
again, he was laid off (the 17th time in 18 years).

This time, finally, I came to the certain conclusion that my hus-
band suffered from a neurological problem. It had become impera-
tive that he be correctly diagnosed and somehow taught to adapt to
his handicap.

My conversations with George, like everyone else's, were difficult
to impossible. Either he said nothing but yes or no to questions that
would normally require elaboration, or he would go on and on and
on about whatever topic had grabbed his interest at the moment,
with no desire for input from the person who was listening to him. If
I expressed disinterest even with just a look, he would become de-
fensive.

I concluded that his disorder was very much analogous to being
deaf as he seemed to not perceive other human beings' nonverbal
language and expectations.

The changes in George's behavior in the two and a half years he's
been on Ritalin are as hard to describe as it is to describe the disor-
der. They are very subtle but the children and I can tell as soon as he
opens his mouth whether or not he's taken the medication.

Mainly, he isn't so defensive; he doesn't get his dander up at every
little thing that doesn't go his way. He listens, and he shuts up when

he perceives that no one wants to listen to him. He is more sponta-neous and invites me to share in some of his activities. He is accept-ing when I decline.

He has always worked very hard and was phenomenally ener-getic. He never seemed to tire. Whereas before he dissipated his energy going from one project to another, focusing on his interests rather than on results, now he completes project after project: gar-dening, remodeling the house, writing, and of course his professional duties.

In summary, I really can't find the words to express what a differ-ence George's treatment with Ritalin has made in my life. The very first pill was more effective than 26 years of love and patience and understanding and seven years of psychotherapy.

I have a Master's degree in neurophysiology and have worked for nearly 30 years in neuroscience or as a teacher of disturbed adoles-cents. I am an expert on Freud. I would never have believed that a drug could have such a profound effect on someone's behavior.

First of all, I thought that a drug's action would be too global to be effective. Secondly, I thought George's problems stemmed from hav-ing been brought up in a dysfunctional family and that he needed to learn new behaviors.

Now I am convinced that Ritalin affects the firing of neurons such that perception of the outside world is different than it is without the medication.

I hope these few pages succeed in showing my gratitude to Dr. Wender and his research team.

NOTES

1. The names and some of the identifying details have been disguised.

2. Her diagnosis was based on the terminology at the time. She did and does meet full criteria for ADHD with hyperactivity, attentional problems, and impulsivity.

3. Sonia is now able to take her last dose of D-amphetamine at 5 or 6 P.M. so that she can control her symptoms throughout the day. When she takes 10 to 20 milligrams of thioridazine (Mellaril®) an hour or two before going to bed, she falls asleep easily and sleeps without interruptions for 7 to 8 hours.

8

Conclusion

■

In this volume I have tried to demonstrate that a substantial portion of children with Attention-deficit Hyperactivity Disorder—perhaps one third, or even more—reaches adulthood with persisting symptoms of the syndrome. Adults with such lingering handicaps as inability to concentrate, impulsivity, explosive temper, and procrastination can be noticeably hampered in achieving career goals and in relationships with others. Accumulated evidence indicates that most such symptoms of ADHD are genetically transmitted and probably derive from monoaminergic malfunctioning. As in children with ADHD, the symptoms in adults can be usefully ameliorated through drug treatment.

Although these highly plausible generalizations lead to medical practice that can be helpful to sufferers from ADHD, they are supported by inadequate and often contradictory research. Further investigation of genetic background, "spectrum" disorders, other therapeutic drugs, and specific biochemical malfunctions might clarify the prevention and treatment of ADHD. In identifying below what I consider interesting research tacks, I recognize the possibility that the proposed projects might yield results that would negate my previous conclusions. I am here reminded of the experimental psychologist Clark Hull, who once observed that he could effectively stimulate research by making declarative assertions that would motivate others to try to invalidate them.

GENETIC STUDIES

■

The further study of the occurrence of ADHD in the children, siblings, and parents of adults with ADHD would bolster our knowledge of the inheritance patterns of the syndrome. With ADHD identified in adults, a next useful study would be a high-risk study of psychopathology in the offspring of ADHD adults. Any such study should aim at a stricter research design in order to avoid some of the confusions of past studies. First, the investigator should ascertain the presence of other psychopathology in the ADHD parent—that is, whether the ADHD parent's psychopathology is "pure" or mixed with such other disorders as Antisocial Personality Disorder or depression. Second, the researcher must determine the psychiatric status of the co-parent. In many high-risk studies the psychiatric status of the co-parent is not ascertained, an oversight that can obviously make it impossible to trace the role of genetic factors in the offspring. The diagnoses of the descendants in turn should distinguish among "pure" ADHD, ADHD in combination with Conduct Disorder, Learning Disorders, alcoholism, depression, and so forth. Of particular interest is the presence or absence of non-ADHD psychopathology in the daughters of the ADHD parent—for instance, in such daughters is there an increased risk for depression (and depression spectrum disorder), somatization disorder, and other disorders linked to Conduct Disorder such as ASPD and substance abuse? Another interesting question is whether daughters of ADHD fathers who do not express the symptoms of ADHD (that is, the penetrance is reduced) transmit the genetic diathesis. This could be studied by comparing the appearance of the ADHD/CD related disorders in the grandsons who are the children of either sons or daughters of ADHD adults (that is, the study would determine the prevalence and nature of psychopathology in these two groups of sons). In still another variation of the above kinds of studies, one might start with the presence of a disorder other than ADHD in adults, such as alcoholism, and attempt to identify apparently related disorders, including ADHD, in the subjects' children and grandchildren.

"SPECTRUM" STUDIES

■

Examining the first-degree relatives of ADHD individuals, one is impressed with the apparently increased frequency of ADHD symptoms that are not sufficient to meet the diagnostic criteria for full-fledged ADHD. "Spectrum" studies of ADHD, a further refinement of the above genetic studies, would seek to determine the incidence of ADHD-like symptoms and signs—not full-fledged ADHD—in first-degree relatives of ADHD adults. Analogous to schizotypal relatives of schizophrenics, such persons might, for example, manifest chronic inattentiveness, volatile mood, or explosive temper. The chronically inattentive are the most interesting. We have excluded patients in whom inattention is the primary symptom from our studies because inattention is a nonspecific symptom that can be seen in mild schizophrenia, anxiety disorders, and depression. However, some chronically inattentive children and some inattentive but not fully ADHD patients show a good response to treatment with stimulant drugs. Thus, recognizing the possibility that such trace symptoms may be related to ADHD may increase the opportunity to provide patients with helpful treatment.

THERAPEUTIC TRIALS

■

DRUG TRIALS

In addition to the constant quest for more efficacious drugs for ADHD treatment, researchers could usefully turn their attention to specific drugs that might be especially helpful to, for example, the primarily inattentive, alcoholics with ADHD symptoms, and ADHD adults with Antisocial Personality Disorder. For alcoholics and ASPD adults, stimulants cannot be employed because even if they are not abused by the patient (and they may be) they are readily "dealt on the street" in exchange for other, more desired substances. Researchers might look into the effectiveness of less abusable or nonabusable drugs such as pemoline, the MAO inhibitors, or bupropion with such persons. Another subcategory requiring specific medications includes patients with major symptoms of ADHD—for example, affective lability, impulsivity, and overreactivity as manifested by anger—in the presence of other psychiatric disorders. Individuals with such ADHD symptoms who are receiving appropriate drug treatments for other psychiatric conditions might also respond to the drugs most effective in ADHD.

DRUG THERAPY PLUS GROUP PSYCHOEDUCATIONAL THERAPY

A particular treatment combination that is in need of additional investigation is medication plus attendance at a group that provides didactic information on the nature of ADHD symptoms and on the benefits and limitations of medication. At the same time, such a group provides positive support, showing the patients that they are not unique or alone, and demonstrating how others are learning to live with ADHD.

DIRECT TESTS OF THE DOPAMINE HYPOTHESIS

■

Although fragmentary data implicate dopamine inadequacy in the development of ADHD, additional research is necessary to identify with certainty the nature of the biochemical malfunction. Examples of such research would be imaging studies showing the binding of dopamine agonists in the brains of normal controls and patients. Such studies might also help us to understand the variable responses among patients: seemingly similar patients may respond better to D-amphetamine than to methylphenidate, or vice versa, and some may not respond at all. More exact understanding of the numerous steps involved in any biochemical process might reveal that various patients are deficient in different groups of steps. Such patient differences might reflect either genetic heterogeneity or individual differences in response to a particular genetic abnormality (penetrance and expression).

Attention-deficit Hyperactivity Disorder holds many problems waiting to be solved by eager researchers. Epidemiology, genetic patterns and structures, brain chemistry, and responses to medication all await further refinement. I fervently hope and expect that young(er) investigators will be motivated to venture down some of these alluring avenues to seek the answers to the multitudinous questions that remain. This syndrome that seriously impairs function and produces distressing symptoms remains—for the nonce—a relatively uninvestigated *terra incognita*, but already developed techniques can be applied and expected to produce new and informative results. To quote the words of one of the founders of quantum mechanics, Niels Bohr, "Prediction is difficult, especially of the future."

APPENDIXES

■

A

Evaluation Measures Frequently Used in Studies

■

Child Behavior Checklist (CBCL). Achenbach and Edelbrock (1981). 20 social competence items, 118 related to behavioral problems.

Child Behavior Checklist. Ontario Child Health Study. Boyle et al. (1987). This measure is used with parents, teachers, and adolescents ages 12 to 16. Items chosen to operationalize DSM-III criteria for ADD, CD, and somatization.

Children's Global Assessment Scale (CGAS). This scale of adaptive functioning is derived by Shaffer et al. (1983) from the Global Assessment Scale.

Clinical Global Impression (CGI). Global improvement which is assessed on a 7-point scale (from very improved to very much worse).

Conners Parent and Teacher Rating Scales and Questionnaires. Conners (1969, 1970, 1973). There are various full and abbreviated versions of these popular measures.

Diagnostic Interview for Children and Adolescents—Parent Version (DICA-P). Herjanic and Campbell (1977); Herjanic and Reich (1982); Reich et al. (1982).

Diagnostic Interview Schedule for Children (DISC). DISC-C = Child Version; DISC-P = Parent Version. National Institute of Mental Health (Costello et al., 1984).

Global Assessment of Functioning Scale (GAF). In DSM-III-R. Based on Global Assessment Scale.

Global Assessment Scale (GAS). Endicott et al. (1976). Forerunner of Global Assessment of Functioning Scale.

Parents' Rating Scale (PRS). Retrospective childhood ratings by parents of possible ADHD adults. See Appendix B, based on Conners Abbreviated Rating Scale.

Profile of Mood States (POMS). McNair et al. (1971).

Quay-Peterson Problem Checklist. Werry and Quay (1971).

Research Diagnostic Criteria (RDC). Spitzer et al. (1975).

Rutter Teacher and Parent Questionnaires. Rutter (1967); Rutter et al. (1970).

Social Adjustment Scale. Weissman (1976).

Symptom Checklist 90 (SCL-90). Derogatis et al. (1973).

Targeted Attention Deficit Disorder Symptoms Rating Scale (TADDS). See Appendix E.

Tarter-Wender Rating Scale. Tarter et al. (1977).

Utah Criteria. Used for diagnosis of ADHD in adults. See Appendix C.

Wender Utah Rating Scale (WURS). Ratings by possible ADHD adults of their childhood behavior. See Appendix D. Ward et al. (1993).

Wide Range Achievement Test. Jastak and Jastak (1978).

B

Parents' Rating Scale

■

The Parents' Rating Scale (PRS) is filled out by the patient's mother or by the adult responsible for his upbringing. The score is determined by the examiner or psychological technician using the following scale: 0 = not at all; 1 = just a little; 2 = pretty much; and 3 = very much.

Parents' Rating Scale

Patient's name _____ # _____ Date _____ Physician _____

To be filled out by the *mother* of the subject (or father only if mother is unavailable).

Instructions: Listed below are items concerning children's behavior and the problems they sometimes have. Read each item carefully and decide how much you think your child was bothered by these problems when he/she was between *six* and *ten* years old. Enter the amount of the problem by putting a check in the column that describes your child at that time.

		NOT AT ALL	JUST A LITTLE	PRETTY MUCH	VERY MUCH
1.	RESTLESS (OVERACTIVE)				
2.	EXCITABLE, IMPULSIVE				
3.	DISTURBS OTHER CHILDREN				
4.	FAILS TO FINISH THINGS STARTED (SHORT ATTENTION SPAN)				
5.	FIDGETING				
6.	INATTENTIVE, DISTRACTIBLE				
7.	DEMANDS MUST BE MET IMMEDIATELY; GETS FRUSTRATED				
8.	CRIES				
9.	MOOD CHANGES QUICKLY				
10.	TEMPER OUTBURSTS (EXPLOSIVE AND UNPREDICTABLE BEHAVIOR)				

Connors Parents Rating Scale *reproduced by permission of Multi-Health Systems, Inc., 908 Niagara Falls Blvd., North Tonawanda, NY, 14120–2060, 1-800-456-3003.*

Percentile Ranks of Adult Controls

Score	Controls ($N = 460$), Percentile
0	20
1	33
2	43
3	52
4	61
5	68
6	76
7	81
8	83
9	88
10	93
11	94
12	95
13	96
14	98
15	98
≥ 16	99

C

Utah Criteria for ADHD in Adults

■

I. CHILDHOOD CHARACTERISTICS
Childhood history consistent with ADHD in childhood. Obtaining reliable historical data usually requires input from the individual's parents or older siblings. The following are our diagnostic criteria for ADHD in childhood:

A. Narrow Criteria (DSM-III)
That the individual met DSM-III-R criteria (now DSM-IV criteria) for ADHD in childhood.

B. Broad Criteria
Both characteristics 1 and 2, and at least one characteristic from 3 through 6.

 1. *Hyperactivity:* More active than other children, unable to sit still, fidgetiness, restlessness, always on the go, talking excessively.
 2. *Attention deficits*: Sometimes described as having a "short attention span," distractibility, unable to finish school work.
 3. *Behavior problems in school.*
 4. *Impulsivity.*
 5. *Overexcitability.*
 6. *Temper outbursts.*

II. ADULT CHARACTERISTICS

A. The presence in adulthood of both characteristics 1 and 2—which the patient observes or says others observe in him—together with two of characteristics 3 through 7.

1. *Persistent motor hyperactivity:* Manifested by restlessness, inability to relax, "nervousness" (meaning inability to settle down—not anticipatory anxiety), inability to persist in sedentary activities (e.g., watching movies, TV, reading the newspaper), being always on the go, dysphoric when inactive.

2. *Attentional difficulties:* Manifested by an inability to keep mind on conversations, distractibility (being aware of other stimuli when attempts are made to filter them out); difficulty keeping mind on reading materials or task; frequent "forgetfulness"; often losing or misplacing things, forgetting plans, car keys, purse, etc.; "mind frequently somewhere else."

3. *Affective lability:* Usually described as antedating adolescence and in some instances beginning as far back as the patient can remember. Manifested by definite shifts from a normal mood to depression or mild euphoria or—more often—excitement; depression described as being "down," "bored," or "discontented"; mood shifts usually last hours to at most a few days and are present without significant physiological concomitants; mood shifts may occur spontaneously or be reactive.

4. *Disorganization, inability to complete tasks:* The subject reports lack of organization in job, running household, or performing school work; tasks frequently not completed; subject switches from one task to another in haphazard fashion; disorganization in activities, problem solving, organizing time, lack of "stick-to-it-tiveness."

5. *Hot temper, explosive short-lived outbursts:* Subject reports he may have transient loss of control and be frightened by his own behavior. Easily provoked or constant irritability. Temper problems interfere with personal relationships.

6. *Emotional overreactivity:* Subject cannot take ordinary stresses in stride and reacts excessively or inappropriately with depression, confusion, uncertainty, anxiety, or anger. Emotional responses interfere with appropriate problem solving. Subject experiences repeated crises in dealing with routine life stresses. Describes self as easily "hassled" or "stressed out."

7. *Impulsivity:* Minor manifestations include talking before thinking things through; interrupting others' conversations; impatience (e.g., while driving); impulse buying. Major manifestations may be similar to those seen in mania and Antiso-

cial Personality Disorder and include, to varying degrees, poor occupational performance; abrupt initiation or termination of relationships (e.g., multiple marriages, separations, divorces); antisocial behavior such as joy-riding, shop-lifting; excessive involvement in pleasurable activities without recognizing risks of painful consequences (e.g., buying sprees, foolish business investments, reckless driving). Subject makes decisions quickly and easily without reflection, often on the basis of insufficient information, to his own disadvantage; inability to delay acting without experiencing discomfort.

B. Absence of the following disorders:
   1. Antisocial Personality Disorder
   2. Major Affective Disorder

C. Absence of signs and symptoms of the following disorders:
   1. Schizophrenia
   2. Schizo-affective Disorder

D. Absence of Schizotypal or Borderline Personality Disorders or traits

E. Associated features:
   Marital instability; academic and vocational success less than expected on the basis of intelligence and education; alcohol or drug abuse; atypical responses to psychoactive medications; family histories of ADHD in childhood, alcoholism, drug abuse, Antisocial Personality Disorder and Briquet's syndrome.

F. Child Temperament Questionnaire
   (Conners Abbreviated Rating Scale.) Although not necessary for diagnosis, a score of 12 or greater as rated by the patient's mother is helpful for diagnostic purposes and may be predictive of treatment response.

D

WENDER UTAH RATING SCALE

PATIENT'S
INITIALS _____

PATIENT'S
NUMBER _____ DATE _____

M.D.'s
INITIALS _____

AS A CHILD I WAS (OR HAD):	Not at all or very slightly	Mildly	Moder- ately	Quite a Bit	Very Much
1. Active, restless, always on the go					
2. Afraid of things					
3. Concentration problems, easily distracted					
4. Anxious, worrying					
5. Nervous, fidgety					
6. Inattentive, daydreaming					
7. Hot or short tempered, low boiling point					
8. Shy, sensitive					
9. Temper outbursts, tantrums					
10. Trouble with stick-to-it-tiveness, not following through, failing to finish things started					
11. Stubborn, strong willed					
12. Sad or blue, depressed, unhappy					
13. Uncautious, dare-devilish, involved in pranks					
14. Not getting a kick out of things, dissatisfied with life					
15. Disobedient with parents, rebellious, sassy					
16. Low opinion of myself					
17. Irritable					
18. Outgoing, friendly, enjoy company of people					
19. Sloppy, disorganized					
20. Moody, have ups and downs					
21. Feel angry					
22. Have friends, popular					
23. Well organized, tidy, neat					
24. Acting without thinking, impulsive					
25. Tend to be immature					
26. Feel guilty, regretful					
27. Lose control of myself					
28. Tend to be or act irrational					
29. Unpopular with other children, didn't keep friends for long, didn't get along with other children					
30. Poorly coordinated, did not participate in sports					

AS A CHILD I WAS (OR HAD):	Not at all or very slightly	Mildly	Moder-ately	Quite a Bit	Very Much
31. Afraid of losing control of self					
32. Well coordinated, picked first in games					
33. (for women only) Tomboyish					
34. Ran away from home					
35. Get in fights					
36. Teased other children					
37. Leader, bossy					
38. Difficulty getting awake					
39. Follower, lead around too much					
40. Trouble seeing things from someone else's point of view					
41. Trouble with authorities, trouble with school, visits to principal's office					
42. Trouble with the police, booked, convicted					
MEDICAL PROBLEMS AS A CHILD:					
43. Headaches					
44. Stomachaches					
45. Constipation					
46. Diarrhea					
47. Food allergies					
48. Other allergies					
49. Bedwetting					
AS A CHILD IN SCHOOL:					
50. Overall a good student, fast					
51. Overall a poor student, slow learner					
52. Slow reader					
53. Slow in *learning* to read					
54. Trouble reversing letters					
55. Problems with spelling					
56. Trouble with mathematics or numbers					
57. Bad handwriting					
58. Though I could read pretty well, I never really enjoyed reading					
59. Did not achieve up to potential					
60. Repeated grades (which grades?) _____					
61. Suspended or expelled (which grades?) _____					

Source: Paul H. Wender, M.D., University of Utah School of Medicine, Salt Lake City, UT 84132.

Scoring: Not at all = 0.
Mildly   = 1.
Moderately = 2.
Quite a bit = 3.
Very much = 4.

Wender Utah Rating Scale Ratings of Adults with Attention Deficit Hyperactivity Disorder, Normal Comparison Subjects, and Depressed Comparison Subjects

WURS Item	Adults with Attention Deficit Hyperactivity Disorder (N = 81)		Normal Comparison Subjects (N = 100)		Depressed Comparison Subjects (N = 70)	
	Mean	SD	Mean	SD	Mean	SD
Individual Items						
Concentration problems, easily distracted	3.3	0.9	0.7	0.9	1.3	1.4
Anxious, worrying	2.8	1.1	1.1	1.0	2.1	1.3
Nervous, fidgety	3.1	0.9	0.6	0.9	1.7	1.4
Inattentive, daydreaming	3.2	1.0	0.6	0.8	1.7	1.4
Hot-or short-tempered, low boiling point	2.7	1.3	0.8	1.0	1.0	1.2
Temper outbursts, tantrums	2.4	1.2	0.6	0.9	1.0	1.5
Trouble with stick-to-it-tiveness	3.0	1.1	0.7	0.9	1.3	1.3
Stubborn, strong-willed	3.1	1.1	1.4	1.2	1.7	1.2
Sad or blue, depressed, unhappy	2.2	1.2	0.4	0.7	2.0	1.4
Disobedient, rebellious, sassy	2.4	1.4	0.5	0.7	0.7	1.1
Low opinion of myself	2.6	1.3	0.7	0.8	2.2	1.5
Irritable	2.4	1.1	0.4	0.6	1.2	1.1
Moody, ups and downs	2.8	1.0	0.8	0.8	1.8	1.3
Angry	2.5	1.2	0.6	0.8	1.4	1.3
Trouble seeing things from someone else's point of view	2.3	1.1	0.8	1.2	1.0	0.8
Acting without thinking, impulsive	2.9	1.1	0.8	0.9	1.4	1.2
Tendency to be immature	2.8	1.6	0.7	0.9	1.1	1.1
Guilty feelings, regretful	2.6	1.1	0.6	0.8	1.8	1.4
Losing control of myself	2.2	1.3	0.3	0.6	0.8	1.0
Tendency to be or act irrational	2.0	1.2	0.2	0.5	0.9	1.1
Unpopular with other children	1.8	1.3	0.2	0.5	0.8	1.0
Trouble with authorities, trouble with school, visits to principal's office	1.8	1.6	0.2	0.6	0.4	0.8
Overall a poor student, slow learner	1.4	1.4	0.1	0.3	0.5	0.7
Trouble with mathematics or numbers	2.1	1.5	0.5	1.0	1.1	1.4
Not achieving up to potential	3.2	1.0	1.1	1.2	1.8	1.5
Total scores						
Men	60.3	14.2	17.9	11.0	34.2	18.0
Women	65.8	14.3	15.0	8.5	30.5	15.8
All subjects	62.2	14.6	16.1	10.6	31.7	17.4

E

Targeted Attention-deficit Disorder Symptoms Rating Scale

Patient Identification _____ Date _____ Rater _____

Circle Time Interval Covered by This Rating
Baseline · Week · Month · Other (specify) _____

    This scale is designed for outpatients and the anchor points for "O" (none) and "4" (very much) do **NOT** refer to the full range of psychopathology on the Global Assessment of Functioning Scale (of 0 to 100). A score of "0" should correspond roughly to a GAF score of 70–80 while a score of "4" would correspond on the TADDS to a GAF score of about 40–50. Scores below 40 describe individuals with very severe psychopathology and/or impaired reality testing or communication. For individuals with such scores, the diagnosis of ADHD is probably not appropriate. Code for overall severity, rating subjective distress, problems in functioning, and problems caused to others.

    The function of the Individual Item Ratings is only to ensure that the areas specified are queried about and rated. The Global Ratings should not be based on the score of the Individual Items but should be based on a weighing of the Items and other information.

General Probes: Depending on context and time period covered (since last visit, the past month, your entire life) introduce questions with:

        Do you have ....
        Are you ....
        Have you been ....
        Do you have trouble with "X"?
        How much of a problem has this been for you?
        Has anyone commented about this?
        What did they say?
        How much (often, long, severe) has this been a problem for you?
        Has this led to difficulties with other people, school, work, family? How?

Rate Frequency & Severity
Global Ratings: 0 - Not at all or rarely true
        1 - Somewhat or sometimes true
        2 - Moderate or true moderately often
        3 - Quite a bit or true quite a bit of the time
        4 - Very true or true very much of the time

Individual Item Ratings: 0 - None or slight
        1 - Somewhat or sometimes true
        2 - Very true or often true

1.   ATTENTION DIFFICULTIES: Global Rating 0-4 _____

Do you have difficulty concentrating, mind wandering, distractibility, do you find your mind is somewhere else? Specify _____	0	1	2
Do people complain that you don't pay attention to them when they're talking? (Who?) _____	0	1	2
Do you have difficulty keeping your mind on reading materials?	0	1	2
Do you misplace things such as your car keys, purse, wallet, watch? Are you forgetful?	0	1	2
Clear inattentiveness, tangentiality in office	0	1	2

2. HYPERACTIVITY/RESTLESSNESS: Global Rating 0-4 _____
Are you overactive, restless?

Are you fidgety?	0	1	2
Things such as drumming with your fingers, kicking or tapping with your foot.	0	1	2
Are you restless, can't sit still, always on the go?	0	1	2
Do you talk too much? Do other people feel you talk too much?	0	1	2
Do you have difficulty relaxing?	0	1	2
Can you sit still through a movie or TV show? Do you get up from the table immediately after dinner?	0	1	2

By observation in office [or reported observation]: fidgetiness, foot tapping

3. TEMPER: Global Rating 0-4 _____
Have you had difficulties controlling your temper? Do you have a "short fuse" or "a low boiling point"? Are you irritable? Do you "keep your anger in"?

Irritable	0	1	2
Contained anger	0	1	2
Outbursts (short fuse, low boiling point)	0	1	2

How frequently?
A few times a day _____ 1× week _____
Daily _____ Occasionally _____
2–3× week _____

With whom do you have problems with your temper?
Spouse or other _____ Other relatives (specify) _____
Friends _____ Co-workers _____
Children _____ Supervisors _____

With anger do you lose control?

Verbally	0	1	2
Physically	0	1	2

How long does it take to cool down after you get angry?

Immediately _____
Within an hour _____
Within a day _____
2–3 days _____
Longer _____

4. MOOD INSTABILITY: Global Rating 0-4 _____

[Help patient to discriminate between mood = "sad" or "happy"
  vs. mood = "irritable or hot tempered"]

How has your mood been?

Are you (have you been) depressed, sad, blue, down in the dumps? Do you have periods when you get excited, "flying," going too fast?	0	1	2
Does your mood change up and down like a roller coaster?	0	1	2
Do you feel "down on yourself," self critical, have low self-esteem?	0	1	2

5. OVERREACTIVITY: Global Rating 0-4 _____

Do you get feelings of being overwhelmed, overloaded, over-stimulated, pressured?

Do you over-react to pressure? Do you feel easily stressed, flustered, easily hassled, discombobulated, depressed, angry?	0	1	2
Do you have problems with overstimulation or going too fast?	0	1	2
Do you make "mountains out of molehills," blow things up out of proportion?	0	1	2

6. DISORGANIZATION: Global Rating 0-4 _____

[How well organized have you been?]

Do you have problems with organization? At work, home or school?
Do you plan out things ahead of time? Money, tasks?
Do you have trouble scheduling things, getting to places on time?
Do you do things systematically or do you jump from [Do you jump from] one task to
  another before finishing the first?

How much stick-to-it-tive-ness do you have?	0	1	2
Do you have trouble planning/organizing your time/money/work?	0	1	2
Do you misplace things, are you forgetful?	0	1	2
Do you have problems starting difficult projects, or do you keep on putting things off, procrastinate?	0	1	2

7. IMPULSIVITY: Global Rating 0-4 _____

[Have you had problems because of doing things without thinking?]
Do you have trouble because you are impulsive?

Have you had problems because of saying or doing things before you've thought things out?	0	1	2
Do you interrupt others when they are talking?	0	1	2
Impetuous decisions, based on angry feelings (such as overly restrictive discipline, quitting jobs, ending relationships)	0	1	2
Are you reckless?	0	1	2

Do others regard you or do you regard yourself as impatient, for example, while driving, with children, others?   0   1   2

Do you act first and think later—make decisions too quickly and without thinking them through, for example, impulse buying?   0   1   2

Have you made any impulsive decisions (e.g., impulse buying) recently or since the last visit?
Rater specify: _____

Patient Name _____ Date _____ Open _____ Mo_____

Rater_____ Double Blind

Week 1 2 3 4 5

ADD TARGET SYMPTOMS	Not at all	Slight	Moderate	Quite a bit	Very much
TADDS	0	1	2	3	4
Concentration problems					
Hyperactivity					
Mood instability or depression					
Temper					
Over-reactivity					
Disorganization					
Impulsivity					

PATIENT/OTHER GLOBAL RATING
(Compared to Baseline)

SEVERITY OF "HYPERACTIVITY"
0 - Superior - better than average
1 - None   - "average" for the general population
2 - Mild
3 - Moderate
4 - Quite a Bit
5 - Very Much

MD		
		1 - Very Much Improved
		2 - Moderately improved
		3 - Mildly improved
		4 - No change
		5 - Mildly worse
		6 - Moderately worse
		7 - Very much worse

SIDE EFFECTS*

1 - Just a little   2 - Pretty much   3 - Very much

_____ Appetite loss _____ Drowsiness _____ Headache

_____ Insomnia _____ Involuntary movements (tics)

_____ Irritability _____ Nervousness _____ Other

Detail _____

_____

BP (sit) _____ **HR** _____ **WT** _____

Time of last dose _____ **Amount of last dose** _____ **mg**

Current dose _____

Dose for next period _____

*This side effect list has been employed in our studies of stimulant drugs. It should not be employed in assessing the side effects of other classes of drugs.

---

8. FEELINGS OF BEING BORED: Global Rating 0-4 _____
Likes excitement. Life is uninteresting.

9. ANXIETY: Global Rating 0-4 _____
Tension, worrying, anticipation.

10. SOMATIC ANXIETY SYMPTOMS: Global Rating 0-4 _____

Do you have headaches, backaches, neckaches, upset stomach, diarrhea, muscular tension or other physical symptoms? (Specify)

11. SLEEP DIFFICULTIES: Global Rating 0-4 _____

Difficult in falling asleep, broken sleep, unsatisfying sleep and fatigue on wakening, dreams, nightmares.

**12. EXCESSIVE OR COMPULSIVE USE OF DRUGS, ALCOHOL, FOOD:
      Global Rating 0-4** _____

Specify _____

---

13. SEVERITY OF "HYPERACTIVITY"
　　　0 - Superior - better than normal
　　　1 - None   - "average" for the general population
　　　2 - Mild
　　　3 - Moderate
　　　4 - Quite a Bit
　　　5 - Very Much

14. IMPAIRMENT IN ROLE FUNCTIONING:

	Superior	Normal	Slight	Moderate	Quite a bit	Very Much	Severe
Work	NA	0	1	2	3	4	5
Academic	NA	0	1	2	3	4	5
Marital or Relational	NA	0	1	2	3	4	5
Household Management/Maintenance, Administrative Tasks (paying bills, etc.)	NA	0	1	2	3	4	5
Parental	NA	0	1	2	3	4	5
Friends and Extended Family	NA	0	1	2	3	4	5
Economic Problems	NA	0	1	2	3	4	5

15. GLOBAL ROLE FUNCTIONING:
(may assign intermediate values, e.g., 3.5): _____

0 = Excellent - no maladjustment, excellent rating in most areas. Handles problems well, good interpersonal relationships, happy with adjustment

1 = Good - adequate adjustment but because of deficiencies cannot be called excellent

2 = Mild maladjustment - definite areas of maladjustment, but limited in severity, pervasiveness, or time manifest

3 = Moderate maladjustment - greater deficiencies (moderate maladjustment includes subjects with good adjustment in some areas but marked maladjustment in others)

4 = Marked maladjustment - relatively persistent, pervasive and severe difficulties

5 = Severe maladjustment - marked or severe maladjustment in most areas

F

ADHD Symptoms and Other Psychiatric Symptoms in Families of Representative Patients from the Utah Studies

■

ADHD patients (unless adopted) typically come from families whose members may have many ADHD characteristics although they do not meet diagnostic criteria for ADHD or related psychiatric disorders. This is akin to Kretschmer's observation that schizophrenics and manic depressives are characterized by specific "family characterology" (1936, p. 115). That kind of familial "flavor" can be seen in the following families of representative ADHD patients in the Utah studies.

MIXTURE OF ADHD AND PROBABLE BIPOLAR AFFECTIVE DISORDER

■

Patient—ADHD, Learning Disorders, high school dropout, period of substance abuse.
Father—periodic depression and a recovered alcoholic.
Mother—restless, a chatterbox, disorganized.
Paternal grandfather—alcoholic.
Paternal grandmother—periodic depressions.

Maternal grandfather—no psychiatric problems.
Maternal grandmother—"menopausal depression."
Brother—no psychiatric problems.
Brother—ADHD with temper problems.
Sister—bipolar mood disorder which responds to lithium.
Sister—inattentive and restless.
Sisters (2)—no psychiatric disorders.
Wife—no psychiatric problems.
Daughter—age 12, no psychiatric problems or learning problems.
Son—age 8, diagnosed as ADHD.
Son—age 3, "beginning to show same symptoms as his brother."

ADHD AND SUBSTANCE ABUSE
(ALCOHOL AND NICOTINE)

■

Patient—ADHD, underachiever, hot-tempered, fired as football coach for verbal abuse of players, religious Latter Day Saint, does not drink.
Father—alcoholic and heavy smoker; died of emphysema.
Mother—alcoholic who quit drinking, heavy smoker.
Paternal grandfather—alcoholic.
Paternal grandmother—no psychiatric problems.
Maternal grandfather—alcoholic.
Maternal grandmother—no psychiatric problems.
Sister—very obese, no self-confidence, 3 marriages and 3 divorces.
Sister—recovering alcoholic, most severely disturbed of siblings.
Brothers (2)—stable and doing well.
Wife—normal.
Son—age 18, "outgrew hyperactivity," is starting to develop self-control.
Son—age 8, "flies off the handle," always talking too much.

ADHD AND LEARNING DISORDERS

■

Patient—ADHD, disorganized, labile mood, easily upset, no Learning Disorders.
Father—8th grade dropout, policeman, alcoholic, "never really learned to read or spell."

Mother—excellent student, "blows up easily."

Sister—ADHD, disorganized, a chatterbox, overbearing.

Wife—inattentive with labile affect.

Son—adult, Learning Disorders.

Daughter—adult, "immature," slow in learning arithmetic and reading.

Daughter—adult, Learning Disorders, very moody, hot temper.

ADHD WITH CONDUCT DISORDER TRAITS

■

Patient—ADHD, delinquent in school; problems in military, got demoted, drank heavily; after discharge got General Education Diploma, returned to religion of childhood.

Father—ADHD, volatile temper, always on the go.

Mother—anxious, depressive, "too sensitive," fidgety.

Paternal grandfather—multiple arrests for driving while intoxicated, appreciable delinquency before entering the military.

Paternal grandmother—alcoholic, emphysema.

Maternal grandfather—hot tempered.

Maternal grandmother—hot tempered, alcoholic.

Brother—"dangerous...hits walls and bloodies his hands."

Brother—bad temper, explosive, poor social skills, "probably ADD," hostile, poor self-esteem.

Brother—alcoholic, died in motorcycle accident.

Other brothers (4)—no psychiatric problems.

Sister—impulsive buyer, flighty, "a bit hyper," temper problems.

Other sisters (2)—no psychiatric problems.

Wife—inattentive, labile affect.

Son—age 16, ADHD, Learning Disorders, on medication.

Daughter—age 15, no psychiatric problems.

Son—age 13, ADHD, Learning Disorders, on medication.

Son—age 11, Learning Disorders.

Daughter—age 9, ADHD, on medication.

ADHD AND ALCOHOL ABUSE

■

Patient—ADHD, Learning Disorders, former alcoholic who converted to fundamentalist religion and became sober.

Father—authoritarian, violent temper, controlling, strict fundamentalist.

Mother—chronically dysthymic.

Paternal grandfather—alcoholic, heavy smoker.

Paternal grandmother—quiet, self-abasing.

Maternal grandfather—violent temper, alcoholic.

Maternal grandmother—no psychiatric problems.

Brother—not ADHD but several ASPD traits, probable "white collar criminal."

Brother—ADHD, heavy drinker.

Brother—no psychiatric problems.

Sister—no psychiatric problems.

Sister—married 4 times, "promiscuous," heavy drinker, successful businesswoman.

Wife—no psychiatric problems.

Daughter—age 13, no psychiatric problems.

Son—age 11, Learning Disorders, no behavior problems.

Daughter—age 10, hyperactive, "slightly hysterical."

Son—age 8, Oppositional Defiant Disorder.

References

■

Abikoff, H. (1987). An evaluation of cognitive behavior therapy for hyperactive children. In B. Lahey and A. Kazdin (Eds.), *Advances in clinical child psychology, Vol. 10.* New York: Plenum.

Abikoff, H., and Klein, R. G. (1992). Attention-deficit hyperactivity and conduct disorder: Comorbidity and implications for treatment. *Journal of Consulting and Clinical Psychology, 60,* 881–892.

Achenbach, T. M., and Edelbrock, C. (1981). Behavioral problems and competencies reported by parents of normal and disturbed children aged four through sixteen. *Monographs of the Society for Research in Child Development, 46,* 1–82.

Akiskal, H. S. (1983). Dysthymic disorder: Psychopathology of proposed chronic depressive subtypes. *American Journal of Psychiatry, 140,* 11–20.

Alberts-Corush, J., Firestone, P., and Goodman, J. T. (1986). Attention and impulsivity characteristics of the biological and adoptive parents of hyperactive and normal control children. *American Journal of Orthopsychiatry, 56,* 413–423.

Allport, G. W. (1937). *Personality, a psychological interpretation.* New York: Holt.

Alterman, A. I., Tarter, R. E., Baughman, T. G., Bober, B. A., and Fabian, S. A. (1985). Differentiation of alcoholics high and low in childhood hyperactivity. *Drug and Alcohol Dependence, 15:* 111–121.

American Heart Association (1984). Jones criteria (revised for guidance in the diagnosis of rheumatic fever). *Circulation, 69,* 204A.

American Psychiatric Association (1980). *Diagnostic and Statistical Manual of Mental Disorders (third edition).* Washington DC: Author.

American Psychiatric Association (1987). *Diagnostic and Statistical Manual of Mental Disorders (third edition, revised)*. Washington, DC: Author.

American Psychiatric Association (1994). *Diagnostic and Statistical Manual of Mental Disorders (fourth edition)*. Washington, DC: Author.

Anderson, J. C., Williams, S., McGee, R., and Silva, P. A. (1987). DSM-III disorders in preadolescent children. *Archives of General Psychiatry*, 44, 69–76.

Arkonac, O., and Guze, S. B. (1963). A family study of hysteria. *New England Journal of Medicine*, 268, 239–242.

Arnold, L. E., Strobl, D., and Weisenbert, A. (1972). Study of the "paradoxical" amphetamine response. *Journal of the American Medical Association*, 222, 693–694.

August, G. J., and Stewart, M. A. (1982). Is there a syndrome of pure hyperactivity? *British Journal of Psychiatry*, 140, 305–311.

August, G. J., and Stewart, M. A. (1983). Familial subtypes of hyperactivity. *Journal of Nervous and Mental Disease*, 171, 362–368.

Bareggi, S. R., Becker, R. E., Ginsburg, B. E., and Genovese, E. (1979). Neurochemical investigation of an endogenous model of the "hyperkinetic syndrome" in a hybrid dog. *Life Sciences*, 24, 481–488.

Barkley, R. A. (1990). *Attention-deficit hyperactivity disorder: A handbook for diagnosis and treatment*. New York: Guilford.

Barkley, R. A., Fischer, M., Edelbrock, C. S., and Smallish, L. (1990). The adolescent outcome of hyperactive children diagnosed by research criteria. I. An 8-year prospective follow-up study. *Journal of the American Academy of Child and Adolescent Psychiatry*, 29, 546–557.

Barrett, R. E., and Balch, T. (1971). Uptake of catecholamines into serotonergic nerve-cells as demonstrated by fluorescence histochemistry. *Experientia*, 27, 663.

Bartholini, G., DaPrado, M., and Pletscher, A. (1968). Decrease of cerebral 5-hydroxytryptamine by 3,4 dihydroxyphenylalanine after inhibition of extra-cerebral decarboxylase. *Journal of Pharmacy and Pharmacology*, 20, 228.

Bell, R. Q. (1968). A reinterpretation of the direction of effects in studies of socialization. *Psychological Review*, 75, 81–95.

Bennett. L. A., Wolin, S. J., and Reiss, D. (1988). Cognitive, behavioral, and emotional problems among school-age children of alcoholic parents. *American Journal of Psychiatry*, 145, 185–190.

Bhatia, M. S., Nigam, V. R., Bohra, N., and Malik, S. C. (1991). Attention deficit disorder with hyperactivity among paediatric outpatients. *Journal of Child Psychology and Psychiatry*, 32, 297–306.

Biederman, J., Munir, K., Knee, D., Habelow, W., Armentano, M., Autor, S., Hoge, S. K., and Waternaux, C. (1986). A family study of patients with attention deficit disorder and normal controls. *Journal of Psychiatric Research*, 20, 263–274.

Biederman, J., Munir, K., and Knee, D. (1987). Conduct and oppositional disorder in clinically referred children with attention deficit disorder: A controlled family study. *Journal of the American Academy of Child and Adolescent Psychiatry*, 26, 724–727.

Biederman, J., Munir, K., Knee, D., Armentano, M. Autor, S., Waternaux, C., and Tsuang, M. (1987). High rate of affective disorders in probands with attention deficit disorder and in their relatives: A controlled family study. *American Journal of Psychiatry*, 144, 330–333.

Biederman, J., Baldessarini, R. J., Wright, V., Knee, D., and Harmatz, J. S. (1989). A double-blind placebo controlled study of desipramine in the treatment of ADD: I. Efficacy. *Journal of the American Academy of Child and Adolescent Psychiatry*, 28, 777–784.

Biederman, J., Faraone, S. V., Keenan, K., Knee, D., and Tsuang, M. T. (1990). Family-genetic and psychosocial risk factors in DSM-III attention deficit disorder. *Journal of the American Academy of Child and Adolescent Psychiatry*, 29, 526–533.

Biederman, J., Faraone, S. V., Keenan, K., Steingard, R., and Tsuang, M. T. (1991). Familial association between attention deficit disorder and anxiety disorders. *American Journal of Psychiatry*, 148, 251–256.

Biederman, J., Newcorn, J., and Sprich, S. E. (1991). Comorbidity of attention deficit hyperactivity disorder (ADHD). *American Journal of Psychiatry*, 148, 564–577.

Biederman, J., Faraone, S. V., Keenan, K., Benjamin, J., Krifcher, B., Moore, C., Sprich-Buckminster, S., Ugaglia, K., Jellinek, M. S., Steingard, R., Spencer, T., Norman, D., Kolodny, R., Kraus, I., Perrin, J., Keller, M. B., and Tsuang, M. T. (1992). Further evidence for family-genetic risk factors in attention deficit hyperactivity disorder. Patterns of comorbidity in probands and relatives in psychiatrically and pediatrically referred samples. *Archives of General Psychiatry*, 49, 728–738.

Bird, H. R., Gould, M. S., Yager, T., Staghezza, B., and Canino, G. (1989). Risk factors for maladjustment in Puerto Rican children. *Journal of the American Academy of Child and Adolescent Psychiatry*, 28, 847–850.

Bleuler, E. (1950). *Dementia praecox or The group of schizophrenias* [1911]. Trans. Joseph Zinkin. New York: International Universities Press.

Bohman, M. (1978). Some genetic aspects of alcoholism and criminality. *Archives of General Psychiatry*, 35, 269–276.

Bohman, M., Sigvardsson, S., and Cloninger, C. R. (1981). Maternal inheritance of alcohol abuse. *Archives of General Psychiatry*, 38, 965–969.

Bohman, M., Cloninger, C. R., Sigvardsson, S., and von Knorring, A-L. (1982). Predisposition to petty criminality in Swedish adoptees: I. Genetic and environmental heterogeneity. *Archives of General Psychiatry*, 39, 1233–1241.

Bohman, M., Cloninger, C. R., von Knorring, S-L., and Sigvardsson, S. (1984). An adoption study of somatoform disorders. III. Cross-fostering analysis and genetic relationship to alcoholism and criminality. *Archives of General Psychiatry*, 41, 872–878.

Bond, E. D., and Smith, L. H. (1935). Post-encephalitic behavior disorders: A ten-year review of the Franklin school. *American Journal of Psychiatry*, 92, 17–33.

Borison, R. L. (1974). Biosynthesis of brain 2-phenylethylamine: Influence of decarboxylase inhibitors and d-amphetamine. *Life Sciences*, 15, 1837–1848.

Boyle, M. H., Offord, D. R., Hofmann, H. G., Catlin, G. P., Byles, J. A., Cadman, D. T., Crawford, J. W., Links, P. S., Rae-Grant, N. I., and Szatmari, P. (1987). Ontario Child Health Study. I. Methodology. *Archives of General Psychiatry*, 44, 826–831.

Bradley, C. (1937). The behavior of children receiving benzedrine. *American Journal of Psychiatry* 94, 577–585.

Breese, G. R., Cooper, B. R., and Hollister, A. S. (1975). Involvement of brain monoamines in the stimulant and paradoxical inhibitory effects of methylphenidate. *Psychopharmacologia*, 44, 5–10.

Cadoret, R. J., Cunningham, L., Loftus, R., and Edwards, J. (1975). Studies of adoptees from psychiatrically disturbed biologic parents. II. Temperament, hyperactive, antisocial, and developmental variables. *Pediatrics*, 87, 301–306.

Cadoret, R. J., and Gath, A. (1980). Biologic correlates of hyperactivity: Evidence for a genetic factor. In S. B. Sells, R. Crandall, M. Roff, J. S. Strauss, and W. Pollin (Eds.), *Human functioning in longitudinal perspective*. Baltimore: Williams and Wilkins.

Cadoret, R. J., and Stewart, M. (1991). An adoption study of attention deficit/ hyperactivity/aggression and their relationship to adult antisocial personality. *Comprehensive Psychiatry* 32:73–82.

Cantwell, D. P. (1972). Psychiatric illness in the families of hyperactive children. *Archives of General Psychiatry*, 27, 414–417.

Cantwell, D. P. (1975). Genetic studies of hyperactive children: Psychiatric illness in biological and adopting parents in genetic research in psychiatry. In R. R. Fieve, D. Rosenthal, and H. Brill (Eds.), *Genetic research in psychiatry*. Baltimore: Johns Hopkins University Press.

Cardon, L. R., Smith, S. D., Fulker, D. W., Kimberling, W. J., Pennington, B. F., and DeFries, J. C. (1994). Quantitative trait locus for reading disability on chromosome 6. *Science*, 266, 276–279.

Carlson, G. A., and Cantwell, D. P. (1979). A survey of depressive symptoms in a child and adolescent population. *Journal of the American Academy of Child Psychiatry*, 18, 587–598.

Carlson, G. A., and Cantwell, D. P. (1980). Unmasking masked depression in children and adolescents. *American Journal of Psychiatry*, 137, 445–449.

Carnoy, P., Soubrie, P., Puech, A. J., and Simon, P. (1986). Performance deficit induced by low doses of dopamine agonists in rats. Towards a model for approaching the neurobiology of negative schizophrenic symptomatology? *Biological Psychiatry,* 21, 11–22.

Cavanagh, R., Clifford, J. S., and Gregory, L. (1989). The use of bromocriptine for the treatment of attention deficit disorder in two chemically dependent patients. *Journal of Psychoactive Drugs,* 21, 217–220.

Chiarello, R. J., and Cole, J. O. (1987) The use of psychostimulants in general psychiatry. *Archives of General Psychiatry,* 44, 286–295.

Chiodo, L. A., and Antelaman, S. M. (1980). Tricyclic antidepressants induce subsensitivity of presynaptic dopamine autoreceptors. *European Journal of Pharmacology,* 64, 203–204.

Clarkin, J. F., and Kendall, P. C. (1992). Comorbidity and treatment planning: Summary and future directions. *Journal of Consulting and Clinical Psychology.* 60, 904–908.

Cleckley, H. (1976). *The mask of sanity (Fifth edition).* St. Louis: C. V. Mosby Co.

Cloninger C. R. (1985). Schizophrenia: Genetic etiological factors. In H. I. Kaplan, and B. J. Sadock (Eds.), *Comprehensive textbook of psychiatry.* Baltimore: Williams and Wilkins.

Cloninger, C. R., and Guze, S. B. (1970). Psychiatric illness and female criminality: The role of sociopathy and hysteria in the antisocial woman. *American Journal of Psychiatry,* 127, 303–311.

Cloninger, C. R., and Guze, S. B. (1973). Psychiatric illness in the families of female criminals: A study of 288 first-degree relatives. *British Journal of Psychiatry,* 122, 697–703.

Cloninger, C. R., Reich, T., and Guze, S. B. (1975). The multifactorial model of disease transmission: III. Familial relationship between sociopathy and hysteria (Briquet's syndrome). *British Journal of Psychiatry,* 127, 23–32.

Cloninger, C. R., Bohman, M., and Sigvardsson, S. (1981). Inheritance of alcohol abuse: Cross-fostering analysis of adopted men. *Archives of General Psychiatry,* 38, 861–868.

Cloninger, C. R., Sigvardsson, S., Bohman, M., and von Knorring, A-L. (1982). Predisposition to petty criminality in Swedish adoptees: II. Cross-fostering analysis of gene-environment interaction. *Archives of General Psychiatry,* 39, 1242–1247.

Cloninger, C. R., Sigvardsson, S., von Knorring, A-L., and Bohman, M. (1984). An adoption study of somatoform disorders. II. Identification of two discrete somatoform disorders. *Archives of General Psychiatry,* 41, 863–871.

Cocores, J. A., Patel, M. D., Gold, M. S., and Pottash, A. C. (1987). Cocaine abuse, attention deficit disorder, and bipolar disorder. *Journal of Nervous and Mental Disease,* 175, 431–432.

Conacher, G. N., and Workman, D. G. (1989). *American Journal of Psychiatry* Vol. 146, 679.

Conners, C. K. (1969). A teacher rating scale for use in drug studies with children. *American Journal of Psychiatry*, 126, 884–888.

Conners, C. K. (1970). Symptom patterns in hyperkinetic, neurotic, and normal children. *Child Development*, 41, 667–682.

Conners, C. K. (1973). Rating scales for use in drug studies with children. *Psychopharmacology Bulletin* [Special issue: Pharmacotherapy with children] 9, 24–84.

Cooper, B. R., Hester, T. J., and Maxwell, R. A. (1980). Behavioral and biochemical effects of the antidepressant bupropion (Wellbutrin): Evidence for selective blockade of dopamine uptake in vivo. *Journal of Pharmacology and Experimental Therapy*, 215, 127–134.

Corson, S. A., Corson, E. O., Arnold, L. E., and Knopp, W. (1976). Animal models of violence and hyperkinesis. In G. Serban, and A. Kling (Eds.), *Animal models in human psychobiology*. New York: Plenum Press.

Coryell, W. (1980). A blind family history study of Briquet's syndrome. Further validation of the diagnosis. *Archives of General Psychiatry*, 37, 1266–1269.

Costello, E. J. (1989) Child psychiatric disorders and their correlates: A primary care pediatric sample. *Journal of the American Academy of Child and Adolescent Psychiatry*, 28, 851–855.

Costello, E. J., Edelbrock, C. S., Kalas, R., Kessler, M., and Klaric, S. (1982). *The NIMH Diagnostic Interview Schedule for Children (DISC)*. Pittsburgh: Authors.

Cox, A., Rutter, M., Yule, B., and Quinlan, B. (1977). Bias resulting from missing information: Some epidemiological findings. *British Journal of Preventive Social Medicine*, 31, 131–136.

Creese, I. (1987). Biochemical properties of CNS dopamine receptors. In H.Y. Meltzer (Ed.), *Psychopharmacology: The third generation of progress*. New York: Raven Press.

Crow, T. J. (1986). The continuum of psychosis and its implication for the structure of the gene. *British Journal of Psychiatry*, 149, 419–429.

Crowe, R. R. (1972). The adopted offspring of women criminal offenders: A study of their arrest records. *Archives of General Psychiatry*, 27, 600–603.

Crowe, R. R. (1974). An adoption study of antisocial personality. *Archives of General Psychiatry*, 31, 785–791.

Cunningham, L., Cadoret, R. J., Loftus, R., and Edwards, J. E. (1975). Studies of adoptees from psychiatrically disturbed biological parents: Psychiatric conditions in childhood and adolescence. *British Journal of Psychiatry* 126, 534–549.

Dannenberg, A. L., Garrison, R. J., and Kannel, W. B. (1988). Incidence of hypertension in the Framingham study. *American Journal of Public Health*, 78, 676–679.

DeObaldia, R., Parsons, O. A., and Yohman, R. (1983). Minimal brain dysfunction symptoms claimed by primary and secondary alcoholics: Relation to cognitive functioning. *International Journal of Neuroscience*, 20, 173–182.

DeObaldia, R., and Parsons, O. A. (1984). Relationship of neuropsychological performance to primary alcoholism and self-reported symptoms of childhood minimal brain dysfunction. *Journal of Studies of Alcohol*, 45, 386–392.

Derogatis, L. R., Lipman, R. S., and Covi, L. (1973). The SCL-90: An outpatient psychiatric rating scale. *Psychopharmacology Bulletin*, 9, 13–28.

Deutsch, C. K., Swanson, J. M., Bruell, J. H., Cantwell, D. P., Weinberg, F., and Baren, M. (1982). Over-representation of adoptees in children with the attention deficit disorder. *Behavioral Genetics*, 12, 231–238.

Deutsch, C. K. (1983). Dissertation for the degree of Doctor of Philosophy. The University of Texas at Austin.

Deutsch, C. K., Matthysse, S., Swanson, J. M., and Farkas, L. G. (1990). Genetic latent structure analysis of dysmorphology in attention deficit disorder. *Journal of the American Academy of Child and Adolescent Psychiatry*, 29, 189–194.

Dren, A. T., Jochimsen, W. G., and Plotnikoff, N. P. (1971). Comparison of pemoline, cocaine, methamphetamine, and methylphenidate self-administration in monkeys. *Pharmacologist*, 13, 281.

Endicott, J., Spitzer, R. L., and Fleiss, J. L. (1976). The global assessment scale: A procedure for overall severity of psychiatric disturbance. *Archives of General Psychiatry*, 33, 766–771.

Eyre, S., Rounsaville, B., and Kleber, H. (1982). History of childhood hyperactivity in a clinic population of opiate addicts. *Journal of Nervous and Mental Disease*, 170, 522–529.

Faraone, S. V., Biederman, J., Keenan, K., and Tsuang, M. T. (1991). A family-genetic study of girls with DSM-III attention deficit disorder. *American Journal of Psychiatry* 148:112–117.

Faraone, S. V., Biederman, J., Chen, W. J., Krifcher, B., Keenan, K., Moore, C., Sprich, S., and Tsuang, M. T. (1992). Segregation analysis of attention deficit hyperactivity disorder. *Psychiatric Genetics*, 2, 257–275.

Firestone, P., Lewy, F., and Douglas, V. I. (1976). Hyperactivity and physical anomalies. *Canadian Psychiatric Association Journal*, 21, 23–26.

Firestone, P., Peters, S., Rivier, M., and Knights, R. M. (1978). Minor physical anomalies in hyperactive, retarded, and normal children and their families. *Journal of Child Psychology and Psychiatry*, 19, 155–160.

Fischer, M., Barkley, R. A., Edelbrock, C. S., et al. (1990). The adolescent outcome of hyperactive children diagnosed by research criteria, II. Academic, attention, and neuropsychological status. *Journal of Consulting and Clinical Psychology*, 58, 580–588.

Fitzgerald, F. S. (1925). *The Great Gatsby*. New York: Scribner's Sons.

Gardner, R. A. (1979). *The objective diagnosis of minimal brain dysfunction.* New Jersey: Creative Therapeutics.

Gelenberg, A. J., Wojcik, J. D., Growdon, J. H., et al. (1980). Tyrosine for the treatment of depression. *American Journal of Psychiatry*, 137, 622–623.

Geschwind, N., and Galaburda, A. M. (1985). Cerebral lateralization. Biological mechanisms, associations, and pathology: I. A hypothesis and a program for research. *Archives of Neurology*, 42, 428–458.

Geschwind, N., and Galaburda, A. M. (1985). Cerebral lateralization. Biological mechanisms, associations, and pathology: II. A hypothesis and a program for research. *Archives of Neurology*, 42, 521–551.

Geschwind, N., and Galaburda, A. M. (1985). Cerebral lateralization. Biological mechanisms, associations, and pathology: III. A hypothesis and a program for research. *Archives of Neurology*, 42, 634–544.

Geschwind, N. (1986). Dyslexia, cerebral dominance, autoimmunity, and sex hormones. In G. T. Pavlidis, and D. F. Fisher (Eds.), *Dyslexia: Its neuropsychology and treatment.* Chichester: Wiley.

Giedd, J. N., Castellanos, X., Casey, B. J., Kozuch, P., King, A. C., Hamburger, S. D., and Rapoport, J. L. (1994). Quantitative morphology of the corpus callosum in attention deficit hyperactivity disorder. *American Journal of Psychiatry*, 151, 665–669.

Gilger, J. W., Pennington, B. F., and DeFries, J. C. (1992). A twin study of the etiology of comorbidity: attention-deficit hyperactivity disorder and dyslexia. *Journal of the American Academy of Child and Adolescent Psychiatry*, 31, 343–348.

Gillberg, C., and Rasmussen, P. (1982). Perceptual, motor and attentional deficits in seven-year old children: Background factors. *Developmental Medicine and Child Neurology*, 24, 752–770.

Ginsburg, B. E., Becker, R. E., Trattner, A., and Bareggi, S. (1984). A genetic taxonomy of hyperkinesis in the dog. *International Journal of Developmental Neuroscience*, 2, 313–322.

Gittelman, R., Mannuzza, S., Shenker, R., and Bonagura, N. (1985). Hyperactive boys almost grown up. I. Psychiatric status. *Archives of General Psychiatry*, 42, 937–947.

Gittelman-Klein, R. (1980). In D. F. Klein, R. Gittelman, F. Quitkin, and A. Rifkin, (Eds.), *Diagnosis and drug treatment of adults and children. (second edition).* New York: Williams and Wilkins.

Goldberg, I. K. (1980). ʟ-Tyrosine in depression (letter). *Lancet*, 2, 364–365.

Goldfarb, W., and Botstein, A. (1956). Physical stigmata in schizophrenic children. Unpublished manuscript. Brooklyn, New York: Henry Ittelson Institute for Child Research.

Golinko, B. E., Rennick, P. M., and Glaros, A. G. (1981). Tolerance to dextroamphetamine sulfate in hyperactive children: Assessment using an empirical neuropsychological paradigm—A pilot study. *Progress in Neuro-Psychopharmacology*, 4, 601–606.

Goodman, R., and Stevenson, J. (1989a). A twin study of hyperactivity—I. An examination of hyperactivity scores and categories derived from Rutter teacher and parent questionnaires. *Journal of Child Psychology and Psychiatry*, 30, 671–689.

Goodman, R., and Stevenson, J. (1989b). A twin study of hyperactivity—II. The aetiological role of genes, family relationships, and perinatal adversity. *Journal of Child Psychology and Psychiatry*, 30, 691–709.

Goodwin, D. W., Schulsinger, F., Hermansen, L., Guze, S. B., and Winokur, G. (1973). Alcohol problems in adoptees raised apart from alcoholic biological parents. *Archives of General Psychiatry*, 28, 238–243.

Goodwin, D. W., Schulsinger, F., Hermansen, L., Guze, S. B., and Winokur, G. (1975). Alcoholism and the hyperactive child syndrome. *Journal of Nervous and Mental Disease*, 160, 349–353.

Goodwin, D. W., Schulsinger, F., Knop, J., Mednick, S., and Guze, S. B. (1975). Alcoholism and depression in adopted-out daughters of alcoholics. *Archives of General Psychiatry*, 34, 751–755.

Goodwin, D. W., Schulsinger, F., Knop, J., Mednick, S., and Guze, S. B. (1977a). Alcoholism and depression in adopted-out daughters of alcoholics. *Archives of General Psychiatry*, 34, 751–755.

Goodwin, D. W., Schulsinger, F., Knop, J., Mednick, S., and Guze, S. B. (1977b). Psychopathology in adopted and nonadopted daughters of alcoholics. *Archives of General Psychiatry*, 34, 1005–1009.

Goodwin, D. W., Schulsinger, F., Knop, J., Mednick, S., and Guze, S. B. (1978). Psychopathology in adopted and nonadopted daughters of alcoholics. *Archives of General Psychiatry*, 34, 1005–1009.

Goodwin, F. K., and Jamison, K. R. (1990) *Manic-depressive illness*. New York: Oxford University Press.

Goyer, P. F., David, G. C., and Rapoport, J. L. (1979). Abuse of prescribed stimulant medication by a 13-year-old hyperactive boy. *Journal of the American Academy of Child Psychiatry*, 18, 170–175.

Greenhill, L. L., Rieder, R. O., Wender, P. H., Buchsbaum, M., and Zahn, R. (1973). Lithium carbonate in the treatment of hyperactive children. *Archives of General Psychiatry*, 28, 636–640.

Gualtieri, C. T., Ondrusek, M. G., and Finley, C. (1985). Attention deficit disorders in adults. *Clinical Neuropharmacology*, 8, 343–356.

Guze, S. B., Wolfgram, E. D., McKinney, J. K., and Cantwell, D. P. (1967). Psychiatric illness in the families of convicted criminals: A study of 519 first-degree relatives. *Disorders of the Nervous System*, 28, 651–659.

Guze, S. B., Goodwin, D. W., and Crane, J. B. (1969). Criminality and psychiatric disorders. *Archives of General Psychiatry*, 20, 583–591.

Guze, S. B., Woodruff, R. A., Jr., and Clayton, P. J. (1971). Hysteria and antisocial behavior: Further evidence of an association. *American Journal of Psychiatry*, 127, 957–960.

Guze, S. B., and Goodwin, D. W. (1972). The consistency of the drinking history and the diagnosis of alcoholism. *Quarterly Journal of Studies of Alcohol* 33, 111–116.

Haenlein, M., and Caul, W. F. (1987). Attention deficit disorder with hyperactivity: A specific hypothesis of reward dysfunction. *Journal of the American Academy of Child and Adolescent Psychiatry*, 26, 356–362.

Hagnell, O., Lanke, J., Rorsman, B., and Ojesjo, L. (1982). Are we entering an age of melancholy? Depressive illnesses in a prospective epidemiological study over 25 years: the Lundaby study, Sweden. *Psychological Medicine*, 12, 279–289.

Hechtman, L., Weiss, G., and Perlman, T. (1984). Hyperactives as young adults: Past and current substance abuse and antisocial behavior. *American Journal of Orthopsychiatry*, 54, 415–425.

Heiman, E. M. (1983). Use of stimulants for alcoholic patients with attention deficit disorder. Letters to the editor. *American Journal of Psychiatry*, 140, 1272.

Herjanic, B., and Campbell, W. (1977). Differentiating psychiatrically disturbed children on the basis of a structured interview. *Journal of Abnormal Child Psychology*, 5, 127–134.

Herjanic, B., and Reich, W. (1982). Development of a structured psychiatric interview for children: Agreement between child and parent on individual symptoms. *Journal of Abnormal Child Psychology*, 10, 307–324.

Heston, L. L., Denney, D. D., and Pauly, I. B. (1966). The adult adjustment of persons institutionalized. *British Journal of Psychiatry*, 112, 1103–1110.

Hill, D. (1947). Amphetamine in psychopathic states. *British Journal of Addiction*, 44, 50–54.

Hill, R. T. (1972). Animal models of the euphorigenic action of amphetamine-like psychomotor stimulant drugs. Invited address presented at the annual meeting of the American Psychological Association (Div. 28), Honolulu, Hawaii.

Hill, T. R. (1928). The problem of juvenile behaviour disorders in chronic epidemic encephalitis. *Journal of Neurology and Psychopathology*, 9, 1–10.

Hinshaw, S.P. (1987). On the distinction between attentional deficits/hyperactivity and conduct problems/aggression in child psychopathology. *Psychological Bulletin*, 101, 443–463.

Hoffman, B. B., and Lefkowitz, R. J. (1990). Adrenergic receptor antagonists. In A. G. Goodman, T. W. Rall, A. S. Nies, and P. Taylor, (Eds.), *Goodman and Gilman's: The pharmacological basis of therapeutics. (Eighth edition)*. New York: Pergamon Press.

Hohman, L. B. (1922). Post-encephalitic behavior disorders in children. *Johns Hopkins Hospital Bulletin*, 380, 372–375.

Hollingshead, A. B., and Redlich, F. C. (1958). *Social class and mental illness: A community study*. New York: John Wiley.

Holmes, T. H., and Rahe, R. H. (1967). The social readjustment rating scale. *Journal of Psychosomatic Research*, 11, 213–218.

Holt, W. J. (1937). Epidemic encephalitis: A follow-up study of two hundred and sixty-two cases. *Archives of Neurology and Psychiatry*, 38, 1135–1144.

Horn, J. M., Green, M., Carney, R., and Erickson, M. T. (1975). Bias against genetic hypotheses in adoption studies. *Archives of General Psychiatry*, 32, 1365–1367.

Hornykiewicz, O. (1973). Dopamine in the basal ganglia. *British Medical Bulletin*, 29, 172–178.

Huessy, H. R. (1974). The adult hyperkinetic. Letters to the editor. *American Journal of Psychiatry*, 131, 724–725.

Huessy, H. R, and Gendron, R. M. (1970). Prevalence of the so-called hyperkinetic syndrome in public school children of Vermont. *Acta Paedopsychiatrica*, 37, 243–248.

Huessy, H., Metoyer, M., and Townsend, M. (1973). Eight-ten year follow-up of children treated in rural Vermont for behavior disorder. *American Journal of Orthopsychiatry*, 43, 236–238.

Huessy, H. R., Cohen, S. M., Blair, C. L., and Rood, P. (1979). Clinical explorations in adult minimal brain dysfunction. In L. Bellak (Ed.), *Psychiatric aspects of minimal brain dysfunction in adults*. New York: Grune and Stratton.

Hunt, R. D. (1987). Treatment effects of oral and transdermal clonidine in relation to methylphenidate. *Psychopharmacology Bulletin*, 23, 111–114.

Hunt, R. D., Minderra, R. B., and Cohen, D. J. (1985). Clonidine benefits children with attention deficit disorder and hyperactivity: Report on a double-blind placebo-controlled crossover study. *Journal of the American Academy of Child Psychiatry*, 24, 617–629.

Hunt, R. D., Capper, L., and O'Connell, P. (1990). Clonidine in child and adolescent psychiatry. *Journal of Child and Adolescent Psychopharmacology*, 1, 87–102.

Hutchings, B., and Mednick, S. A. (1975). Registered criminality in the adoptive and biological parents of registered male criminal adoptees. In R. R. Fieve, D. Rosenthal, and H. Brill (Eds.), *Genetic research in psychiatry*. Baltimore: Johns Hopkins University Press.

Hutt, C. S., Snider, S. R., and Fahn, S. (1977). Interaction between bromocriptine and levodopa: Biochemical basis for an improved treatment for Parkinsonism. *Neurology*, 27, 505.

Jaffe, S. L. (1991). Intranasal abuse of prescribed methylphenidate by an alcohol and drug abusing adolescent with ADHD. *Journal of the American Academy of Child and Adolescent Psychiatry*, 30.

James, W. (1890). *The principles of psychology*. Cambridge: Harvard University Press.

Jankovic, J. (1993). Deprenyl in attention deficit associated with Tourette's syndrome. *Archives of Neurology*, 50, 286–288.

Jastak, J., and Jastak, S. (1978). *A wide-range achievement test manual,* Wilmington, DE: Jastak Associates.

Johnson, A. B. (1959). *A treatise on language: Or the relation which words bear to things* [1836]. Ed. David Rynin. Berkeley: University of California Press.

Johnston, J. P. (1968). Some observations upon a new inhibitor of monoamine oxidase in brain tissue. *Biochemical Pharmacology*, 17, 1285.

Jones, K. L., Smith, D. W., Ulleland, C. N., and Streissguth, A. P. (1973). Pattern of malformation in offspring of chronic alcoholic mothers. *Lancet*, 1, 1267–1271.

Kaij, L., and Dock, J. (1975). Grandsons of alcoholics. A test of sex-linked transmission of alcohol abuse. *Archives of General Psychiatry*, 32, 1379–1381.

Kanner, L. (1962). *Child psychiatry (third edition).* Springfield, Il: Charles C Thomas.

Kashani, J., Chapel, J. L., Ellis, J., and Shekim, W. O. (1979). Hyperactive girls. *Journal of Operational Psychiatry*, 10, 145–148.

Kaplan, S. L., Busner, J., Kupietz, S., Wassermann, E., and Segal, B. (1990). Effects of methylphenidate on adolescents with aggressive conduct disorder and ADDH: A preliminary report. *Journal of the American Academy of Child and Adolescent Psychiatry*, 29, 719–723.

Kendall, P. C., and Clarkin, J. F. (1992). Introduction to special section: Comorbidity and treatment implications. *Journal of Consulting and Clinical Psychology*, 60, 833–834.

Kety, S. S., Rosenthal, D., Wender, P. H., and Schulsinger, F. (1968). The types of prevalence of mental illness in the biological and adoptive families of adopted schizophrenics. In D. Rosenthal and S. S. Kety, (Eds.), *The transmission of schizophrenia.* New York: Pergamon Press.

Kety, S. S., Rosenthal, D., Wender, P. H., and Schulsinger, F. (1971). Mental illness in the biological and adoptive families of adopted schizophrenics. *American Journal of Psychiatry*, 128, 302–306.

Kety, S. S., Rosenthal, D., Wender, P. H., Schulsinger, F., and Jacobsen, B. (1975). Mental illness in the biological and adoptive families of adopted individuals who have become schizophrenic: A preliminary report based on psychiatric interviews. In R.R. Fieve, D. Rosenthal, and H. Brill (Eds.), *Genetic research in psychiatry.* Baltimore: The Johns Hopkins University Press.

Khantzian, E. J. (1983). An extreme case of cocaine dependence and marked improvement with methylphenidate treatment. *American Journal of Psychiatry*, 140, 784–785.

Klein, D. F. (1974). Endogenomorphic depression: A conceptual and terminological revision. *Archives of General Psychiatry*, 31, 447–454.

Klein, D. F., Gittelman, R., Quitkin, F., and Rifkin, A. (1980). *Diagnosis and drug treatment of psychiatric disorders: Adults and children (second edition)*. Baltimore/London: Williams and Wilkins.

Klerman, G. L., Lavori, P. W., Rice, J., Reich, T., Endicott, J., Andreasen, N. C., Keller, M. B., and Hirschfield, R. M. A. (1985). Birth-cohort trends in rates of major depressive disorder among relatives of patients with affective disorder. *Archives of General Psychiatry*, 42, 689–693.

Klorman, R., Brumaghim, J. T., Fitzpatrick, P. A., and Borgstedt, A. D. (1990). Clinical effects of a controlled trial of methylphenidate on adolescents with attention deficit disorder. *Journal of the American Academy of Child and Adolescent Psychiatry*, 29, 702–709.

Kretschmer, E. (1936). *Physique and character. (second edition)*. Trans. W. J. H. Sprott. London: Kegan Paul, Trench, Trubner and Co., Ltd.

Krouse, J. P., and Kauffman, J. M. (1982). Minor physical anomalies in exceptional children: A review and critique of research. *Journal of Abnormal Child Psychology*, 10, 247–264.

Lahey, B. B., Piacentini, J. C., McBurnett, K., Stone, P., Hartdagen, S., and Hynd, G. (1988). Psychopathology in the parents of children with conduct disorder and hyperactivity. *Journal of the American Academy of Child and Adolescent Psychiatry*, 27, 163–170.

Lapouse, R., and Monk, M. (1958). An epidemiological study of behavior characteristics in children. *American Journal of Public Health* 48, 1134–1144.

Lasagna, L., von Felsinger, J. M., and Beecher, H. K. (1955). Drug-induced mood changes in man. 1. Observations on healthy subjects, chronically ill patients, and "postaddicts." *Journal of the American Medical Association*, 157, 1006–1020.

Laufer, M. W., and Denhoff, E. (1957). Hyperkinetic behavior syndrome in children. *Journal of Pediatrics*, 50, 463–474.

Lerer, R. J., Artner, J., and Lerer, M. P. (1979). Handwriting deficits in children with minimal brain dysfunction: Effects of methylphenidate (Ritalin) and placebo. *Journal of Learning Disabilities*, 12, 450–455.

Levy, S. (1959). Post-encephalitic behavior disorder—a forgotten entity: A report of 100 cases. *American Journal of Psychiatry*, 115, 1062–1067.

Lindahl, E. L., and Michelsson, K. (1986). Neurodevelopmental significance of minor and major congenital anomalies in neonatal high risk children. *Neuropediatrics*, 17, 86–93.

Lipper, S., Murphy, D. L., Slater, S., and Buchsbaum M. S. (1979). Comparative behavioral effects of clorgyline and pargyline in man: A preliminary evaluation. *Psychopharmacology*, 62, 123–128.

Loeber, R., Lahey, B. B., and Thomas, C. (1991). Diagnostic conundrum of oppositional defiant disorder and conduct disorder. *Journal of Abnormal Psychology*, 100, 379–390.

Loney, J., Langhorne, J. E., and Paternite, C. E. (1978). An empirical basis for subgrouping the hyperkinetic/minimal brain dysfunction syndrome. *Journal of Abnormal Psychology, 87*, 431–441.

Loney, J., and Milich, R. S. (1981). Hyperactivity, inattention, and aggression in clinical practice. In M. Wolraich, and D. K. Routh, (Eds.), *Advances in behavioral pediatrics, Vol. 2*, Greenwich, CT: JAI Press.

Loney, J., and Milich, R. (1982). Hyperactivity, inattention and aggression in clinical practice. In M. Wolraich and D. Routh (Eds.), *Advances in developmental and behavioral pediatrics, Vol 3*. Greenwich, CT: JAI Press.

Loney, J., Kramer, J., and Milich, R. S. (1981). The hyperactive child grows up: predictors of symptoms, delinquency and achievement at follow-up. In K. D. Gadow and J. Loney (Eds.), *Psychosocial aspects of drug treatment of hyperactivity.* Boulder, CO: Westview.

Lopez, R. (1965). Hyperactivity in twins. *Canadian Psychiatric Association Journal, 10*, 421.

Mann, H., and Greenspan, S. (1976). The identification and treatment of adult brain dysfunction. *American Journal of Psychiatry, 133*, 1013–1017.

Mannuzza, S., and Gittelman, R. (1984). The adolescent outcome of hyperactive girls. *Psychiatry Research, 13*, 19–29.

Mannuzza, S., Klein, R. G., Bonagura, N., Malloy, P., Giampino, T. L., and Addalli, K. A. (1991). Hyperactive boys almost grown up. V. Replication of psychiatric status. *Archives of General Psychiatry, 48*, 77–83.

Mannuzza, S., Klein, R. G., Bessler, A., Malloy, P., and LaPadula, M. (1993). Adult outcome of hyperactive boys: Educational achievement, occupational rank, and psychiatric status. *Archives of General Psychiatry, 50*, 565–576.

Matochik, J. A., Nordahl, T. E., Gross, M., Semple, W. E., King, A. C., Cohen, R. M., and Zametkin, A. J. (1993). Effects of acute stimulant medication on cerebral metabolism in adults with hyperactivity. *Neuropsychopharmacology, 8*, 377–386.

Mattes, J. A. (1986). Propranolol for adults with temper outbursts and residual attention deficit disorder. *Journal of Clinical Psychopharmacology, 6*, 299–302.

Mattes, J. A., Boswell, L., and Oliver, H. (1984). Methylphenidate effects on symptoms of attention deficit disorder in adults. *Archives of General Psychiatry, 41*, 1059–1063.

May, P. R. A. (1968). *The treatment of chronic schizophrenia.* New York: Science House.

McGee, R., Feehan, M., Williams, S., Partridge, F., Silva, P. A., and Kelly, J. (1990). DSM-III disorders in a large sample of adolescents. *Journal of the American Academy of Child and Adolescent Psychiatry, 29*, 611–619.

McKusick, V. A. (1969). On lumpers and splitters, or the nosology of genetic disease. *Perspectives in biology and medicine.* Chicago: The University of Chicago Press.

McNair, D. M., Lorr, M., and Droppleman, L. F. (1971). *Manual: Profile of mood states.* San Diego: Educational and Industrial Testing Service.

Medical Research Council Working Party on Phenylketonuria. (1993). Phenylketonuria due to phenylalanine hydroxylase deficiency: An unfolding story. *British Medical Journal,* 306, 115–119.

Mednick, S. A., and Schulsinger, F. (1968). Some premorbid characteristics related to breakdown in children with schizophrenic mothers. In D. Rosenthal and S. S. Kety (Eds.), *The transmission of schizophrenia.* New York: Pergamon Press.

Miles, T. R. (1983). *Dyslexia.* Springfield, IL: Charles C Thomas.

Morrison, J. (1980). Adult psychiatric disorders in parents of hyperactive children. *American Journal of Psychiatry,* 137, 825–827.

Morrison, J. R., and Stewart, M. A. (1971). A family study of the hyperactive child syndrome. *Biological Psychiatry,* 3, 189–195.

Morrison, J. R., and Stewart, M. A. (1973). The psychiatric studies of the legal families of adopted hyperactive children. *Archives of General Psychiatry* 28, 888–891.

Morrison, J. R., and Stewart, M. A. (1974). Bilateral inheritance as evidence for polygenicity: The hyperactive child syndrome. *Journal of Nervous and Mental Disease,* 158, 226–228.

Murphy, D. L. (1978). Substrate-selective monoamine oxidase: Inhibitor, tissue, species and functional differences. *Biochemical Pharmacology,* 27, 1889–1893.

Murphy, D. L., Lipper, S., Slater, S., and Shiling, D. (1979). Selectivity of clorgyline and pargyline as inhibitors of monoamine oxidases A and B in vivo in man. *Psychopharmacology,* 62, 129–32.

Murphy, D. L., Aulakh, C. S., Garrick, N. A., and Sunderland, T. (1987). Monoamine oxidase inhibitors as antidepressants: Implications for the mechanism of action of antidepressants and the psychobiology of the affective disorders and some related disorders. In H. Y. Meltzer (Ed.), *Psychopharmacology: The third generation of progress.* New York: Raven Press.

Nimitkitpaisan, Y., Bose, S., Kumar, R., and Pradhan, S. N. (1977). Effects of L-dopa on self-stimulation and brain biogenic amines in rats. *Neuropharmacology,* 16, 557.

Offord, D. R., Boyle, M. H., Szatmari, P., Rae-Grant, N., Links, P. S., Cadman, D. T., Byles, J. A., Crawford, J. W., Munroe Blum, H., Byrne, C., Thomas, H., and Woodward, C. (1987). Ontario Child Health Study: Six-month prevalence of disorder and rates of service utilization. *Archives of General Psychiatry,* 44, 832–836.

Offord, D. R., Boyle, M. H., Fleming, J. E., Blum, H. M., and Rae-Grant, N. I. (1989). Ontario Child Health Study: Summary of selected results. *Canadian Journal of Psychiatry,* 34, 483–491.

O'Leary, K. D., Vivian, D., and Nisi, A. (1985). Hyperactivity in Italy. *Journal of Abnormal Child Psychology,* 13, 485–500.

Oliver, J. E., and Buchanan, A. H. (1979). Generations of maltreated children and multi-agency care in one kindred. *British Journal of Psychiatry*, 135, 289–303.

Omenn, G. S. (1973). Genetic issues in the syndrome of minimal brain dysfunction. *Seminars-in-Psychiatry*, 5, 5–17.

O'Reilly, R. A. (1987). Warfarin metabolism and drug-drug interactions. *Advance Experiments in Medical Biology*, 214, 205–212.

Paternite, C., and Loney, J. (1980). Childhood hyperkinesis: Relationships between symptomatology and home environment. In C. K. Whalen and B. Henker (Eds.), *Hyperactive children: The social economy of identification and treatment*. New York: Academic Press.

Pauls, D. L., Shaywitz, S. E., Kramer, P. L., et al. (1983). Demonstration of vertical transmission of attention deficit disorder. *Annals of Neurology*, 14, 363.

Pelham, W. E., Jr., Gnagy, E. M., Greenslade, K. E., and Milich, R. (1992). Teacher ratings of DSM-III-R symptoms for the disruptive behavior disorders. *Journal of the American Academy of Child and Adolescent Psychiatry*, 31, 210–218.

Perley, M. J., and Guze, S. B. (1962). Hysteria—the stability and usefulness of clinical criteria. *New England Journal of Medicine*, 266, 421–426.

Phillips, N. R. (1923). Clinical psychiatry. *Journal of Mental Science*, 69, 245–247.

Piacentini, J. C., McBurnett, K., Stone, P., Hartdagen, S., and Hynd, G. (1988). Psychopathology in the parents of children with conduct disorder and hyperactivity. *Journal of the American Academy of Child and Adolescent Psychiatry*, 27, 163–170.

Pickar, D., Murphy, D. L., Cohen, R. M., Campbell, I. C., and Lipper, (1982). Selective and nonselective monoamine oxidase inhibitors. *Archives of General Psychiatry*, 39, 535–540.

Post, R. M., and Goodwin, F. K. (1978). Approaches to brain amines in psychiatric patients: A reevaluation of cerebrospinal fluid studies. In L. L. Iversen, S. D. Iverson, and S. H. Snyder (Eds.), *Handbook of psychopharmacology, Vol. 13: Biology of mood and antianxiety drugs*. New York: Plenum.

Pritchard, J. E. (1835). *A treatise on insanity*. London: Sherwood, Gilbert and Piper.

Quinn, P. O., and Rapoport, J. L. (1974). Minor physical anomalies and neurological status in hyperactive boys. *Pediatrics*, 53, 742–747.

Rapoport, J. L., Buchsbaum, M. S., Weingartner, H., Zahn, T. P., Ludlow, C., and Mikkelsen, E. J. (1980). Dextroamphetamine. *Archives of General Psychiatry*, 37, 933–943.

Ratey, J. J., Greenberg, M. S., and Lindem, K. J. (1991). Combination of treatments for attention deficit hyperactivity disorder in adults. *Journal of Nervous and Mental Disease*, 179, 699–701.

Reich, T., Rice, J. P., Cloninger, C. R., and Suarez, B. K. (1982). The detection of major genes in clinical populations. *Progress in Neuro-Psychopharmacology and Biological Psychiatry*, 6, 663.

Reimherr, F. W., Wood, D. R., and Wender, P. H. (1980). An open trial of L-dopa and carbidopa in minimally brain dysfunctioned adults. *American Journal of Psychiatry*, 137, 73–75.

Reimherr, F. W., Wender, P. H., Ebert, M. H., and Wood, D. R. (1984). Cerebrospinal fluid homovanillic acid and 5-hydroxyindole acetic acid in adults with attention deficit disorder, residual type (ADD,RT). *Psychiatry Research*, 11, 71–78.

Reimherr, F. W., Wender, P. H., Wood, D. R., and Ward, M. (1987). An open trial of l-tyrosine in the treatment of attention deficit disorder, residual type. *American Journal of Psychiatry*, 144, 1071–1073.

Rifkin, A. (1980). *Diagnosis and drug treatment of psychiatric disorders: Adults and children.* (second edition). Baltimore: Williams and Wilkins.

Rifkin, A., Quitkin, F., Carrillo, C., Blumberg, A. G., and Klein, D. F. (1972). Lithium treatment in emotionally unstable character disorder. *Archives of General Psychiatry*, 27, 519–523.

Robins, L. (1966). *Deviant children grown up.* Baltimore: Williams and Wilkins.

Robins, L. N. (1985). Epidemiology: Reflections on testing the validity of psychiatric interviews. *Archives of General Psychiatry*, 42, 918–924.

Robins, L. N., and Price, R. K. (1991). Adult disorders predicted by childhood conduct problems: Results from the NIMH Epidemiologic Catchment Area project. *Psychiatry*, 54, 116–32.

Rosenthal, D. (1970). *Genetic theory and abnormal behavior.* McGraw-Hill, New York.

Rosenthal, D., Wender, P. H., Kety, S. S., Schulsinger, F., Welner, J., and Ostergaard, L. (1968). Schizophrenics' offspring reared in adoptive homes. *Journal of Psychiatry Research*, 6, 377–391.

Rosenthal, D., Wender, P. H., Kety, S. S., Welner, S., and Schulsinger, F. (1971). The adopted-away offspring of schizophrenics. *American Journal of Psychiatry*, 128, 307–311.

Rounsaville, B. J., Anton, S. F., Carroll, K., Budde, D., Prusoff, B. A., and Gawin, F. (1991). Psychiatric diagnoses of treatment-seeking cocaine abusers. *Archives of General Psychiatry*, 48, 43–51.

Rutter, M. (1967). A children's behavioural questionnaire for completion by teachers: Preliminary findings. *Journal of Child Psychology and Psychiatry*, 8, 1–11.

Rutter, M. (1978). Prevalence and types of dyslexia. In A. L. Benton and D. Pearl (Eds.), *Dyslexia: An appraisal of current knowledge.* New York: Oxford University Press.

Rutter, M., and Yule, W. (1970). Reading retardation and antisocial behavior—the nature of the association. In M. Rutter, J. Tizard, and K. Whitmore (Eds.), *Education, health, and behavior.* London: Longmans.

Safer, D. J. (1973). A familial factor in minimal brain dysfunction. *Behavior Genetics*, 3, 175–186.

Safer, D. J., and Allen, R. P. (1989). Absence of tolerance to the behavioral effects of methylphenidate in hyperactive and inattentive children. *Journal of Pediatrics*, 115, 1003–1008.

Sandberg, S., Rutter, M., and Taylor, E. (1978). Hyperkinetic disorder in psychiatric clinic attenders. *Developmental Medicine in Child Neurology*, 20, 279–299.

Sandberg, S., Wieselberg, M., and Shaffer, D. (1980). Hyperkinetic and conduct problem children in a primary school population: Some epidemiological considerations. *Journal of Child Psychology and Psychiatry*, 21, 293–311.

Satel, S. L., and Southwick, S. (1987). Consequences of abrupt reduction of chronic symptoms. *American Journal of Psychiatry*, 144, 1362.

Satin, M. S., Winsberg, B. G., Monetti, C. H., Sverd, J., and Foss, D. A. (1985). A general population screen for attention deficit disorder with hyperactivity. *Journal of the American Academy of Child Psychiatry*, 24, 756–764.

Satterfield, J. H., Hoppe, C. M., and Schell, A. M. (1982). A prospective study of delinquency in 100 adolescent boys with attention deficit disorder and 88 normal adolescent boys. *American Journal of Psychiatry*, 139, 797–798.

Satterfield, J. H., and Schell, A. M. (1984). Childhood brain function differences in delinquent and non-delinquent hyperactive boys. *Electroencephalography and Clinical Neurophysiology*, 57, 199–207.

Scarr, S. (1966). Genetic factors in activity motivation. *Child Development*, 37, 663–667.

Schachar, R., and Wachsmuth, R. (1990). Hyperactivity and parental psychopathology. *Journal of Child Psychology and Psychiatry*, 31, 381–392.

Schachar, R. J., Rutter, M., and Smith, A. (1981). The characteristics of situationally and pervasively hyperactive children: Implications for syndrome definition. *Journal of Child Psychology and Psychiatry*, 22, 375–392.

Schecter, M. D., Carlson, P. V., Simmons, J. Q. III, and Work, H. H. (1964). Emotional problems in the adoptee. *Archives of General Psychiatry* 10, 37–45.

Schneider, K. (1958). *Psychopathic personalities*. Trans. M. W. Hamilton. London: Cassell.

Schulsinger, F. (1972). Psychopathy: Heredity and environment. *International Journal of Mental Health*, 1, 190–206.

Schulz, S. C., Cornelius, J., Schulz, P. M. and Soloff, P. H. (1988). The amphetamine challenge test in patients with borderline disorder. *American Journal of Psychiatry*, 145, 809–814.

Schuster, C. R., Woods, J. H., and Seevers, M. H. (1969). Self-administration of central stimulants by the monkey. In F. Sjoqvist and M. Tottie (Eds.), *Abuse of central stimulants.* New York: Raven Press.

Semrud-Clikeman, M., Biederman, J., Sprich-Buckminster, S., Lehman, B. K., Faraone, S. V., and Norman, D. (1992). Comorbidity between ADDH and learning disability: A review and report in a clinically referred sample. *Journal of the American Academy of Child and Adolescent Psychiatry,* 3,439–448.

Shaffer, D., Gould, M. S., Brasic, J., Ambrosini, P., Fisher, P., Bird, H., and Aluwahlia, S. (1983). A children's global assessment scale (CGAS). *Archives of General Psychiatry,* 40, 1228–1231.

Shapiro, S. K., and Garfinkel, B. D. (1986). The occurrence of behavior disorders in children: The interdependence of attention deficit disorder and conduct disorder. *Journal of the American Academy of Child Psychiatry,* 25, 809–819.

Shaywitz, B. A., Cohen, D. J., and Bowers, M. B. (1977). CSF monoamine metabolites in children with minimal brain dysfunction: Evidence for alteration of d\brain dopamine. *Journal of Pediatrics,* 90, 67–71.

Shaywitz, S. E., Cohen, D. J., and Shaywitz, B. A. (1980). Behavior and learning difficulties in children of normal intelligence born to alcoholic mothers. *Journal of Pediatrics,* 96, 978–982.

Shekim, W. O., Kashani, J., Beck, N., Cantwell, D. P., Martin, J., Rosenberg, J., and Costello, A. (1985). The prevalence of attention deficit disorders in a rural midwestern community sample of nine-year-old children. *Journal of the American Academy of Child Psychiatry,* 24, 765–770.

Shekim, W. O., Masterson, A., Cantwell, D. P., Hanna, G. L., and McCracken, J. T. (1989). Nomifensine maleate in adult attention deficit disorder. *Journal of Nervous and Mental Disease,* 177, 296–299.

Shekim, W. O., Asarnow, R. F., Hess, E., Zaucha, K., and Wheeler, N. (1990). A clinical and demographic profile of a sample of adults with attention deficit hyperactivity disorder, residual state. *Comprehensive Psychiatry,* 31, 416–425.

Shen, Y-c., Wang, Y-f., and Yang, X-l. (1985). An epidemiological investigation of minimal brain dysfunction in six elementary schools in Beijing. *Journal of Child Psychology and Psychiatry,* 26, 777–787.

Shetty, T., and Chase, T. N. (1976). Central monoamines and hyperkinesis of childhood. *Neurology,* 26, 1000–1002.

Sigvardsson, S., von Knorring, A.-L., Bohman, M., and Cloninger, C. R. (1984). An adoption study of somatoform disorders. I. The relationship of somatization to psychiatric disability. *Archives of General Psychiatry,* 41, 853–859.

Silver, L. B. (1981). The relationship between learning disabilities, hyperactivity, distractibility and behavioral problems: A clinical analysis. *Journal of the American Academy of Child Psychiatry,* 20, 385–390.

Simeon, J. G., Ferguson. H. B., and Van Wyck Fleet, J. (1986). Bupropion effects in attention deficit and conduct disorders. *Canadian Journal of Psychiatry*, 31, 581–585.

Smith, D. W. (1982). *Recognized patterns of human malformation (third edition)*. Philadelphia: Saunders.

Spitzer, R., Endicott, J., and Robins, E. (1975). *Research diagnostic criteria for a selected group of functional disorders*. New York: Biometrics Research.

Sprague, R., Cohen, M. N., and Werry, J. (1974). *Normative data on the Conners Teacher Rating Scale and Abbreviated Scale*. Unpublished manuscript, University of Illinois.

Stangl, D., Pfohl, B., Zimmerman, M., Bowers, W., and Corenthal, C. (1985). A structured interview for the DSM-III personality disorders. *Archives of General Psychiatry*, 42, 591–596.

Stewart, M. A. (1970). Hyperactive children. *Scientific American*, 222, 94–98.

Stewart, M. A., and Morrison, J. R. (1973). Affective disorder among the relatives of hyperactive children. *Journal of Child Psychology and Psychiatry*, 14, 209–212.

Stewart, M. A., deBlois, C. S., and Cummings, C. (1980). Psychiatric disorder in the parents of hyperactive boys and those with conduct disorder. *Journal of Child Psychology and Psychiatry*, 21, 283–292.

Stewart, M. A., Cummings, C., Singer, S., and deBlois, C. S. (1981). The overlap between hyperactive and unsocialized aggressive children. *Journal of Child Psychology and Psychiatry*, 22, 35–45.

Still, G. F. (1902). The Coulstonian lectures on some abnormal psychical conditions in children. *Lancet*, i, 1008–1012, 1077–1082, 1163–1168.

Strange, P. G. (1993). Dopamine receptors in the basal ganglia: Relevance to Parkinson's disease. *Movement Disorders*, 8, 263–270.

Streissguth, A. P., Martin, D. C., Barr, H. M., Sandman, B. M., Kirchner, G. L., and Darby, B. L. (1984). Intrauterine alcohol and nicotine exposure: Attention and reaction time in 4-year-old children. *Developmental Psychology*, 20, 533–541.

Sturge, C. (1982). Reading retardation and antisocial behavior. *Journal of Child Psychology and Psychiatry*, 23, 21–31.

Sullivan, H. S. (1954). *The Psychiatric Interview*. New York: Norton.

Summers, C., DeVries, J. B., and Horn, A. S. (1981). Behavioural and neurochemical studies on apomorphine-induced hypomotility in mice. *Neuropharmacology*, 20, 1203–1208.

Szatmari, P., Offord, D. R., and Boyle, M. H. (1989). Ontario Child Health Study: Prevalence of attention deficit disorder with hyperactivity. *Journal of Child Psychology and Psychiatry*, 30, 219–230.

Tarter, R. E. (1982). Psychosocial history, minimal brain dysfunction and differential drinking patterns of male alcoholics. *Journal of Clinical Psychology*, 38, 867–873.

Tarter, R. E., McBride, H., Buonpane, N., and Schneider, D. U. (1977). Differentiation of alcoholics: Childhood history of minimal brain dysfunction, family history, and drinking pattern. *Archives of General Psychiatry*, 34, 761–768.

Thorley, G. (1984). Review of follow-up and follow-back studies of childhood hyperactivity. *Psychological Bulletin*, 96, 116–132.

Trites, R. L., Dugas, E., Lynch, G., and Ferguson, H. B. (1979). Prevalence of hyperactivity. *Journal of Pediatric Psychology*, 4, 179–188.

Tsuang, M. T., and Faraone, S. V. (1990). *The genetics of mood disorders.* Baltimore: The Johns Hopkins University Press.

Turnquist, K., Frances, R., Rosenfield, W., and Mobarak, A. (1983). Pemoline in attention deficit disorder and alcoholism: A case study. *American Journal of Psychiatry*, 140, 622–624.

Ullman, R. K., Sleator, E. K., and Sprague, R. L. (1985). A change of mind: The Conners abbreviated rating scales reconsidered. *Journal of Abnormal Child Psychology*, 13, 553–565.

Vandenberg, S. G., Singer, S. M., and Pauls, D. L. (1986). *The heredity and behavior disorders in adults and children.* New York: Plenum.

Velez, C. N., Johnson, J., and Cohen, P. (1989). A longitudinal analysis of selected risk factors for childhood psychopathology. *Journal of the American Academy of Child and Adolescent Psychiatry*, 28, 861–864.

Vogel, F., and Motulsky, A. G. (1986). *Human genetics: Problems and approaches.* Berlin: Springer-Verlag.

von Economo, C. (1930). *Encephalitis lethargica: Its sequelae and treatment.* Trans. K. O. Newman. London. Oxford University Press.

von Felsinger, J. N., Lasagna, L., and Beecher, H. K. (1955). Drug-induced mood changes in man. II. Personality and reactions to drugs. *Journal of the American Medical Association*, 157, 113–119.

Waddington, J. L., and O'Boyle, K. M. (1989). Drugs acting on brain dopamine receptors: A conceptual re-evaluation five years after the first selective D-1 antagonist. *Pharmacology Therapeutics*, 43, 1–52.

Waldrop, M. F., Pedersen, F. A., and Bell, R. Q. (1968). Minor physical anomalies and behavior. *Child Development*, 39, 391–400.

Waldrop, M. F., Bell, R. Q., McLaughlin, B., and Halverson, C. F., Jr. (1978). Newborn minor physical anomalies predict short attention span, peer aggression, and impulsivity at age 3. *Science*, 199, 563–564.

Ward, M. F., Wender, P. H., and Reimherr, F. W. (1993). The Wender Utah Rating Scale: An aid in the retrospective diagnosis of attention deficit hyperactivity disorder. *American Journal of Psychiatry*, 150, 885–890.

Weiss, G., and Hechtman, L. T. (1993). *Hyperactive children grown up: ADHD in children, adolescents, and adults (Second edition).* New York: Guilford.

Weiss, G., Hechtman, L., Milroy, T., and Perlman, T. (1985). Psychiatric status of hyperactives as adults: A controlled prospective 15-year follow-up of

63 hyperactive children. *Journal of the American Academy of Child Psychiatry*, 23, 211–220.

Weiss, R. D., and Mirin, S. M. (1986). Subtypes of cocaine abusers. *Psychiatric Clinics of North America*, 9, 491–501.

Weissman, M. M., and Bothwell, S. (1976). Assessment of social adjustment by patient self-report. *Archives of General Psychiatry*, 33, 1111–1115.

Welner, Z., Welner, A., Stewart, M., Palkes, H., and Wish, E. (1977). A controlled study of siblings of hyperactive children. *Journal of Nervous and Mental Disease*, 165, 110–117.

Wender, P. H. (1968). Vicious and virtuous circles: The role of deviation amplifying feedback in the origin and perpetuation of behavior. *Psychiatry*, 31, 309–324.

Wender, P. H. (1971). *Minimal brain dysfunction in children*. New York: Wiley.

Wender, P. H. (1972). The minimal brain dysfunction syndrome in children: I. The syndrome and its relevance for psychiatry; II. A psychological and biochemical model for the syndrome. *Journal of Nervous and Mental Disease*, 155, 55–71.

Wender, P. H. (1976). An hypothesis for a possible biochemical basis of minimal brain dysfunction. In R. M. Knights and D. Bakker (Eds.), *The neuropsychology of learning*. Baltimore: University Park Press.

Wender, P. H. (1978). Minimal brain dysfunction: An overview. In M. A. Lipton, A. DiMascio, and K. F. Killan (Eds.), *Psychopharmacology: A generation of progress*. New York: Raven Press.

Wender, P. H. (1987). *The hyperactive child, adolescent, and adult*. New York: Oxford University Press.

Wender, P. H., Rosenthal, D., Kety, S. S., Schulsinger, F., and Welner, J. (1973). Social class and psychopathology in adoptees: An experimental method for separating the roles of genetic and experiential factors. *Archives of General Psychiatry*, 28, 318–325.

Wender, P. H., Rosenthal, D., Kety, S. S., Schulsinger, F., and Welner, J. (1974). Crossfostering: A research strategy for clarifying the role of genetic and experiential factors in the etiology of schizophrenia. *Archives of General Psychiatry*, 30, 121–128.

Wender, P. H., Rosenthal, D., Rainer, J. D., Greenhill, L. and Sarlin, M. B. (1977). Schizophrenics' adopting parents. *Archives of General Psychiatry*, 34, 777–784.

Wender, P. H., Reimherr, F. W., and Wood, D. R. (1981). Attention deficit disorder ('minimal brain dysfunction') in adults: A replication study of diagnosis and drug treatment. *Archives of General Psychiatry*, 38, 449–456.

Wender, P. H., Wood, D. R., Reimherr, F. W., and Ward, M. (1983). An open trial of pargyline in the treatment of attention deficit disorder, residual type. *Psychiatry Research*, 9, 329–336.

Wender, P. H., Reimherr, F. W., Wood, D., and Ward, M. (1985). A controlled study of methylphenidate in the treatment of attention deficit disorder, residual type, in adults. *American Journal of Psychiatry*, 142, 547–552.

Wender, P. H., and Reimherr, F. W. (1990). Bupropion treatment of attention-deficit hyperactivity disorder in adults. *American Journal of Psychiatry*, 147, 1018–1020.

Werry, J. S., and Quay, H. C. (1971). The prevalence of behavior symptoms in younger elementary school children. *American Journal of Orthopsychiatry*, 41, 136–143.

Willerman, L. (1973). Activity level and hyperactivity in twins. *Chid Development*, 44, 288–293.

Wilson, M. C., and Hitomi, M. (1969). Further studies of the self-administration of psychomotor stimulants in the rhesus monkey. *Common Problems in Drug Addiction*, 31, 6056–6063.

Woerner, P. I., and Guze, S. B. (1968). A family and marital study of hysteria. *British Journal of Psychiatry*, 114, 161–168.

Wood, D. R., Reimherr, F. W., Wender, P. H., and Johnson, G. E. (1976). Diagnosis and treatment of minimal brain dysfunction in adults. *Archives of General Psychiatry*, 33, 1453–1460.

Wood, D. R., Reimherr, F. W., and Wender, P. H. (1982). Effects of levodopa on attention deficit disorder, residual type. *Psychiatry Research*, 6, 13–20.

Wood, D. R., and Reimherr, F. W. (1983). Minimal brain dysfunction (attention deficit disorder) in adults. In S. Akhtar (Ed.), *New psychiatric syndromes: DSM-III and beyond.* New York: Jason Aronson.

Wood, D. R., Reimherr, F. W., and Wender, P. H. (1983). The use of L-deprenyl in the treatment of attention deficit disorder, residual type (ADD,RT). *Psychopharmacology Bulletin*, 19, 627–629.

Wood, D., Wender, P. H., and Reimherr, F. W. (1983). The prevalence of attention deficit disorder, residual type, or minimal brain dysfunction, in a population of male alcoholic patients. *American Journal of Psychiatry*, 140, 95–98.

Wood, D. R., Reimherr, F. W., and Wender, P. H. (1985). The treatment of attention deficit disorder with DL-phenylalanine. *Psychiatry Research*, 16, 21–26.

Wurtman, R. J. Hefti, F., and Melamed, E. (1980). Precursor control of neurotransmitter synthesis. *Pharmacological Reviews*, 32, 315.

Yao, K.-n., Solanto, M. V., and Wender, E. H. (1988). Prevalence of hyperactivity among newly immigrated Chinese-American children. *Developmental and Behavioral Pediatrics*, 9, 367–374.

Zametkin, A., Rapoport, J. L., Murphy, D. L., Linnoila, M., and Ismond, D. (1985). Treatment of hyperactive children with monoamine oxidase inhibitors. *Archives of General Psychiatry*, 42, 962–966.

Zametkin, A. J., and Rapoport, J. L. (1987). Neurobiology of attention deficit disorder with hyperactivity: Where have we come in 50 years? *Journal of* the *American Academy of Child and Adolescent Psychiatry, 26,* 676–686. [Erratum, (1988). *Journal of the American Academy of Child and Adolescent Psychiatry, 27,* 338.]

Zametkin, A. J., Nordahl, T. E., Gross, M., King, A. C., Semple, W. E., Rumsey, J., Hamburger, S., and Cohen, R. M. (1990). Cerebral glucose metabolism in adults with hyperactivity of childhood onset. *New England Journal of Medicine, 323,* 1361–1366.

Zimmerman, F., and Burgemeister, (1958). Action of methyl-phenidylacetate (Ritalin) and reserpine in behavior disorders in children and adults. *American Journal of Psychiatry, 115,* 323–328.

Zubin, J., Burdock, E. I., Sutton, S., and Cheek, F. (1959). Epidemiological aspects of prognosis in mental illness. In *Epidemiology of mental disorder.* Washington DC: American Association for the Advancement of Science.

Zuckerman, M. (1985). Biological foundations of the sensation-seeking temperament. In J. Strelau (Ed.), *The biological bases of personality and behavior:* I. Washington, DC: Hemisphere.

Name Index

■

Abikoff, 89
Akiskal, 129, 133
Alberts-Corush, 97
Allport, G., 146
Alterman, 61
Anderson, 54
Aristotle, 11
Arkonac, 100
Arnold, 154
August, 37, 85

Balch, 109
Bareggi, 107
Barkley, 31, 39, 63
Barrett, 109
Bartholini, 109
Beck, 51
Bell, 24
Bennett, 79
Bhatia, 57
Biederman, 86–89, 113, 130, 165
Bird, 56
Bleuler, 11, 44
Blum, 53
Bohman, 100–101, 103
Bohra, 57
Bond, 80
Borison, 109
Boyle, 53, 59

Bradley, 154
Buchanan, 137
Burgemeister, 154
Byles, 53
Byrne, 53

Cadman, 53
Cadoret, 98
Canino, 56
Cantwell, 27, 51, 83, 96, 98, 133
Cardon, 120
Carlson, 27, 133
Carnoy, 114
Catlin, 53
Cavanagh, 173
Chase, 105
Clarkin, 92
Cleckley, 37, 103
Cloninger, 100–101, 103, 134
Cocores, 62
Cohen, 56
Cooper, 163
Costello, 51, 55
Cox, 65
Crawford, 53
Creese, 114
Crow, 101–102
Crowe, 100
Cunningham, 98

Dannenberg, 46
Denhoff, 26–27
DeObaldia, 61, 101
Deutsch, 33, 96, 99, 139
Dock, 113
Dren, 157

Eyre, 101

Faraone, 86–87, 92, 113
Feehan, 57
Fineman, 139
Firestone, 32–33
Fischer, 63
Fitzgerald, F. S., 20
Fleming, 53
Foss, 52
Freud, S., 137

Gardner, 18
Garfinkel, 52
Gath, 98
Gelenberg, 110
Gendron, 48
Giedd, 112
Gilger, 92
Gillberg, 32
Ginsberg, 107
Gittelman, 38, 63, 65, 113
Gittelman-Klein, 174
Gnagy, 58
Goldberg, 110
Goodman, 55, 59, 89, 91–92, 102
Goodwin, 61, 97, 100, 105
Gould, 56
Goyer, 171
Greenhill, 175
Greenslade, 58
Greenspan, 155
Gualtieri, 160–161
Guze, 100

Hagnell, 46
Hauser, 78
Hechtman, 63, 67–68
Heiman, 184
Heston, 94–95
Hill, 80, 154

Hinshaw, 38
Hitomi, 157
Hoffman, 177
Hofmann, 53
Hohman, 80
Holt, W., 81
Horn, 99
Hornykiewicz, 105
Huessy, H., 38, 48, 65, 155, 164, 174
Hull, C., 228
Hunt, 175
Hutchings, 100–101
Hutt, 109

Jaffe, 171, 180
James, W., 15
Jankovic, 111, 162
Johnston, 56, 111
Jones, 33

Kaij, 113
Kanner, L., 82
Kaplan, 165
Kashani, 51, 113
Kauffman, 32
Kelly, 57
Kendall, 92
Kety, 44, 90, 94, 97, 184
Khantzian, 62
Klein, D., 27, 116, 132
Klein, R. G., 39, 63, 66, 68–69, 86, 89, 130
Klerman, 47
Klorman, 165
Kretschmer, 44, 253
Krouse, 32

Lahey, 88
Lapouse, 47
Laufer, 26–27
Leech, 99
Lerer, 32
Levy, 81
Lindahl, 33
Links, 53
Loeber, 38, 65
Loney, 7, 86
Lopez, 91

McGee, 54, 57
McKusick, 11, 43, 118
Malik, 57
Mann, 155
Mannuzza, 38, 63, 65–66, 68–69, 86, 89, 113, 130
Martin, 51
Matochik, 111
Mattes, 115, 160–161
Mednick 100–101, 170
Michelsson, 33
Milich, 7, 58, 86
Mirin, 62
Monetti, 52
Monk, 47
Morrison, 83–84, 96, 98, 112
Motulsky, 93
Murphy, 111, 117, 162

Nigram, 57
Nimitkitpaisan, 109
Nonne, 81

O'Boyle, 113
Offord, 53, 59
O'Leary, 51
Oliver, 137
Omenn, 113
O'Reilly, 115
Orwell, G., 17

Partridge, 57
Paternite, 96
Pauls, 113
Pelham, 58
Perley, 100
Phillips, 80
Pickar, 162
Popper, K., 116
Post, 105
Price, 125
Pritchard, 80

Quay, 48
Quinn, 32
Quitkin, 175

Rae-Grant, 53

Rapoport, 114
Rasmussen, 32
Ratey, 114, 177
Reimherr, F., 106, 108–109, 113, 117, 163, 166, 172
Rifkin, 175
Robins, 43–45, 88, 125
Rosenberg, 51
Rosenthal, D., 95
Rounsaville, 101
Rutter, 18, 35, 50

Safer, 94
Sandberg, 36, 49
Satel, 196
Satin, 52
Satterfield, 36, 63, 69
Scarr, 92
Schachar, 50, 59
Schecter, 99
Schell, 36
Schneider, 133
Schulsinger, 103, 170
Schulz, 170
Schuster, 157
Semrud-Clikeman, 92
Shaffer, 49
Shapiro, 52
Shaywitz, 79, 105
Shekim, 61, 173
Shen, 50
Shetty, 105
Sigvardsson, 100
Silva, 54, 57
Simeon, 172
Smith, 33, 50
Solanto, 54
Southwick, 196
Sprague, 58
Staghezza, 56
Stangl, 140
Stevenson, 55, 59
Stewart, 21, 37, 83–85, 88, 96, 98, 112
Still, 81
Strange, 113
Streissguth, 79
Strobl, 154

Sullivan, H. S., 146
Sverd, 52
Swanson, 99
Szatmari, 53

Tarter, 61, 101
Thomas, 53
Thorley, 62
Trites, 43, 49
Tsuang, 93
Turnquist, 184

Ullmann, 58

Vandenberg, 92
Velez, 56
Vogel, 93
Von Economo, 80–82

Waddington, 113
Waldrop, 32
Wang, 50
Weisenbert, 154

Weiss, 62–63, 65–69, 130
Welner, 84
Wender, P. H., 3, 9, 24, 54, 94, 105,
     113, 122, 138, 156–157, 159,
     161–163, 172
Werry, 48
Wieselberg, 49
Willerman, 91
Williams, 54, 57
Wilson, 157
Winsberg, 52
Wood, D., 61, 108–109, 113, 155,
     162–163
Woodward, 53
Wurtman, 107

Yager, 56
Yang, 50
Yao, 54

Zametkin, 111, 114, 162
Zimmerman, 154
Zuckerman, 28

Subject Index

Academic and vocational under-
achievement, 136–138
ADD (Attention Deficit Disorder,
without hyperactivity), 4, 10,
125, 185–186
ADD/CD, 87–88. See also Conduct
Disorder
ADD-H (Attention Deficit Dis-
order, with hyperactivity), 4,
10
DSM-III criteria for, 4–5, 125
ADD in adults (Attention Deficit
Disorder, Residual Type), 5, 8–
9, 19
ADD/OPD, 87–88
ADHD. See Attention-Deficit/
Hyperactivity Disorder
ADHD-like disorder. See von
Economo's encephalitis
ADHD spectrum disorders, 103
proposed research on, 230
treatment of, 184–188
Adoption studies
adoptive parents method, 95–96
of alcohol abuse, 101
Copenhagen adoption register
(NIMH), 97
of criminality, 100
critical features of, 94

and etiology of ADHD, 83, 93–
100
of Minimal Brain Dysfunction,
94–95
and nature-nurture debate, 93–
94, 96
problems of, 98
rate of ADHD in adoptees, reasons for, 99
in schizophrenia, 44
Adrenergic drugs, 175–177
Adrenergic factors, ADHD and,
176
Adult diagnostic criteria, 9
Affective lability, 26–28, 127
response to medication, 182
Alcohol and substance abuse
ADHD and, 3, 28, 101, 139, 154,
193
adoption study of, 101
in biological parents of subjects,
83–84, 96–98, 113, 190–191
cocaine users with ADHD, 62
effect of maternal alcohol use,
33
gender difference, 101
"hyperactivity" in adults and,
33, 83
Amantadine, 173

Amine metabolites in cerebrospinal fluid, 104–107
Amitriptyline, 174
Amphetamines
problems as Schedule II drugs, 166
side effects of, 169–170
in studies of ADHD adults, 154, 162–163
D-Amphetamine (Dexedrine), 167–168
and HVA reduction, 105
in study of adult ADHD, 162–163
Antidepressant and mood-stabilizing drugs, 163, 171–178. *See also specific drugs and drug groups*
Antisocial Personality Disorder (ASPD)
vs. ADHD, differential diagnosis, 137
as adult version of CD, 37–39, 64, 66, 68, 125
in relatives of ADHD probands, 88–89
symptoms of, 37
ASPD. *See* Antisocial Personality Disorder
Attention Deficit Disorder, Residual Type, (ADD in adults)
DSM-III criteria for, 5–6, 19
problems with the description, 8–9
Attention Deficit Disorder (ADD), 4, 10, 125, 185–186
Attention-Deficit/Hyperactivity Disorder
Combined Type, 7
comorbidities of, 39–40, 52, 54, 89, 92, 102, 125. *See also specific disorders*
gender difference, 112–113
heterogeneity of symptoms, 10–11
polythetic definition of, 9–10
Predominantly Hyperactive-Impulsive Type, 7

Predominantly Inattentive Type, 7
"pure" *vs.* ADHD with CD, 89
symptoms and signs, 13–40. *See also specific symptoms*
as syndrome, 11
Attention difficulties
of adulthood, 15–16. *See also* Impaired concentration
of childhood, 13–15

Biological studies of ADHD, 103–112
administration of dopamine precursors, 107–110, 163
amine metabolites in cerebrospinal fluid, 104–107
imaging, 111–112
monoamine oxidase inhibitors, therapeutic trials of, 110–111, 162–163
neurotransmitters, measuring activity of, 104
Borderline Personality Disorder (BPD)
vs. ADHD, 131–132
exclusion of subjects with, 129–130
response to anti-ADHD medication, 187–188
symptoms, 129
BPD. *See* Borderline Personality Disorder
Briquet's syndrome, ADHD and, 3, 100, 134, 139
Bromocryptine, 173
Bupropion, 117
antidepressant, 163, 172–173
dopaminergic action, 163
practical considerations, 172–173

Canadian studies, 49, 53, 59
Catecholaminergic activity
and ADHD, 113–114
and Minimal Brain Dysfunction, 76–77
CATRS. *See* Conners Abbreviated Teacher Rating Scale

CD. *See* Conduct Disorder
Cerebrospinal fluid
  amine metabolies in, 104–107
  study of, in adults, 106
Child Behavior Checklist, 53, 55–56
Childhood depression rating scale, 96
Child rearing
  of child with ADHD, 137
  for woman with ADHD, 137
Children's Global Assessment Scale, 56
Chinese study, 50–51
Clinical Global Impression, 108
Clonidine, 175–176
Clorgyline, 162
Comorbidities of ADHD, 39–40, 52, 54, 89, 92, 102, 125. *See also specific disorders*
Concentration, impaired. *See* Impaired concentration
Conduct Disorder (CD)
  and ADHD, 3, 4, 6, 7, 38, 52, 59, 89, 102, 125
  Antisocial Personality Disorder and, 37–39, 64, 66, 68, 125
  in childhood, 36–38
  DSM criteria for, 37
  gender difference, 59
  Group Type, 37
  noncompliance in, 23
  Solitary Aggressive Type, 37
Conners Abbreviated Rating Scale, 123
Conners Abbreviated Teacher Rating Scale (CATRS), 54, 58
Conners parent questionnaire, 50, 96
Conners Teacher Rating Scale (CTRS), 49–52, 54
Coordination, impaired, 17–20
Copenhagen adoption register (NIHM), 97
Couple treatment, 193, 196
Criminality, studies of, 100–101
Cross-sectional studies, 60–62

Deprenyl (now selegiline), 111, 162, 171
Depression, ADHD and, 29, 30, 186–187
Desipramine, 165
Developmental reading disorder, 16
Deviation amplifying feedback, 24
"Diagnosis" in psychiatry, 41–42
  categorical technique, 42–44
  dimensional technique, 42–44
  sensitivity and specificity of criteria, 45
Diagnosis of ADHD in adults, 122–143
  and academic, vocational, homemaking performance, 136–138
  "bell ringers" for ADHD, 135–140
  and current complaints, 135–136
  differential diagnosis, 130–134, 137
  exclusionary criteria, 129
  and family history, 138–139
  inclusionary criteria, 123–128
  informant, necessity of, 140
  and "marital" functioning, 138
  number of symptoms for diagnosis, 141–142
  pharmcological history, 139
  physical signs, 139–140
  psychological consequences of, 188–189
  rationale for inclusionary and exclusionary criteria, 129–134
  reasons for being missed, 134
  specific approaches, 134–140
  Utah Criteria, 124–128
Diagnostic heterogeneity, 77
Diagnostic Interview for Children and Adolescents (DICA), 52
Diagnostic Interview for Children and Adolescents-Parent Version (DICA-P), 86–87
Diagnostic Interview Schedule for Children and for Parents (DISC-P), 51, 55–56, 87

Diagnostic Interview Schedule for Children (DISC-C), 44, 51, 54–56

Differential diagnosis, 130–134, 137

DISC-C. See Diagnostic Interview Schedule for Children

DISC-P. See Diagnostic Interview Schedule for Children and for Parents

Disorder of Written Expression, 33–34

Disorganization
in adulthood, 22–23, 128
in childhood, 22
response to medication, 183

Disruptive Behavior Disorders, 6, 38

Dizygotic (DZ) twins, 90–92

L-Dopa, 108, 163

Dopaminergic drugs, 153, 163, 172–173

Dopaminergic etiology of ADHD, 3. See also Biological studies of ADHD
ADHD and decreased dopaminergic function, 105, 107, 110, 114, 120, 153
and effect of bupropion, 163

Dopamine turnover, homovanillic acid and, 105

Drug treatment. See also specific drugs and drug groups
abuse potential, 150, 179–180
in adolescents, 165–166
cost, 179
drug dependence, abusive vs. obligatory, 150
education about, 147–152
evaluation of effects, 181–184
improvements, types of, 158
informant, role of, 178–179
long-term study, 159
possible toxicity, 151
practical considerations, 166–184
pros and cons of, 149–152
quality control, 179
studies of, in adults, 154–165

DSM (Diagnostic and Statistical Manual of Mental Disorders)
ADD-H, criteria for, 4–5, 125
ADD in adults, criteria for, 5–6, 19
Conduct Disorder, criteria for, 37
designations for ADHD, 4–7
Oppositional Defiant Disorder, criteria for, 38
symptoms for diagnosing ADHD, 42

"Dyslexia," 33, 35–36, 39, 124, 184

DZ. See Dizygotic (DZ) twins

Education of adult patient, 144–152
about drug therapy, 147–152
initial consultations, 145–147

Emotional characteristics: temper and mood
in adulthood, 28–29, 127–128
in childhood, 26–28

Encephalitis lethargica (von Economo's encephalitis), 76, 80–81

Epidemiologic Catchment Area Project (ECA), 44

Epidemiologic studies, 44, 47

Etiology of ADHD, 76-121
biological studies, 103–112. See also Biological studies of ADHD
dopaminergic, 3, 105, 107, 110, 114, 120, 153
future studies in molecular genetics, 118–120
and genetic heterogeneity, 10–11, 77–79
genetic studies, 82–103. See also Genetic studies of ADHD
and mechanism of transmission, 112–118
and metabolic heterogeneity of ADHD, 117
nature-nurture debate, 83, 89–90, 93–94, 96
research horizon, 112–120
and variable penetrance or expression, 79, 231

Evaluation measures used in studies, 235–236
Experiences of adult ADHD patients on stimulants, 198–227
  Bruce C, 205–209
  Caroline G, 202–205
  comment by spouse of Bruce C, 206–209
  comment by spouse of George F, 224–227
  Daniel P, 198–202
  George F, 216–227
  Sonia D, 209–216

Family studies in ADHD
  ADD, OD, and major depression in relatives, 86–87
  ADHD and learning disorders in relatives, 254–255
  ADHD and substance abuse in relatives, 254, 255–256
  alcoholism, sociopathy, or hysteria in parents, 83–84, 96, 113
  ASPD and ADHD in biological relatives, 89
  and etiology of ADHD, 82–90
  familial associations of ADD and CD, 88, 255
  mixture of ADHD and bipolar disorder in relatives, 253–254
  possible errors in early studies, 84–85
Fluoxetine, 174–175
Follow-back studies, 62
Foot movements (Wender's sign), 20, 139

Generalized anxiety disorder (GAD), ADHD and, 62
Genetic heterogeneity, 10–11, 77–78, 120, 231
Genetic studies of ADHD, 82–103
  adoption studies, 83, 93–100
  conclusions based on, 100–103
  family studies, 82–90
  problems of early studies, 82
  proposed research, 229

theory of genetic transmission, 3, 65, 100, 112, 228
twin studies, 83, 90–93
Global Assessment Scale, 158, 206
Glucose metabolism (cerebral), imaging studies of, 111–112

Homovanillic acid (HVA)
  and brain dopamine turnover, 105, 114
  and response to methylphenidate, 106–107
HVA. See Homovanillic acid
The Hyperactive Child, Adolescent, and Adult (P. Wender), 169
Hyperactive child syndrome, 4
Hyperactivity
  in adult alcoholics, 61
  in adults (Utah Criteria), 126
  aggressive and nonaggressive, 86
  in children, 17–19, 49
  response to medication, 181
  situational vs. pervasive, 50, 55
Hyperkinesis, 4, 85
"Hyperkinesis Index," 96
Hysteria, in parents of subjects, 83–84, 96

Imaging studies, 104, 111–112
Imipramine, 174
Impaired concentration (in adults), 126–127
  response to medication, 181–182, 185
Impaired coordination, 17–20
Impulsivity
  in adulthood, 21, 128
  in childhood, 20–21
  response to medication, 183
Inattentiveness. See Impaired concentration
Incidence of ADHD, 46
India, ADHD study in, 57
Informed consent, 103
Injuries, frequency of, 21, 28

Interpersonal traits
in adulthood, 25–26
in childhood, 25
Italian study, 51

Kiddie SADS, 44

Learning Disorders, ADHD and, 3
in adulthood, 35–36, 136
in childhood, 33–35, 92, 136
in relatives of patients, 254–255
Lithium, 175
Longitudinal studies, 56 63–64. See
also Prospective studies

Magnetic resonance imaging (MRI),
111–112
Major depression
ADHD and, 27, 89, 134, 175, 186
in relatives of ADD probands,
86–87, 89
MAOIs. See Monoamine oxidase
inhibitors
Maternal alcohol use, ADHD and,
33
Mathematics Disorder
in adulthood, 35
in childhood, 33–34
MBD. See Minimal Brain Dysfunction
Medication, response to. See also
Drug treatment
in adulthood, 31–32
in childhood, 30–31
Methamphetamine (Desoxyn), 167–
168
Methylphenidate (Ritalin), 154,
168–169
accounts by patients treated
with, 198–227
prototype drug for ADHD, 155
side effects of, 169–170
in studies with adults, 106–107,
154–161
Minimal brain damage, 4
Minimal Brain Dysfunction (MBD),
4, 18, 32, 50
adoption studies of, 94–95

in adults, 122–123
and decreased catecholaminergic
activity, 76–77
drug trials on patients with, 164–
165
genetic origin, 76
nongenetic phenocopies, 79
Minor physical anomalies (MPAs),
81
in adulthood, 33, 139
in childhood, 32–33
and maternal alcohol use, 33
as possible markers, 32–33
Molecular genetics
candidate gene method, 119
DNA polymorphisms, 119
and etiology of ADHD, 118–120
use of markers, 119–120
Monoamine oxidase inhibitors
(MAOIs)
practical considerations, 171–
172
side effects of, 162
therapeutic trials of, 110–111,
162–163
Monozygotic (MZ) twins, 90–93
Mood disorders
vs. ADHD, 132–134
biological depression, special
problem of, 134
exclusion of subjects with, 129–
130
in relatives of ADHD children,
130
Mood lability, 26–28
response to medication, 182. See
also Antidepressant and mood-
stabilizing drugs
Mood-stabilizing drugs. See Antidepressant and mood
lability
"Moral insanity," 80
Mothers, interviews with, 47, 123
Motor abnormalities: hyperactivity
and impaired coordination
in adulthood, 19–20, 126
in childhood, 17–19
in Utah Criteria, 126

MPAs. *See* Minor physical anomalies
MZ. *See* Monozygotic (MZ) twins

Natural history of ADHD, 60–74
  critique of prospective studies, 64–69, 74
  cross-sectional studies, 60–62
  follow-back studies, 62
  prospective studies, 63–64
Nature-nurture debate, 83, 90, 93–94, 96
Neurodevelopmental examinations, 18
Neuroleptics, 177–178
Neurotransmitters. *See also specific neurotransmitter effects*
  and hypotheses of ADHD etiology, 115
  measuring activity of, 104
New Zealand studies, 54, 57
Nomifensine, 173
Noncompliance
  in adulthood, 24–25
  in childhood, 23–24
  varying styles of, 23
Noradrenergic activity, ADHD and, 114, 153
"Normal," as ambiguous term, 46
Nosological history of ADHD, 4–8
  DSM designations and criteria, 4–7
  earlier names for ADHD, 4
  subtypes identified in DSM-IV, 7

ODD. *See* Oppositional Defiant Disorder
Ontario Child Health Study, 53, 59
OPD (Oppositional Personality Disorder), 87–88
Oppositional Defiant Disorder (ODD), 125
  ADHD and 6, 7, 38
  DSM-III-R criteria for, 38
  noncompliance in, 23
Oppositional Personality Disorder (OPD), 87–88

Parents' Rating Scale (PRS), 123, 157, 237–239
Pargyline, 111, 162
  taken off the market, 171
Paroxetine, 175
Passive Aggressive Personality Disorder, 38, 125
Patients, types of
  referred by ADHD child's physician, 148
  referred by nonphysician therapist, 149
  unwilling or doubtful, 148–149
Pemoline, 35
  inclusion criteria in study with, 157
  side effects of, 170–171
  in studies with adults, 155–157
Phenelzine (Nardil), 172
Phenethylamine, 109
Phenocopy
  of ADHD, 117. *See also* von Economo's encephalitis
  description of, 79–82
Phenylalanine, 109, 163
Physical abuse, of ADHD child, 191
Physician's Global Assessment of Change, 157
Physician's Global Rating Scale, 158
Physician's Target Symptom Scale, 158
Pleiotropism, 79
Polythetic definition of ADHD, 9–10
Positron emission tomography (PET), 104, 111
Prevalence of ADHD in adults, 41–75
  best estimate, 69, 74, 228
  conclusions from prevalence studies, 58–60
  and diagnostic criteria, 44–45
  major childhood prevalence studies, 47–60, 70–73
  method for estimating, 41
  natural history of ADHD, 60–74

Prevalence of ADHD in adults (*Cont.*)
  purposes of study of, 45–46
  and techniques for diagnosis, 42–44
  variables in a study of, 44
Principles of Psychology (W. James), 15
Probenecid, 105–106
Profile of Mood States (POMS), 158
Prospective studies, 63–64
  critique of, 64–69, 74
PRS. *See* Parents' Rating Scale
Psychological management, 188–196
  consequences of diagnosis and treatment, 188–189
  couple treatment, 193, 196
  psychotherapeutic goals and approaches, 190–193
  self-monitoring, 189–190
  unanswered psychological questions, 196

Quay-Peterson Problem Checklist, 48

Reading Disorder
  in adulthood, 35
  in childhood, 33–34
  developmental reading disorder, 16
Research proposals
  direct tests of dopamine hypothesis, 231
  drug therapy plus group psycho-educational therapy, 231
  drug trials, 230–231
  on etiology of ADHD, 112–120
  genetic studies, 229
  "spectrum" studies, 230
  therapeutic trials, 230–231
Right-left discrimination, problems of, 36
Ritalin. *See* Methylphenidate
Rutter parent questionnaire, 54, 55
Rutter teacher questionnaire, 50, 51, 54, 55

School problems, 13–14, 17, 20–21, 22, 48–50
Selective serotonin reuptake inhibitors (SSRIs), 174–175
Selegiline (formerly deprenyl), 111, 162, 171
Self-esteem, 27
Self-monitoring, in treatment, 189–190
Self-perception, inaccuracy of, 69
Sertraline, 175
Short-term memory, problems of, 16
Social Adjustment Scale, 160, 206
Sociopathy, in parents of subjects, 83–84, 96
Specific Developmental Disorders, 6, 7
Spectrum disorders. *See* ADHD spectrum disorders
Spectrum of severity, notion of, 44
SSRIs (Selective serotonin reuptake inhibitors), 174–175
"St. Louis triad," 100, 120
Stimulant medication, 167–171. *See also* Drug treatment; *specific drugs*
  abuse potential, 171, 179–180
  effectiveness of, 166
  general principles, 167
  and increased dopaminergic activity, 153
  for patients with MBD, 164–165
  problem as Schedule II drugs, 161–162
  response in adults, 31–32
  response in children, 30–31
Stress intolerance, 29-30, 128
  response to medication, 183
Symptoms and signs, in children and adults, 13–40. *See also* *specific symptoms*
  altered emotionality: temper and mood, 26–29
  altered interpersonal relations, 25–26
  altered response to social reinforcement, 23–25

attention difficulties, 13–16
disorganization, 22–23
impulsivity, 20–21
motor abnormalities: hyperactivity and impaired coordination, 17–20
response to medication, 30–32
stress intolerance, 29–30
Syndromes associated with ADHD, 32–39
Conduct Disorder, 36–39. See also Conduct Disorder
Learning Disorder, 3, 33–36, 92, 136
minor physical anomalies (MPAs), 32–33

Targeted Attention Deficit Disorder Rating Scale (TADDS), 181, 247–251
Teacher questionnaire, 48–50, 54, 58
Temper, 26–29, 127–128
response to medication, 182
Tourette's syndrome, ADHD and, 111, 162
Tranylcypromine (Parnate), 162–163, 172
Treatment, in adults, 144–197
of ADHD combined with other diagnoses, 184–188
of ADHD spectrum disorders, 184–188
drug treatment, 153–188, 194–195. See also Drug treatment
education of patient, 144–152
ineffectiveness of psychological intervention, 146
informant, role of 178–179
patients, type of, 148–149
psychological management, 188–196. See also Psychological management

Tricyclic antidepressants (TCAs)
for ADHD adults and children, 173–174
for patients with MBD, 164–165
Twin studies, in ADHD, 55, 83
and etiology of ADHD, 90–93
monozygotic (MZ) vs. dizygotic (DZ), 90–93
and nature-nurture debate, 83, 93
L-Tyrosine, 109–110, 163

Undifferentiated Attention Deficit Disorder, 6
Utah Criteria, for diagnosis of ADHD in adults, 106, 124, 157, 184
adult diagnostic criteria, 126–128, 241–243
BPD traits excluded, 131, 161
childhood history, 124–126, 241
number of symptoms for diagnosis, 141
other exclusions, 161

Variable expression, 79
Variable penetrance, 79
Viral infection and ADHD-like disorder. See von Economo's encephalitis
von Economo's encephalitis (encephalitis lethargica)
and ADHD-like disorder in children, 76, 80–82
and Parkinson's syndrome in adults, 81

Wechsler Adult Intelligence Scale, 35
Wender's sign (foot movements), 20, 139
Wender Utah Rating Scale (WURS), 69, 123, 245–246
Wide-Range Achievement Test (WRAT), 35